a LANGE medical book

Examination & Board Review

Medical Biostatistics & Epidemiology

First Edition

Diane Essex-Sorlie, PhD
Professor of Biometrics
University of Illinois College of Medicine
at Urbana-Champaign

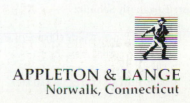

APPLETON & LANGE
Norwalk, Connecticut

95 96 97 98 / 10 9 8 7 6 5 4 3 2 1

Prentice Hall International (UK) Limited, *London*
Prentice Hall of Australia Pty. Limited, *Sydney*
Prentice Hall Canada, Inc., *Toronto*
Prentice Hall Hispanoamericana, S.A., *Mexico*
Prentice Hall of India Private Limited, *New Delhi*
Prentice Hall of Japan, Inc., *Tokyo*
Simon & Schuster Asia Pte. Ltd., *Singapore*
Editora Prentice Hall do Brasil Ltda., *Rio de Janeiro*
Prentice Hall *Englewood Cliffs, New Jersey*

ISBN: 0-8385-6219-1
ISSN: 1079-4883

Acquisitions Editor: John Dolan
Production Editor: Chris Langan
Designer: Elizabeth Schmitz

ISBN 0-8385-6219-1

9 780838 562192

90000

PRINTED IN THE UNITED STATES OF AMERICA

This book is dedicated to individuals who have enriched my life immeasurably.
The late Elsie Bennett Essex, a strong courageous woman.
The late Anthony and Emma Marinangeli, devoted and loving, always.
Edward Minium, an exceptional teacher.
Marten Kernis, a colleague, friend, and mentor.
Daniel K. Bloomfield, a friend, colleague, and mentor.
Lillian and Harold Sorlie, kind, warm, and loving.
AND
William Sorlie, the most extraordinary man I have met.

Table of Contents

Acknowledgments

I am indebted to the staff of Lange Medical Publications because they allowed me to turn a dream into reality. In particular, Stephen Foster, an Appleton & Lange sales representative, introduced me to John Dolan, senior medical editor at Appleton & Lange. I am most fortunate to have had John Dolan's advocacy, support, encouragement, and enthusiasm throughout this project. Gregory Huth and Chris Langan coordinated the production and helped turn my printed pages into a finished product. In addition, I am grateful to John Dinolfo, my developmental editor; words of thanks are inadequate to describe my gratitude for his excellent stylistic suggestions, encouragement, sense of humor, and commitment. If this book serves the audiences for whom it is intended, John Dinolfo deserves much of the credit.

I also wish to thank journal editors, such as *The New England Journal of Medicine,* and textbook publishers, such as *John Wiley, Inc.,* for allowing me to adapt and reproduce material. It is with the kind permission of the *Biometrika* trustees that I am able to adapt and reproduce statistical tables.

Dr. Edward Minium taught the first several statistics courses I took as an undergraduate and master's degree-level student. His enthusiasm for statistics and his dedication to teaching still serve today as my role model. He is a teacher extraordinaire. I am also indebted to my students who, over many years, encouraged me, challenged me to explain concepts clearly, and put up with my continuous experimentation with different teaching techniques. Further, several colleagues encouraged me throughout my writing. I thank Dr. Howard Bers and Dr. Marten Kernis for their constant support. Always in good cheer, Dr. Peter Imrey answered my questions, even when he struggled to cope with his own workload. Dr. H. Bruce Bosmann was generous in providing summer research awards that allowed me to concentrate on my writing. Jeffrey Loftiss in the Library of the Health Sciences helped me secure copies of many articles that were not available on the Urbana-Champaign campus of the University of Illinois. His good humor and efficiency are more than appreciated.

Writing this book has given me great personal and professional joy. I am privileged to share these joys with my husband, William Sorlie, who is my constant support. He quipped just recently, "I hope she finishes the book soon because I would like to see her again." He spent many nights and weekends alone while I wrote and wrote and wrote. . . . Thank you for your never-ending encouragement.

Finally, my beloved grandparents, Emma and Anthony Marinangeli died within two weeks of each other during the early stages of my writing. I owe them a debt I can never repay for their love and belief in me. Elsie Bennet Essex, my paternal grandmother, inspired me when she was alive; her memories continue to inspire me. Thank you for strength and courage.

Preface

Medical Biostatistics & Epidemiology: Examination & Board Review grew out of my intense love of teaching and my commitment to students, as well as to faculty who work diligently to teach biostatistics & epidemiology. It (1) covers many important concepts tested on the United States Licensing Examinations (USMLE) and provides a structured review for individuals preparing for these examinations; (2) presents a sound treatment of basic biostatistics and epidemiology that is highly accessible, even to readers who have not had a basic biostatistics course; (3) addresses the fundamental statistical and epidemiological concepts necessary to read and evaluate much of published medical literature; (4) serves as a resource for students, clinicians, and other health care professionals who would like to refresh their memory about basic statistical or epidemiological concepts or learn about a concept unfamiliar to them; and (5) can be used as a textbook for introductory medical statistics and epidemiology, with little or no supplementation by the instructor.

The key features of this book include the following:

- Each chapter begins with a clinical example that introduces statistical and epidemiological concepts.
- Objectives in each chapter help readers identify key concepts and reach key instructional goals.
- Clinical examples are used extensively to highlight the application and interpretation of statistical and epidemiological concepts.
- Many chapters conclude with a summary table that outlines a statistical test, including formulae, assumptions, relevant distributions and statistical tables.
- Flow charts are included in many chapters to help readers select the appropriate statistical test.
- Boxes summarize the analysis of clinical data and reinforce teaching concepts. These boxes provide a complete overview of an analysis, beginning with hypotheses and ending with interpreting results.
- Chapters include self-study questions with detailed solutions. These exercises are intended to help readers develop and sharpen diverse skills, including reading tables and graphs, interpreting results, formulating conclusions, selecting statistical tests, and conducting small-scale analyses and interpreting their results.
- The book concludes with a chapter on reading and evaluating the medical literature; an evaluation checklist is provided to help individuals use their reading time as effectively as possible.
- Finally, a 122-item comprehensive examination appears in the appendix. The answer key includes for each question: (a) a brief explanation of the correct answer, (b) the concept tested, and (c) reference to the chapter(s) in which the concept is presented. The examination format is similar to those used on course final examinations and licensure exams.

Diane Essex-Sorlie, Ph.D.

Urbana, Illinois
December 1994

Defining Basic Concepts

1

Clinical Example: Primary Invasive Breast Cancer

> To determine whether a relationship exists between tumor angiogenesis and metastatic status (metastases present/metastases absent), oncologists studied tumor specimens from 90 randomly selected women with primary invasive breast cancer. Forty women had metastases and 50 women were without metastases ($n_{WITH} = 40$, $n_{WITHOUT} = 50$). Representative samples of invasive disease were selected from tumor specimen sections stained with hematoxylin and eosin. The number of microvessels per stained section was counted on a 200x field. In women with metastases, the mean number of microvessels per 200x field was 101, with a standard deviation of 49.3. In women without metastases, the mean number of microvessels was 45, with a standard deviation of 21.1. Based on these results, the clinicians concluded that tumor angiogenesis correlates directly with metastatic status in the patients evaluated.

Like all other disciplines, statistics has unique concepts and a specialized vocabulary that we must understand to comprehend the medical literature. Consider the research summarized above. In this hypothetical example based on very real clinical issues, can you distinguish the **independent variable** from the **dependent variable**? Are these variables **quantitative** or **qualitative**? To which patients can these results be extended (**generalized**)—that is, what is the **target population**? Which statistical analyses are appropriate, given the goals of the study and the way in which the variables are measured?

To answer these and other key questions, you must have a good understanding of the statistical and epidemiologic concepts discussed in this chapter. A solid grasp of the following concepts will help you evaluate published reports and determine whether—and to whom—findings may be extended.

OBJECTIVES

When you complete this chapter, you should be able to:

- Define key concepts in statistics and epidemiology.
- Read a brief clinical example and identify the type of study, independent variable, sample population, and other key features.
- Read a brief clinical example and determine if the conclusions extend to the individuals to whom they are being applied.

STATISTICS VERSUS EPIDEMIOLOGY

Statistics is "the science and art of dealing with variation in data through collection, classification, and analysis in such a way as to obtain reliable results" (Last, 1983, p 100). **Biostatistics** and **biometrics** refer to the application of statistics in medicine. For example, a biostatistician used statistical tools to analyze the data in the opening clinical example. The goal was to determine if tumor angiogenesis and metastatic status are related. **Epidemiology** is the study of the development, frequency, distribution, determinants, and consequences of disease in human populations. Epidemiologic research typically seeks to (1) understand the causes of disease, (2) plan treatment, and (3) contribute to the development of public health policies. For example, an epidemiologist may study new cases of AIDS in a 12-month period and compare the findings to results from earlier studies, to detect changing disease patterns. An epidemiologist may also investigate an outbreak of bacterial meningitis in a university to identify disease determinants (eg, exposure and lifestyle patterns). Based on the findings, the university may decide to offer immunizations to all students.

DESCRIPTIVE VERSUS INFERENTIAL STATISTICS

The discipline of statistics is often divided into two branches: descriptive and inferential. The goal of **descriptive statistics** is to organize and summarize data. The goal of **inferential statistics** is to draw inferences and reach conclusions about data, when only a part of a population, or **sample**, has been studied. A **generalization** is a principle deduced from limited information (a sample) and extended to a larger collection of observations (the population). To **generalize** is to make deductions from limited information and extend those deductions to a larger collection of observations.

The **population** is the complete set of observations, patients, entities, measurements, and so forth, about which we would like to draw conclusions. The **sampled population** is the group from which the sample (or subset of the population) is drawn. The **target population** is the group to which we would like to extend our conclusions. Numerical characteristics of populations are **parameters.** Numerical characteristics of samples are **statistics.** For example, the mean microvessel count of the 40 women with primary invasive breast cancer with metastases is a statistic—in this case, 101. Lower-case "n" is frequently used to indicate sample size, that is, the number of entities observed—in this case, the number of patients. Upper-case N is generally used to designate population size.

Consider the research about breast cancer and tumor angiogenesis mentioned at the beginning of the chapter. Two populations were sampled. Forty randomly selected women with primary invasive breast cancer with metastases constitute the first population. Fifty randomly selected women with primary invasive breast cancer without metastases comprise the second population.

VARIABLES

Certain characteristics, attributes, and qualities are of interest to us; as we study them, we draw inferences and conclusions about them. Characteristics that can be measured are called **variables.** The term "variable" is used because its values may change, depending on related factors. Thus, we may measure an individual's blood pressure or heart rate on two separate occasions and find considerable variability, which can be due to many factors, such as the time of day or whether the person has just eaten a meal or smoked a cigarette.

Several types of variables exist in statistics. An **independent variable** is a characteristic or experimental intervention thought to influence a particular event or a manifestation of it. A **dependent variable** is the resulting outcome, event, or manifestation "whose variation we seek to explain or account for by the influences of independent variables" (Last, 1983, p 28). Thus, in our clinical example at the beginning of the chapter, metastatic status is the independent variable; microvessel counts per 200x field is the dependent variable. **Confounding variables** are factors that distort the degree to which the independent variable affects the dependent variable. The distortion may occur because the confounding factor is associated with the independent variable, dependent variable, or both (Masuner & Kramer, 1985, pp 159–160). If not taken into account by study design or statistical analysis, confounding variables may lead to erroneous conclusions.

The following example contains a confounding variable. In some men, workplace exposure to sulfur dioxide (SO_2) has been linked to the development of chronic cough. Cigarette smoking is also associated with chronic cough in some men. If we examine the relationship between SO_2 exposure and chronic cough, we may develop incorrect conclusions, unless we include cigarette smoking history (a confounding variable) in our analysis.

MEASUREMENT OF VARIABLES

One of fours scales may be used to measure variables; these are the nominal, ordinal, interval, and ratio scales. A **nominal scale** uses names, labels, numbers, or other symbols to assign objects to a series of categories. A nominal scale contains a series of *unordered categories* or classes that are mutually exclusive and exhaustive. Labels, numbers, or other symbols are used to differentiate one class from another. Nominal variables are also called categorical or qualitative variables. Qualitative variables describe qualities or attributes that cannot be measured in the same sense as, for example, height, weight, cholesterol, triglyceride level, age, and blood pressure. Observations in a class are qualitatively the same; observations in different classes are qualitatively different. We determine nominal variables by identifying the categories or classes making up the scale and indicating the number or percentage of observations in each class or category. Examples of variables measured on a nominal scale include blood type, type of cancer, race, sex, and handedness. In our opening scenario, metastatic status (with/without) is a qualitative or nominal variable.

An **ordinal scale** contains distinct *ordered* or *ranked* qualitative categories. For this reason, ordinal scales are sometimes called **rank-order scales**. Labels, numbers, or other symbols are used to distinguish ordered categories. Observations that differ from category to category can be ranked according to whether the observation is more or less of some criterion. The categories are qualitative in the sense that the distance between and among them is not measurable numerically. However, the number or percentage of observations in each category can be described. Duke's classification of colorectal cancer (stages A through D) is an ordinal scale. Stage A represents cancer limited to the mucosa and submucosa. Stage B denotes cancer that extends into the muscularis or serosa. Stage C signifies cancer that involves the regional lymph nodes. Stage D represents cancer that has metastasized to the liver, bone, and/ or lung. The categories are ordered because the extent of disease is more limited and prognosis more favorable in stage A than in stage D. In fact, approximately 90% of patients with cancer limited to the mucosa and submucosa (stage A) survive 5 years. In contrast, approximately 5% of patients whose cancer has metastasized to the liver, bone, and/or lung survive 5 years (stage D) (Glickman, 1987, p 1300).

Interval and ratio scales are used to describe quantitative variables. Similar statistical techniques can be applied to data from interval and ratio scales. A **quantitative variable** can be measured according to amount or quantity. Serum cholesterol, body weight, white blood cell count, body temperature, and patient age are quantitative variables. **Interval scales** involve assigning numbers at equal intervals from an arbitrary origin. Objects are ordered by the amount of the characteristic they possess. The arbitrarily selected origin (or zero point) does not imply a true absence of the measured characteristic. Fahrenheit and Celsius temperature scales are examples of an interval scale.

A **ratio scale** is an interval scale with a true zero point that reflects the absence of the measured characteristic. Blood pressure, body weight, time, age, Kelvin temperature, volume, and mass are ratio scales. Because the ratio scale has a true zero point, ratios between values are meaningful. For example, a patient who weighs 80 kg weighs twice as much as a patient who weighs 40 kg.

Interval and ratio scales, sometimes called **quantitative** or **numerical scales,** can be discrete or continuous. **Discrete scales** have integer values. Hospital census (number of beds occupied), number of new cases of AIDS in 12 months, number of patients seen in a family practice clinic in 12 months, and number of angioplasties performed in 6 months are examples of variables measured on a discrete scale. With **continuous scales**, values may have fractional components. Gestational age (eg, 17.6 weeks), body weight (eg, 50.5 kg), body temperature (eg, 97.4 °F), and survival postdiagnosis (eg, 6.3 months) are measured on a continuous scale. Depending on the precision required (as indicated by the number of places to the right of the decimal), continuous data may be reported as integer values. For example, many health surveys report body weight to the nearest kilogram or patient age to the nearest year. Despite such simplification, these variables are still continuous because they can exhibit fractional components, at least in theory. Thus they can be measured on a continuum.

COMMON TYPES OF STUDIES

Investigators design studies in different ways in order to measure variables and use these measurements to learn and draw conclusions about phenomena, such as diseases and treatments. Because different types of studies are appropriate for studying different kinds of questions, it is important that you understand the key elements of common study designs. This understanding will help you read the medical literature, understand the type of conclusions that can be drawn from different types of studies, and evaluate the validity of conclusions.

Research can be divided into *observational studies* or *experiments,* based on whether patients are merely observed or whether some kind of intervention is performed (Dawson-Saunders & Trapp, 1994, p 6). Case reports and case series, case control, cohort (prospective and retrospective), and cross-sectional studies are observational, because one or more groups of patients are observed. Their characteristics are recorded for analysis—for example, exposure to pesticides and subsequent development of cancer, or augmentation mammoplasty with silicone gel breast implants and subsequent development of systemic sclerosis. Clinical trials are experiments because the investigator manipulates or controls an intervention, such as different drugs, drug doses, procedures, or treatments. For example, investigators may conduct a clinical trial to compare the use of zidovudine (AZT) alone to combination therapy with zidovudine, ddI, and pyridinone in patients with AIDS.

Case reports or **case series studies** are careful, detailed descriptions of interesting characteristics in a single patient (case report) or series of patients (case series). A case report and a case series study exclude patients without the characteristic or the disease under investigation. Case series studies may produce hypotheses that lead to more formalized research to identify causes of disease, diagnose disease, or treat disease.

In a **case-control study**, we use data from cases and controls to test theories derived from inferences about previously studied factors, past events, or experiences. *Cases* are persons who have the characteristic or disease of interest *at the outset of the investigation*; *control patients* are disease free. Case-control studies require knowledge of disease status at the beginning of the study. In this kind of study, we examine the experience and history of patients to identify factors present in the history of cases, but absent in the history of controls. Case-control studies are especially useful when investigating relatively rare diseases, such as certain types of brain tumors. Because disease status is known at the beginning of the investigation, researchers can select a sufficient number of diseased and nondiseased individuals in order to reach valid statistical conclusions about the illness. Because they "look back" from disease status to factors that may explain the occurrence of disease, case-control studies are sometimes called retrospective studies. However, an increasing number of investigators now reserve the term *retrospective* for a type of *cohort study* (Hennekens & Buring, 1987, p 23).

Cross-sectional studies provide a "snapshot" of what is happening at a particular point in time, rather than over a period of time. Cross-sectional studies are especially useful for evaluating a new diagnostic procedure and for estimating the frequency (prevalence) of a disease or a characteristic at a point in time. For example, a nationwide health survey may be conducted to describe the number of adults who attempt to control their fat intake, exercise strenuously 3 times per week, or use seatbelts regularly. An investigator might also use a cross-sectional study to evaluate the utility of a technetium-labeled granulocyte scan to diagnose active inflammatory bowel disease, and to compare the results to findings from conventional barium-contrast studies.

Cohort studies involve a carefully defined population that has been or may be exposed to a factor or factors thought to contribute to the occurrence of disease or other outcome. Subsets of the population, called cohorts, are followed over time to see if they develop disease. Thus, the starting point of all cohort studies is exposure status.

Cohort studies are either prospective or retrospective (Hennekens & Buring, 1987, p 23). In a **prospective cohort study,** exposed and unexposed individuals are followed at regular intervals to learn about the development and extent of disease. For example, clinicians might conduct a prospective cohort study to compare the frequency of colds, bronchitis, and other respiratory problems in nonsmokers who are exposed to secondary cigarette smoke in the home, versus nonsmokers who are *not* exposed to secondary cigarette smoke in the home. In this type of study, the researchers would follow individuals for up to a year or more to monitor the incidence of respiratory infections.

In a **retrospective cohort study**, the investigation is initiated at a point in time after the exposure has occurred; however, the outcome of interest may or may not have occurred already by the time the study begins. Investigators begin with exposure status and use medical records, death certificates, and other available information to document disease development. For example, investigators may rely on patient charts to identify women who took diethylstilbestrol (DES) between 1947 and 1971 to treat threatened miscarriage. The objective is to use the medical records of offspring to determine whether fetal exposure to DES is associated with reproductive abnormalities, such as clear cell carcinoma of the vagina in fetal-exposed women and testicular abnormalities in fetal-exposed men. Cohort studies are an ideal way to investigate relatively common diseases or outcomes, such as how the development of breast cancer may differ in women with and without a family history of breast cancer.

Sometimes called intervention or experimental studies, **clinical trials** evaluate the effectiveness of a therapeutic procedure or agent (eg, a new drug). **Controlled clinical trials** compare a therapeutic agent or procedure with another agent or procedure. Patients in one group receive the new agent or procedure, while patients in the control (or reference) group receive a placebo or another drug or procedure. Investigations with one experimental treatment are **uncontrolled clinical trials;** because no control (or reference) group is included, the experimental treatment cannot be compared to another intervention. Without a control or reference group, it is often impossible to separate treatment effects from other factors, such as normal biologic variation within and between patients. Because controlled trials are more likely to permit researchers to decide whether differences are due to a treatment, clinical intervention, or some other factors, medical researchers and clinicians often consider controlled trials more useful than uncontrolled studies (Dawson-Saunders & Trapp, 1994, p 13).

UNDERSTANDING ASPECTS OF STUDY DESIGN

Certain terms are used frequently in the medical literature to describe features of the design of a study. An understanding of these terms will help you evaluate a study and assess the degree to which conclusions can be extended from the patients studied to other individuals.

A **placebo** is an inert medication or procedure intended to be indistinguishable from the experimental or active treatment. Patients are not told whether they receive an active medication or a placebo. The placebo sometimes has a therapeutic effect, which is due to the patient's expectation that he or she will feel better or that the disease will improve after taking medication. Improvement, then, is attributed to the patient's expectation that a treatment or drug is beneficial. This improvement is known as a **placebo** or **halo effect**.

To **replicate** is to administer the same drug or procedure to two or more patients under identical conditions. **Replication** is the act of repeating an investigation to confirm findings or to improve the accuracy of measurements.

To **control** is to minimize extraneous sources of variation, either by study design or statistical analysis. Control in a study design can be accomplished by:

Including a control (or reference) group.
Randomly assigning patients to treatment groups or experimental conditions.
Restricting patients who enroll in the study to reduce variation between patients.
Matching patients (described below).

Statistical control can be achieved through the selection of an appropriate analysis, by mathematical modeling, or by statistical adjustment.

Random assignment of patients to treatment groups or conditions minimizes extraneous variation by helping to ensure that all patients who enroll in the study have an equal chance of receiving the treatment (Fletcher et al, 1988, p 122).

In **matching**, often referred to as **pair matching**, the investigator matches patients as they enter the study, based on characteristics thought to be associated with the outcome of interest. Pair matching is done so that the patients in each pair are as alike as possible with respect to certain factors, such as disease severity, age, smoking history, family history, or sex. One member of the pair is assigned randomly to one group; the pairmate is then placed automatically in the other group. Investigators often match patients according to age or disease severity. As noted earlier, matching is one way to control extraneous variation and increase the likelihood that differences between groups occur because of the treatment or intervention, rather than being due initial differences between the groups.

Bias is any error or effect that causes the results of a study to depart from true values (Last, 1983, p 10). Bias can occur because one or more of the following is inadequate: the measuring instrument, selection of patients, assignment of patients to treatments, or method of measuring outcomes of interest. Suppose researchers want to study the relationship between estrogen replacement therapy in women and subsequent development of breast cancer. For the estrogen replacement group, patients with a family history of breast cancer are selected; for the control group (who receive a placebo), patients without a family history of breast cancer are selected. This example illustrates a *confounding bias* in selecting patients, because the outcome of interest (breast cancer development) is confounded by family history. In this case, the development of breast cancer is more likely to occur in women with a family history of breast cancer than in women without a family history. Keep in mind that bias due to patient assignment can occur when patients with substantial disease are selected for the treatment group and patients whose disease is "mild" are assigned to the placebo group, or vice versa.

Confounding occurs when the effects of one or more variables cannot be separated from each other and from their effect on the dependent variable (Last, 1983, p 21). In the hypothetical research on breast cancer and estrogen use, the effects of family history and estrogen use are not separated to determine their respective impact on the development of breast cancer in the sampled population. Thus, the effect of treatment is confounded by family history. An excellent discussion of confounding and other flaws in the medical literature is presented by Michael and associates (1984).

Validity is the extent to which a device (eg, a test) measures what it purports to measure, or a clinical observation accurately describes a phenomenon. Validity is discussed most frequently in terms of internal and external validity. A study has **internal validity** if the differences between treatment groups can be attributed to the independent variable(s). Sampling procedures, definition of outcomes, measurement of outcomes, statistical analyses, and administration of treatments must all be appropriate for a study to be internally valid. Internal validity is required to extend a finding beyond the patients studied (Fletcher et al, 1988, p 12).

External validity refers to the degree to which research findings can be applied or *generalized* to individuals other than those who were studied. External validity applies only to a specified target population (Last, 1983, p 108). Suppose that after examining the effect of AZT to prolong the life span of 25 AIDS patients with full-blown disease, we try to generalize our findings to asymptomatic, HIV-positive individuals. Our conclusions could be misleading because they may lack sufficient external validity. However, if we generalize our conclusions to AIDS patients whose disease stage and other characteristics closely resemble those of patients in our study group, our findings could have high external validity.

Reliability is another important consideration when evaluating the results of a study. Reliability refers to the degree to which a measuring device or a procedure produces repeatable results on each subsequent use or occasion. **Reproducibility** and **repeatability** are synonyms for reliability. Results may be reliable but not valid, as when a blood pressure cuff produces a diastolic reading that is relatively repeatable for a patient but is substantially higher (or lower) than the patient's true pressure.

SUMMARY

To read and evaluate medical literature, including published studies as well as information distributed by pharmaceutical companies, you must have a good understanding of concepts and vocabulary unique to the discipline of statistics. In addition to discussing the goals of statistics, we define and explain a wide range of statistical concepts in this chapter, including

(1) salient features of samples and populations, (2) main types of variables and scales for measuring them, (3) different kinds of epidemiologic and biomedical studies, and (4) key features of study designs.

Central to statistics and epidemiology are populations and samples. A population is the complete set of observations, patients, or measurements about which we would like to draw conclusions. Toward this end, we obtain one or more samples; study characteristics and responses of individuals in the sample(s); use this information to draw conclusions; and extend the conclusions beyond the persons from whom information was collected. The sampled population is the population from which information is obtained. The target population is the group to which we apply our findings. A sample is a subset of the population.

Characteristics or qualities that can be measured are called variables. An independent variable is a characteristics or experimental intervention thought to influence an event or manifestation of it. A dependent variable is the resulting outcome. Confounding variables are factors that distort the degree to which the independent variable affects the dependent variable. The effect of confounding variables can be minimized by (1) experimental design, (2) careful sampling of patients, and (3) statistical analysis.

To study the effect of the independent variable, we must be able to measure the resulting outcome. To measure variables, we may use one of four scales: nominal, ordinal, interval, or ratio. A nominal scale consists of a series of unordered classes that are mutually exclusive and exhaustive. Labels, numbers, or other symbols are used to differentiate one class from another. We count the number of observations in each class. Nominal variables are called qualitative or categorical variables. Cancer type (eg, lung, prostate, breast, liver) is a nominal variable. An ordinal scale contains distinct ordered or ranked qualitative categories. Labels, numbers, or other symbols are used to distinguish ordered categories. Duke's classification of colorectal cancer is an example of an ordinal scale. An interval scale involves assigning numbers at equal intervals from an arbitrary zero point and ordering quantitative variables, such as Fahrenheit temperature, by the amount of the characteristic they possess. A ratio scale is an interval scale with a true zero point; body weight and mass are examples of variables measured on a ratio scale.

Researchers and statisticians often classify variables as qualitative or quantitative. Qualitative variables describe qualities or attributes that cannot be measured numerically in the same sense as height, total cholesterol, triglyceride level, or age. Qualitative variables are measured on a nominal or ordinal scale. Quantitative variables, such as serum lead level ($\mu g/dL$), can be measured numerically according to the amount or quantity of the characteristic they possess. Quantitative variables are measured on interval and ratio scales. The distinction between qualitative and quantitative variables is important, because different types of statistical analyses are used examine these two types of variables.

Depending on the types of research questions asked, various types of studies can be designed to measure variables; measurements are then used to draw conclusions about phenomena, such as diseases and treatments. Observational studies include case reports, case series, case control, cohort, and cross-sectional studies. In a clinical trial, the investigator manipulates or controls an intervention (eg, different drugs or treatments). Clinical trials can include controlled or uncontrolled experiments. Controlled clinical trials compare a therapeutic agent or procedure to another agent or procedure. Because they involve only one treatment or procedure, uncontrolled clinical trials do not permit comparison of an experimental treatment to another intervention.

Identifying the important demographic and clinical characteristics of the sampled population, and comparing those characteristics to attributes of the target population, is a vital part of determining when—and to what extent—results from a published study may be generalized. External validity is the degree to which findings can be applied to individuals who did not contribute data to the study.

REFERENCES

Dawson-Saunders B, Trapp R: *Basic and Clinical Biostatistics,* 2nd ed. Appleton & Lange, 1994.

Fletcher R, Fletcher S, Wagner E: *Clinical Epidemiology: The Essentials,* 2nd ed. Williams & Wilkins, 1988.

Glickman R: Inflammatory bowel disease: Ulcerative colitis and Crohn's disease. In: *Harrison's Principles of Internal Medicine,* 11th ed. Braunwald E et al (editors). McGraw-Hill, 1987.

Hennekens C, Buring J: *Epidemiology in Medicine.* Little, Brown, 1987.

Last JM (editor): *A Dictionary of Epidemiology.* Oxford University Press, 1983.

Mausner J, Kramer S: *Epidemiology: An Introductory Text,* 2nd ed. Saunders, 1985.

Michael M, Boyce W, Wilcox A: *Biomedical Bestiary: An Epidemiologic Guide to Flaws and Fallacies in the Medical Literature.* Little, Brown, 1984.

Self-study Questions

Part I: Definitions

Define each of the following terms.

Bias	Epidemiology	Qualitative variable
Biostatistics (biometrics)	External validity	Quantitative variable
Case-control study	Generalization	Random assignment
Case report study	Independent variable	Ratio scale of measurement
Case series study	Inferential statistics	Reliability (reproducibility,
Clinical trial	Internal validity	repeatability)
Cohort study	Interval scale of	Replication
Confounding	measurement	Retrospective cohort study
Confounding variable	Matching (pair matching)	Sample
Continuous scale	Nominal scale	Sampled population
Control	Ordinal scale (rank-order	Statistics
Controlled clinical trial	scale)	Target population
Cross-sectional study	Parameter	Uncontrolled clinical trial
Dependent variable	Placebo effect (halo effect)	Validity
Descriptive statistics	Population	Variable
Discrete scale	Prospective cohort study	

Part II: Level of Measurement

Specify for each of the following whether the variable is *qualitative* or *quantitative*.

1. Household income (to the nearest thousand dollars).
2. Type of cancer (eg, breast, lung, colorectal).
3. Infant birthweight (grams).
4. Systolic blood pressure (below normal, within normal range, above normal).
5. Infant birthweight (low birthweight/normal birthweight).
6. Household income (below poverty level, at poverty level, above poverty level).
7. Systolic blood pressure (mm Hg).
8. Parity (number of viable offspring produced by a woman).
9. Drug dose (mg).
10. Cancer staging (eg, Duke's classification scheme).

Part III: Key Elements

Read each of the following clinical examples and identify the type of study design, independent variable, dependent variable, and target population. Identify whether the dependent variable is qualitative or quantitative.

1. Eighty-five immunocompromised patients participated in an early randomized, controlled trial to assess acyclovir's effectiveness to treat mucotaneous herpes simplex virus (HSV) infections. Group A contained 39 HSV-infected patients who received acyclovir for 10 days. HSV-infected group B patients (n_B = 46) received a placebo for 10 days. The clinicians concluded that acyclovir therapy accelerated healing of mucotaneous HSV infections based on the number of lesions that cleared, cessation of lesion formation (yes/no), and time to crusting (days) in immunocompromised patients.

2. Two thousand African-American women, ages 35 to 55 years, were surveyed to determine their adherence to recommended breast and cervical cancer screening schedules. At the time of the survey, each women lived in the inner city of a southern metropolitan area. Twenty-seven percent of the women had a household income under $5000; 32% had not graduated from high school; 68% were unmarried or separated; 20% were unemployed. Forty-eight percent had their most recent Papanicolaou (Pap) smear and 35% had mammography during the 12 months prior to the survey. The investigators concluded that African-American women in this age group who live in the inner city do not adhere to suggested screening schedules.

3. A total of 551 children born to human immunodeficiency virus type 1 (HIV-1) seropositive mothers between 1990 and 1991 were followed from birth to age 15 months. Of these, 101 (18.3%) acquired infection and seroconverted to HIV-1. Fifty percent of the children who acquired infection died by age 13.8 months. Method of delivery (vaginal/cesarean) did not alter the findings. The authors concluded that mother-to-child transmission of HIV-1 infection is a major public health problem.

Part IV: Generalizations

Read each of the following clinical examples and determine if the findings have been extended to the appropriate target population.

1. Oncologists at the National Cancer Institute studied the effect of interleukin-2 (IL-2), an immune system protein, in patients with spreading melanoma or unresponsive, spreading kidney cell cancer. Their goal was to determine if the use of IL-2 spurs the patient's immune system to fight the cancer and halt its spread. In 300 patients treated, 20 experienced total remission and remained in remission for at least 8 years. Additionally, 34 other patients experienced a partial regression of their cancer. The investigators concluded that the use of IL-2 marks a significant advance in the treatment of these two types of cancer.

2. Twenty-five male volunteers, ages 18 to 24 years, participated in a study to compare the effects of small doses of melatonin and a placebo to induce sleep at bedtime. Subjects who took melatonin fell asleep in 5 or 6 minutes; volunteers who received the placebo took 15 minutes or more to fall asleep. The researchers concluded that melatonin in small doses may be an effective sleep aid. They also concluded that it may be an effective agent for treating jet lag.

3. Because shorter hospital stays for cancer patients have shifted the burden of care to family members, the American Cancer Society sponsored a study to examine the effects of caregiving on family members. Three hundred patients undergoing outpatient treatment for breast, prostate, lung, or colorectal tumors were identified. Patients and their families were followed for 12 months to determine how family members were affected. The mean age of patients was 59. The mean age of caregivers was 55; 81% of caregivers were spouses. Primary caregivers spent an average of 4.2 hours per day caring for the patient; many caregivers averaged 8 hours or more per day for patients with advanced disease. Half of the caregivers worked full time outside the home; among these, 11% had to take a leave of absence from work to care for the patient. Fifty-five percent of patients required help dressing, bathing, eating, and using the bathroom. Sixty percent required help with cooking, housework, errands, and transportation. The investigators concluded that at-home care of cancer patients such as the ones studied exacts a heavy toll on the primary caregiver, who is the spouse in most cases.

Solutions

Part II: Level of Measurement

1. Household income (to the nearest thousand dollars): Quantitative.
2. Type of cancer (breast, lung, colorectal, etc.): Qualitative.
3. Infant birth weight (grams): Quantitative.
4. Systolic blood pressure (below normal, normal, above normal): Qualitative.
5. Infant birth weight (low, normal): Qualitative.
6. Household income (below, at, above poverty level): Qualitative.
7. Systolic blood pressure (mm Hg): Quantitative.
8. Parity (number of viable offspring produced by a woman: Quantitative.
9. Drug dose (mg): Quantitative.
10. Cancer staging (eg, Duke's classification scheme): Qualitative.

Part III: Key Elements

1. Herpes simplex virus infections.
   Study design: Controlled clinical trial.
   Independent variable: Drug (acyclovir versus placebo).
   Dependent variables and measurement. Cessation of lesion formation (yes/no): Qualitative. Time to lesion crusting (days): Quantitative. Number of lesions that cleared: Quantitative.
   Target population: Immunocompromised patients with HSV infections.
2. Breast and cervical cancer screening.
   Study design: Cross-sectional.
   Independent variable: There is no clearly defined independent variable.
   Dependent variables and measurement. Participated in cervical cancer screening in the 12 months prior to the study (yes/no): Qualitative. Participated in breast cancer screening in the 12 months prior to the study (yes/no): Qualitative.
   Target population: African-American women, 35 to 55 years of age, who live in an inner city (note that the investigators do not restrict their conclusion to a specific geographic area, eg, metropolitan area in the South).
3. HIV-1 positive mothers and their children.
   Study design: Prospective cohort.
   Independent variable: HIV-1 infection of mother (which is a constant) method of delivery is a *confounding variable*.
   Dependent variables and measurement. Infection acquisition and seroconversion (yes/ no): Qualitative. Life span from birth to end of study (months): Quantitative.
   Target population: Children born to mothers who are HIV-1 seropositive during pregnancy.

Part IV: Generalizations

1. IL-2 and immune system functioning. The investigators extended their findings to the treatment of patients with spreading melanoma or unresponsive, spreading kidney cell cancer. The sampled and target populations appear to be the same. Thus, the clinicians generalized their findings to the appropriate patients.
2. Melatonin as a sleep aid. The sampled population consists of male volunteers, ages 18 to 24 years. The findings about the effectiveness of melatonin as a sleep aid are applied without restrictions, such as the individual's age, general health, or sex. It is inappropriate at this point to extend these findings so broadly. In addition, the conclusions about the treatment of jet lag are unfounded because it does not appear that the investigators included any subjects with jet lag.
3. Caregiving and cancer patients. The investigators temper their conclusions by applying

them to the "at home care of cancer patients such as the ones studied." It appears, then, that the sampled and target populations are sufficiently similar to support the investigators' generalizations.

Summarizing Data in Tables and Graphs   2

Clinical Example: Alcohol and Trauma

To determine whether alcohol is an important risk factor in trauma, Meyers and Zepeda (1990) studied 2262 patients admitted to a trauma center between January 1985 and December 1987. Blood alcohol levels were measured on 2095 of patients (93%); alcohol was present in the blood of 855 (41%). Among these 855 trauma patients, 274 (32%) had blood alcohol levels higher than 100 mg/dL. The investigators concluded that "the level of alcohol involvement in trauma is high and this involvement must be addressed by the medical community and health care system" (p 149).

In this study, Meyers and colleagues helped to clarify an important issue in public health. Their data support the widespread clinical impression that alcohol is an important risk factor in trauma. Greenberg (1933, p 133) defines **risk factor** as an attribute or agent that is thought to be related to the occurrence of a particular outcome, such as a disease. For example, cigarette smoking is a risk factor for lung cancer. In our clinical example, injury is the outcome and alcohol is the agent. Meyers and Zepeda collected demographic data, including the patient's age, the time of day, and the day of the week when the trauma patient was seen; and information about the type and severity of the injury (eg, gunshot wound, stabbing, motorcycle accident). The clinicians then *organized* and *summarized* their data to identify key features and patterns. Recall from Chapter 1 that organization and summarization are the goals of descriptive statistics. In their study, Meyers and Zepeda could have listed each piece information for each of the 2262 trauma patients. This approach, however, does not allow us to locate salient information easily or quickly. For example, how many trauma patients were seen on Saturdays? Was a greater percentage of patients seen on Saturdays or another day of the week? Was a greater number of blood alcohol tests positive in a particular age group? Answers to these and similar questions can be obtained readily if data are summarized in a table or graph.

Tables and graphs are central to descriptive statistics because they allow investigators to communicate efficiently and economically. In this chapter, we will discuss commonly encountered formats for tables and graphs. We will also illustrate how easily data can be distorted if a table or graph is constructed incorrectly.

OBJECTIVES

When you complete this chapter, you should be able to:

- Differentiate various kinds of tables and graphs according to their key features.
- Discuss the appropriate use of different tables and graphs in light of the research questions and the corresponding variables.
- Read tables and graphs and identify key trends and other features of the data.

Table 2–1. Unordered array containing systolic blood
pressure (mm Hg) of 8 women.

127	102
140	137
125	139
117	140

PRESENTING DATA IN TABLES

Tables are often used to present qualitative and quantitative variables. The unordered array, ungrouped frequency distribution, grouped frequency distribution, and relative frequency distribution are described below. Tables that are inappropriate for the questions asked or the information displayed can lead to erroneous conclusions. Therefore, we provide the rules for constructing and common statistical tables in the next several sections.

Unordered Array

An **unordered array** is a listing of observations without regard to their order of magnitude or frequency of occurrence. Researchers use this tabular format to display quantitative and qualitative data. If the number of events or entities (eg, patients) is small, this format may be useful. Table 2–1 gives an example of an unordered array. The systolic blood pressures (mm Hg) of 8 women, ages 30 to 40 years, are listed; these readings were obtained during a routine gynecologic visit.

Occasionally, a clinician may want to construct a similar table to summarize data from a case series investigation. With some modification in format, a display appropriate to a case series study can be developed. An example is presented in Table 2–2, which summarizes quantitative and qualitative data from a case series investigation by Varga and co-workers (1989). The investigators describe 4 women who presented with systemic sclerosis after augmentation mammoplasty (breast enlargement) with silicone-gel implants. Systemic sclerosis "is a multisystem disorder of unknown etiology characterized by fibrosis of the skin, blood vessels, and kidneys" (Gilliland, 1991, p 1443). Age at the time of the procedure and other variables of interest are listed on the left of the table; these variables form the rows. Patients are identified across the top of the table and form the columns. Patient data appear in the intersection of the appropriate row and column. For example, patient 1 was 32 years of age when she had breast enlargement. Fifteen years elapsed between the procedure and development of systemic sclerosis. Note that patients are not ordered on any variable (eg, age) when the procedure was done or the length of time between the procedure and development of the disorder. Whether the variables of interest form the rows and patients form the columns is a matter of personal preference. Row-by-column tables are discussed in more detail in Chapters 7 and 15.

Table 2–2. Clinical characteristics of women who developed systemic sclerosis after augmentation mammoplasty.

	Patient			
Variable	**1**	**2**	**3**	**4**
Age at mammoplasty (years)	32	50	34	37
Interval between mammoplasty and systemic sclerosis (years)	15	9	10	6
Raynaud phenomenon	Yes	No	Yes	Yes
Extent of scleroderma	Diffuse	Diffuse	Limited	Diffuse
Joint or tendon sheath involvement	Yes	Yes	Yes	Yes
Lymphadenopathy	Yes	Yes	Yes	No
Esophageal dysfunction	No	No	Yes	Yes
Pulmonary involvement	Yes	Yes	Yes	No

Adapted with permission from Varga J, Schumacher H, Jimenez S: Systemic sclerosis after augmentation mammoplasty with silicone implants. *Ann Intern Med* 1989;111:377.

Table 2–3. Ungrouped frequency distribution of FEV_1 measurements of 97 pediatric patients.

$FEV_1{}^a$	Freq	$FEV_1{}^a$	Freq	$FEV_1{}^a$	Freq	$FEV_1{}^a$	Freq	$FEV_1{}^a$	Freq	$FEV_1{}^a$	Freq
132	1	112	0	92	4	72	0	52	2	32	0
131	0	111	1	91	2	71	1	51	0	31	0
130	0	110	1	90	3	70	1	50	0	30	0
129	0	109	1	89	5	69	0	49	0	29	1
128	0	108	3	88	4	68	1	48	0	Total	97
127	1	107	0	87	0	67	1	47	1		
126	0	106	2	86	0	66	0	46	0		
125	0	105	2	85	0	65	3	45	0		
124	0	104	1	84	0	64	1	44	0		
123	0	103	1	83	2	63	1	43	0		
122	1	102	2	82	5	62	1	42	0		
121	0	101	4	81	1	61	0	41	1		
120	0	100	4	80	2	60	1	40	1		
119	1	99	0	79	5	59	2	39	0		
118	0	98	1	78	1	58	0	38	0		
117	0	97	0	77	0	57	0	37	0		
116	0	96	3	76	0	56	0	36	0		
115	0	95	2	75	1	55	1	35	0		
114	1	94	1	74	1	54	1	34	0		
113	2	93	1	73	3	53	0	33	0		

^{a}Expressed as percentage of predicted values.

Ungrouped Frequency Distribution (Ordered Array)

Another type of table is the **ungrouped frequency distribution**, also known as **ordered array**. An ungrouped frequency distribution is used only for quantitative data. A distribution is a table or graph in which all values of a variable of interest are displayed with their corresponding frequency (Last, 1983, p 29). In an ungrouped frequency distribution, observations are arranged in order of magnitude, along with their frequency of occurrence. Table 2–3 contains FEV_1 (forced expiratory volume in 1 second) measurements of 97 patients, ages 6 to 18 years, seen in the office by a pediatric allergist. FEV_1, the volume of gas exhaled during the first second of expiration, is one of several measurements of pulmonary function (Weinberger & Drazen, 1991, p 1033). Pulmonary function tests objectively measure "the ability of the respiratory system to perform gas exchange by assessing its ventilation, diffusion, and mechanical properties" (Stauffer, 1988, p 133). A mathematical equation was used to standardize the data in Table 2–3 by age, height, race, and sex. The data are expressed as a percentage of predicted values. Thus, a value of 100% has the same meaning regardless of the age, height, race, or sex of the patient. Put another way, a value of 100% indicates that, in the first second of the test, a patient expelled 100% of the volume of air expected for an individual of his or her age, height, sex, and race. A value of 80% indicates that, in the first second of the test, a patient expelled 80% of the volume expected for an individual of his or her age, sex, height, and race. According to Weinberger and Drazen (1991, p 1035), pulmonary function is considered normal if predicted values range between 80% and 120%.

A researcher constructs an ungrouped frequency distribution by ranking observations from highest to lowest, as in Table 2–3; alternately, observations may be ranked from lowest to highest. After observations are tallied, the number of times each observation occurs is converted to a *count* or *frequency*. Keep in mind that every value between the largest and smallest observation is listed, regardless of whether the value actually occurred. A zero frequency is recorded for values that were not observed (such as 131, 115, 107, 99, in Table 2–3). Note that the table is assigned a number and title, appropriate column headings are included, and the total number of observations is noted.

Regardless of the number of observations in an ungrouped frequency distribution, this type of table makes it easy to identify the largest and smallest observation and determine the *range,* that is, the difference between the largest and smallest observation. The largest observation in

Table 2–3 is 132 and the smallest is 29; thus the range is 103 ($132 - 29 = 103$). The range, which is used primarily in descriptive statistics, is discussed further in Chapter 3. As the number of observations in an ungrouped frequency distribution increases, it becomes more difficult to identify trends in the data. In this case, the usefulness of the ungrouped frequency distribution decreases.

Grouped Frequency Distribution

By contrast, the **grouped frequency distribution** becomes more useful as the number of observations increases. Like the ungrouped frequency distribution, the grouped frequency distribution is appropriate for quantitative data. Observations in a grouped frequency distribution are organized into **class intervals**; the frequency of occurrence in each interval is then recorded. Table 2–4 shows a grouped frequency distribution constructed from the data in Table 2–3.
To construct a grouped frequency distribution, follow these steps:

1. Locate the largest and smallest observation.

2. Compute the range.

3. Use the range as a guide to determine the number of class intervals.

4. Construct the class intervals.

5. Tally the number of observations in each class interval and convert the tallies to counts (frequencies).

6. Organize the table. Number it and give it a title. List class intervals in the left column and corresponding frequencies in the right column. Label each column clearly. Include the number of observations in the table.

Because the salient characteristics of data can be altered by the choice of the number of class intervals, rules-of-thumb for constructing a grouped frequency distribution have been suggested. Some statisticians recommend using between 10 and 20 intervals (Minium et al, 1993, p 31). Others advise using between 6 and 14 (Dawson-Saunders & Trapp, 1994, p 26) or between 6 and 15 intervals (Daniel, 1991, p 7). If the number of intervals is too small, excessive **grouping error** can occur. Grouping error is the loss of identity of individual observations. The effect of grouping error is easier to visualize in a graph (see Figure 2–5) than a

Table 2–4. Grouped frequency distribution of FEV$_1$ measurements of 97 pediatric patients.

FEV$_1$ Measurements[a]	Frequency	True Limits
125–132	2	124.5–132.5
117–124	2	116.5–124.5
109–116	6	108.5–116.5
101–108	15	100.5–108.5
93–100	12	92.5–100.5
85–92	18	84.5–92.5
77–84	16	76.5–84.5
69–76	7	68.5–76.5
61–68	8	60.5–68.5
53–60	5	52.5–60.5
45–52	3	44.5–52.5
37–44	2	36.5–44.5
29–36	1	28.5–36.5
Total number of observations (n)	97	

[a]Expressed as percentage of predicted values.

table; therefore, it is discussed later in this chapter (see "The Effect of Grouping Error"). If the number of intervals is too large, it may not be possible to summarize data.

The "6-to-14" rule-of-thumb was used to construct the grouped frequency distribution presented in Table 2–4. This is done as follows. After locating the largest and smallest observation, calculate the range. Next, divide the range by 6 and then by 14. Use these results to identify a convenient class interval width. If we wish to construct a grouped frequency distribution with approximately 6 intervals, we would choose an interval width of 17 units (range = 103; 103/6 = 17.17); for 14 intervals, the class interval width would be 7 units (103/14 = 7.36). Table 2–4, which contains 13 intervals, was constructed using an interval width of 8 units. Given the moderately large range in FEV_1 measurements, 6 or 7 intervals would have produced too much grouping error. Therefore, a larger number of class intervals was created.

It may appear from Table 2–4 that the interval width is 7 units (for example $36 - 29 = 7$); however, the width is 8 units. The interval width is based on the **true** or **real limits** of each interval. True limits are one-half the unit of measurement above and below the actual value of an observation. Because the FEV_1 measurements in Tables 2–3 and 2–4 were reported to the nearest integer, the true limits of 29 are 28.5 to 29.5. If we use the true limits of each interval, we obtain the correct interval width of 8 units. For example, the first interval extends from 29 to 36; its true limits are 28.5 to 36.5. The interval width is $36.5 - 28.5 = 8$. Although true limits usually do not appear in tables in the published literature, they are included in Table 2–4 (column 3) to illustrate their "behind-the-scenes" role. True limits are used later in this chapter to construct different types of graphs.

To construct the class intervals, we select a convenient starting point for the lower limit of the first interval. The lowest FEV_1 measurement was chosen in our example. Form the class intervals so that they are *mutually exclusive* and *exhaustive*. Mutually exclusive means that an observation can be categorized in only one interval. For example, the intervals 45 to 55 and 55 to 65 are *not* mutually exclusive because a value of 55 can be counted in both intervals. Exhaustive means that all intervals between the lowest and highest are included, even if no observation occurs in an interval.

Organize the intervals, beginning with the largest or smallest. For example, the intervals in Table 2–4 are arranged in descending order from the top of the table. Each class interval is constructed so that the lower limit is on the left and upper limit is on the right of the interval (eg, 37–44). Class intervals are generally the same width. Occasionally, the top or bottom interval may be open ended (eg, 36 or less, or 125 or more). Researchers use open-ended intervals when a relatively large gap exists between the two or three lowest or two or three highest values. In general, avoid using grouped frequency distributions with open-ended intervals because these open-ended intervals do not allow us to construct some types of graphs and calculate some statistical indices (eg, the range).

RELATIVE FREQUENCY DISTRIBUTION

Many researchers prefer to work with a **relative frequency distribution** which contains percentage or proportionate frequencies, rather than raw frequencies. Percentage and proportionate frequencies are referred to as **relative frequencies** because they are computed in relation to the total number of observations. We obtain a percentage frequency by dividing the frequency in a class interval (f_i) by the total number of observations (sample size, n) and multiplying by 100: $[(f_i/n) \times 100]$, where i indicates the interval number, such as $i = 1$ for the first interval, $i = 2$ for the second interval, and so on. Thus the percentage frequency for the interval 45 to 52 is 6.19% $[(6/97) \times 100 = 6.1856\%$, or 6.19% rounded to two decimals]. We calculate proportionate frequency by dividing the frequency in a class interval by the total number of observations (f_i/n).

GROUPED PERCENTAGE FREQUENCY DISTRIBUTION

We can convert the grouped frequency distribution in Table 2–4 into a grouped percentage frequency distribution by adding a percentage frequency column. Table 2–5 contains percentage frequencies (column 4).

Table 2–5. Grouped percentage frequency distribution of FEV_1 measurements of 97 pediatric patients.

FEV_1 Measurements[a]	Frequency	Midpoint	Percentage Frequency
125–132	2	128.5	2.06
117–124	2	120.5	2.06
109–116	6	112.5	6.19
101–108	15	104.5	15.46
93–100	12	96.5	12.37
85–92	18	88.5	18.56
77–84	16	80.5	16.49
69–76	7	72.5	7.22
61–68	8	64.5	8.25
53–60	5	56.5	5.15
45–52	3	48.5	3.09
37–44	2	40.5	2.06
29–36	1	32.5	1.04
Total number of observations (n)	97		

[a]Expressed as percentage of predicted values.

We learn from Table 2–5 that approximately 1% of the patients had FEV_1 measurements between 29 and 36% of predicted values. Approximately 19% (18.56%) had FEV_1 measurements between 85 and 92% of predicted values. Percentage frequencies allow us to discern quickly whether the reported distribution of measurements resembles those obtained by a clinician from his or her patients.

In many instances, the use of a relative frequency, like percentage frequency, is based on personal preference. An important caveat exists, however. Relative frequency *must* be used when data sets with different sample sizes are compared. Suppose a pediatric allergist wishes to determine whether FEV_1 measurements differ in the fall and spring. In the fall, the clinician collects the 97 measurements presented in Table 2–5. In the spring, she collects FEV_1 measurements from 175 patients who are virtually identical on important demographic and clinical variables to the patients seen in the fall. To compare the two sets of data, the clinician converts the raw frequency in each class interval to a percentage frequency. It is easier now to discuss differences and similarities between the two samples based on the respective percentage frequencies. Because the number of patients is greater in the spring (n_{SPRING} = 175 versus n_{FALL} = 97), we expect a greater number of observations in almost every class interval for the spring sample. Thus, it would be inappropriate to contrast the raw frequencies in the two samples.

DISPLAYING DATA IN GRAPHS

Graphs are used widely to provide a visual display of data, often showing interesting patterns and findings. The bar diagram, histogram, and frequency polygon are three graphic formats discussed below. Because graphs are used so commonly and most word-processing, graphics, and statistical software offer numerous graphic options, with several variations on basic graph types, it is important that you understand when different types of graphs are used and how they should be constructed. An inappropriate format or method of construction can present data in a misleading fashion, no matter how attractive the computer may make it appear. Therefore, it is vitally important that you understand the principles underlying the construction and use of the graphic formats discussed in this chapter. Thus, the impact of constructing too few class intervals, and the effect of manipulating the relationship between the length of the x-axis and height of the y-axis, are illustrated.

Graphed frequency distributions generally have a horizontal and vertical axis. The horizontal axis is referred to as the x-axis or abscissa. The vertical axis is called the y-axis or ordinate. Numerical values of a quantitative variable and categories of a qualitative variable are typically plotted on the x-axis. The frequency, or some function of it, is shown on the y-axis.

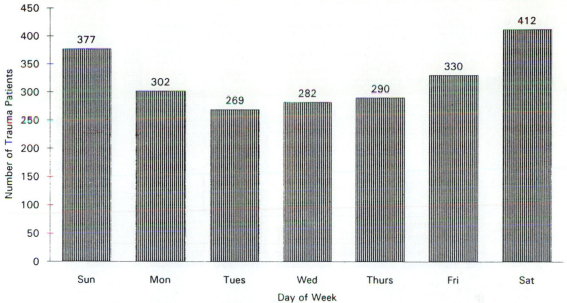

Figure 2–1. Total number of trauma patients by day of week (n = 2262). (Adapted with permission from Meyers H et al: Alcohol and trauma. An endemic syndrome. *West J Med* 1990;**153**:149.)

Bar Diagram

A **bar diagram** consists of a series of nonadjacent bars plotted on the x-axis, with frequency plotted on the y-axis. The bars represent the categories of a *nominal* or *ordinal variable*. Each observation is classified into only one category. The frequency of observations in each category is represented by the length of the corresponding bars. Each axis is labeled clearly. The figure is numbered and titled.

We began this chapter with a clinical example. Recall that Dr. Meyers and her associates sought to determine whether alcohol is an important risk factor in trauma. The bar diagram in Figure 2–1 shows the number of trauma patients by day of the week. For the reader's convenience, the number of patients per day is indicated at the top of each bar. Of the 2262 trauma patients seen in the trauma center, the largest number received treatment on Saturdays (n_{SAT} = 412). The next largest group of patients presented on Sundays (n_{SUN} = 377). The number of patients seen was lowest on Tuesday (n_{TUES} = 269); the number increased on Wednesday, Thursday, and Friday until reaching a high on Saturday.

Figure 2–2 depicts the percentage, rather than number, of trauma patients by day of the week. Horizontal grid lines make it easier for the reader to determine the percentage frequencies. This graphs shows that approximately 17% of trauma patients were brought to the trauma center on Sundays. The highest percentage of trauma patients (approximately 18%) was seen on Saturdays. The fewest number of patients (slightly less than 12%) presented on Tuesdays.

Rather than creating separate bar diagrams to display the number of trauma patients on whom blood alcohol levels (BAL) were determined and the number of these patients with positive tests (BAL+), the investigators constructed one graph. The bar diagram in Figure 2–3 shows the total number of trauma patients by day of the week, number of blood alcohol tests performed, and number of positive tests. Horizontal grid lines have been added. Note that the bars within a given day are adjacent, but the bars for different days are not.

We can determine from Figure 2–3 that the number of blood alcohol tests ranged from approximately 250 on Tuesdays to just over 350 on Sundays. Although the number of trauma victims seen was greatest on Saturdays, more blood alcohol tests were done on Sundays than on any other day. However, the highest percentage of positive tests (BAL+) occurred on Saturdays, when approximately 200 of the 300 tests were positive (or about 67%). In contrast, 250 tests were done on Tuesdays and slightly fewer than 75 (approximately 30%) were positive.

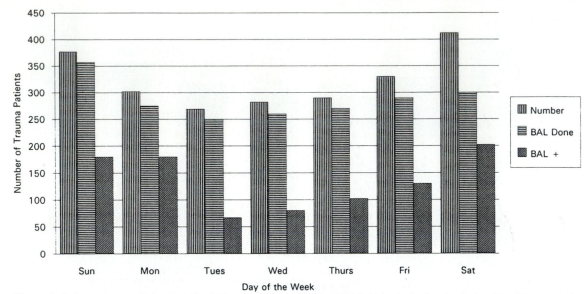

Figure 2–2. Percentage of trauma patients by day of the week (n = 2262). (Adapted with permission from Meyers et al: Alcohol and trauma. An endemic syndrome. *West J Med* 1990;**153**:149.)

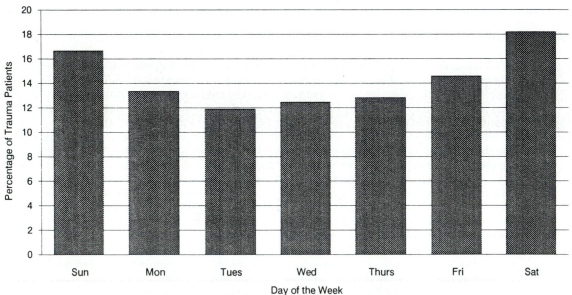

Figure 2–3. Total number of trauma patients by day of week and blood alcohol level. (Adapted with permission from Meyers et al: Alcohol and trauma: An endemic syndrome. *West J Med* 1990;**153**:149.)

Histogram

Like the bar diagram, the **histogram** is frequently used in research. Used to summarize *quantitative* data, a histogram contains a series of adjacent bars; the height of each bar indicates frequency. By convention, the x-axis contains the quantitative values of the variable of interest; the y-axis depicts frequency. However, some statistical software presents information in the opposite way (that is, the x-axis contains frequency). The FEV_1 measurements

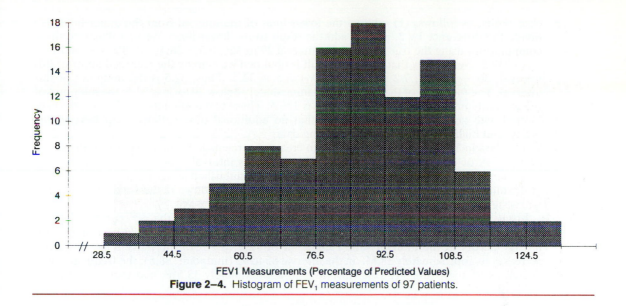

Figure 2–4. Histogram of FEV$_1$ measurements of 97 patients.

summarized in Table 2–5 are displayed in Figure 2–4. A double slash mark (//) appears on the x-axis near the origin to indicate that a portion of the scale of measurement (0 to 28) has been omitted. We can see from Figure 2–4 that relatively few of the FEV$_1$ measurements occur in the lowest or highest intervals. The largest concentration of values occurs between 76.5 and 108.5.

Note that the feet of each bar are plotted at the *true limits* of each class interval. The true limits of each interval appear in Table 2–4. Because the vertical boundaries of each bar coincide with the true limits of a particular interval, adjacent bars touch each other. To illustrate, the rectangle representing the frequency in the first interval (29–36) is plotted at 28.5 to 36.5; the rectangle showing the frequency in the second interval (37–44) has vertical boundaries plotted at 36.5 to 44.5. Thus, the two bars are contiguous because they share the common vertical boundary of 36.5. A gap or space between bars occurs only if a class interval has a zero frequency. The area of each bar is proportional to the percentage of observations in the class interval. For example, 18 observations occur in the interval 85 to 92; these account for 18.56% of the total number of measurements [(18/97) × 100% = 18.56%]. Therefore, 18.56% of the total area occupied by the histogram is covered by the rectangle representing the interval 85 to 92. Thus, a histogram depicts area. According to Dawson-Saunders and Trapp (1994, p 27), "the area concept is one reason the width of the classes should be equal; otherwise, the height of the columns in the histogram must be appropriately modified to maintain the correct area."

Frequency Polygon

Like the histogram, the **frequency polygon** is appropriate for *quantitative* data. The x-axis contains the numeric values of the variable of interest; the y-axis represents frequency. The frequency polygon contains a series of points plotted at the midpoint of each class interval and connected to each other by a straight line. The height of the points corresponds to the frequency in each interval. The **midpoint** of a class interval is a value that occurs halfway between the upper and lower limits of the interval. The polygon is brought down to the x-axis by plotting a zero frequency at the midpoint of the class interval immediately below and above the lowest and highest intervals containing observations. The total area under the frequency polygon is equal to the total area under a histogram (Daniel, 1991, p 12). The interval immediately below the lowest in our FEV$_1$ example is 21 to 28; the interval immediately above the highest one is 133 to 140. We compute the midpoint by using either the true or recorded class limits, as follows: (1) subtract the lower limit of the interval from the upper limit, (2) divide the difference by 2, and (3) add the result to the lower limit. We first illustrate these computations using the true limits of the interval 29 to 36: $36.5 - 28.5 = 8$; $8/2 = 4$; and $28.5 + 4 = 32.5$. Next, show that the same result is obtained we employ the recorded limits of this interval: $36 - 29 = 7$; $7/2 = 3.5$; and $29 + 3.5 = 32.5$. Thus, 32.5 is the midpoint of this interval. The midpoint of the class interval immediately below 29 to 36 is 20.5; the midpoint of the interval immediately above 125 to 132 is 136.5. These two midpoints (20.5 and 136.5) are plotted with zero frequency to indicate that no additional observations occur beyond the lowest and highest class intervals containing data.

The data in Table 2–5 have been used to create a percentage frequency polygon displayed in graph A of Figure 2–5. The midpoint of each class interval appears in Table 2–5, even though midpoints usually do not appear in tables in the published literature. Points are plotted at the midpoint of each class interval; the polygon is brought down to the x-axis; the // on the x-axis signifies the omission of values on the lower end of the x-axis.

From the polygon in graph A of Figure 2–5 we observe that the percentage of FEV_1 measurements increases in each of the lower intervals; a slight decrease in percentage frequency occurs in the interval with a midpoint of 72.5 (69–76). The percentage frequency increases to approximately 18.5% in the interval 85 to 92 (midpoint, 88.5); the frequency then decreases to approximately 12%, increases to approximately 15.5%, and then decreases in

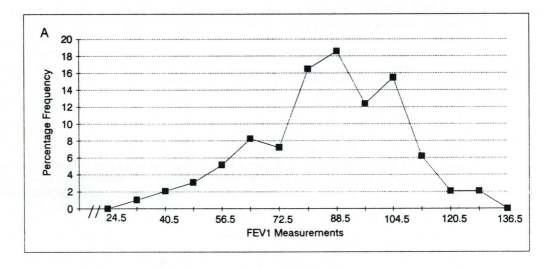

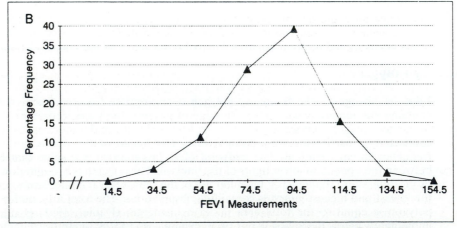

Figure 2–5. The effect of using too few class intervals (data from Table 2–5).

the subsequent interval. The percentage of FEV_1 values in the two highest intervals is relatively small: approximately 2% in each interval.

The Effect of Grouping Error

Grouping error, the loss of identity for one or more observations, occurs whenever data are grouped into class intervals. Grouping error is particularly problematic when too few class intervals are constructed. In such cases, the graph may appear smoother and more regular than it would appear if a more appropriate number of intervals had been used. Rules-of-thumb for graph construction (eg, use between 6 and 14 class intervals) were developed to minimize grouping error.

Figure 2–5 contains two percentage frequency polygons. The polygon in graph A was constructed from Table 2–5 in which the FEV_1 measurements were cast into 13 class intervals. Note the decrease in percentage frequency between the intervals of 61 to 68 (midpoint, 64.5) and 69 to 76 (midpoint, 72.5); and between 85 to 92 (midpoint, 88.5) and 93 to 100 (midpoint, 96.5). Now examine the bottom panel (graph B). The raw data from Table 2–3 were cast into 6 intervals and then used to create a polygon. An interval width of 20 was utilized; the lowest interval containing data is 25 to 44; the highest containing observations is 125 to 144. The data in graph B appear smooth and regular. Percentage frequency increases from the lowest interval to the one containing the observations of 85 to 104 (midpoint, 94.5), and then decreases in each subsequent interval.

Although the number of intervals used to group and graph the raw data in Table 2–3 is at the lower limit of the 6-to-14 rule-of-thumb, 6 intervals are insufficient for these data. In this case, the selection of an appropriate number of intervals is determined by various factors, including:

Awareness of the range (103 for the FEV_1 measurements).
Knowledge of the data being graphed.
Overall experience working with data.

Researchers may often construct three or four versions of the same graph before determining the best version. The "best" graph is one that will not make the data appear more regular than they actually are, or that will not overemphasize relatively minor increases or decreases.

The Effect of Changing the Relationship Between the X- and Y-axes

The appearance and salient features of graphed data can be altered by changing the relationship between the x- and y-axes. Consequently, some statisticians recommend that the height of the y-axis should be approximately 0.6 to 0.8 the length of the x-axis (Minium et al, 1993, p 50).

Figure 2–6 presents three percentage frequency polygons. Each graph contains the same data. However, we have manipulated the relationship between the length of the x-axis and the height of the y-axis. In the top panel (A), we have reduced the height of the y-axis and elongated the x-axis. Note the flat appearance of the top polygon: decreases and increases in percentage frequency appear rather small. This contrasts markedly with the polygon in the left lower panel (B), where the x-axis has been shortened and the y-axis lengthened, making the increases and decreases in percentage frequency appear rather substantial. The third panel (C) contains a percentage frequency polygon constructed according to the 0.6 to 0.8 rule-of-thumb: that is, the height of the y-axis is between 0.6 and 0.8 the length of the x-axis. It is not essential that you follow this rule of thumb in every instance. However, keep in mind its extreme importance: to prevent the distortion of data, a reasonable balance must exist between the height of the y-axis and length of the x-axis. Otherwise, data may be presented in a misleading way.

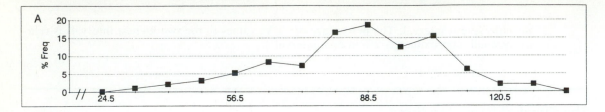

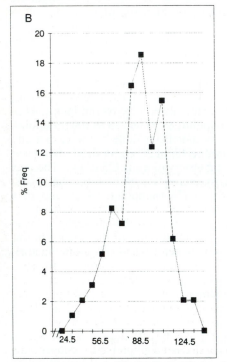

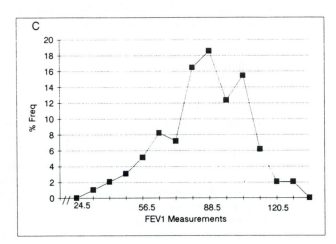

Figure 2–6. Effects of altering the relationship between the x- and y-axis.

Shapes of Distributions

Tables and graphs provide important information about salient characteristics of a set of observations, such as the category or class interval in which the largest number of observations occurred. In addition, graphs can depict how *quantitative* observations distribute themselves throughout the range of values contained in the data. Do observations occur with greater frequency in the middle and with relatively lesser frequency in the extremes? Do the observations occur with greater frequency in the lower range of values and with relatively lesser frequency in the upper extreme? Do observations aggregate more in the upper extreme? These questions focus on the *shape of the distribution* of observations.

The shape of a distribution (symmetric or asymmetric) can be determined readily from a graph of a set of quantitative observations. Shape is a key factor in determining which statistical indices should be used to summarize and interpret data. These indices are discussed in the next chapter. In a **symmetric distribution,** the right and left halves are identical; the right half is the mirror image of the left. In an **asymmetric distribution,** the left and right halves are not identical. Asymmetric distributions are also called **skewed distributions.**

Commonly encountered distributions are graphed in Figure 2–7. Real data seldom produce curves that are as smooth and even as those displayed in this figure. However, many collections of observations, when graphed, approximate a symmetric curve. To help you visualize

A. Symmetric

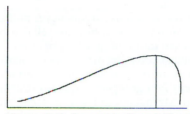

B. Symmetric

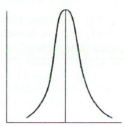

C. Negatively Skewed

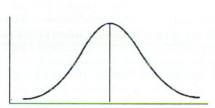

D. Positively Skewed

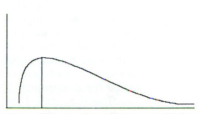

Figure 2–7. Symmetric (A and B) and skewed (C and D) distributions. (The x-axis contains quantitative values; the y-axis contains frequency.)

the halves of a distribution, a perpendicular has been dropped from the highest point on each curve (point of greatest frequency) to the x-axis. Diagrams A and B depict symmetric distributions. Symmetric distributions, or reasonable approximations, tend to result when a relatively large number of quantitative observations are tabled or graphed, (eg, systolic blood pressure, diastolic blood pressure, or height in the general adult population). Diagrams C and D illustrate asymmetric or skewed distributions. Skewed distributions may occur for several reasons, depending on the phenomenon or patient groups studied. For example, the distribution of age at onset of Alzheimer's disease is skewed because the disease tends to occur in the later decades of life. A skewed distribution is named according to the direction in which the thin tail points. If the thin tail points to the left of the perpendicular, the distribution is negatively skewed; if the thin tail points to the right of the perpendicular, the distribution is positively skewed. Look again at the observations in diagram C in Figure 2–7. The observations tend to aggregate at the upper end of the distribution and relatively few observations occur in the lower end; this distribution is negatively skewed. The observations in diagram D are skewed positively; note that the measurements tend to accumulate in the lower portion of the distribution and relatively few values occur in the upper tail.

SUMMARY

Tables and graphs allow efficient and economical communication about the salient characteristics of a set of observations. Because they are so useful for organizing and summarizing data, tables and graphs are central to descriptive statistics.

Tabular arrangements of data include the unordered array, ungrouped frequency distribution, and grouped frequency distribution. An unordered array can be used with qualitative and quantitative data. The ungrouped and grouped frequency distribution are used only for quantitative data. An unordered array lists quantitative or qualitative measurements without regard to order of magnitude or frequency of occurrence. In contrast, the ungrouped frequency distribution lists all quantitative measurements between the largest and smallest observed values, arranged according to order of magnitude; the frequency of each observation is also included. The grouped frequency distribution contains mutually exclusive and exhaustive class intervals for quantitative data, plus the frequency of occurrence of observations in each interval.

The bar diagram, histogram, and frequency polygon are three graphic formats that are commonly used to present medical data. The bar diagram is used appropriately with qualitative data. The histogram and frequency polygon are used to represent quantitative data. The bar diagram contains nonadjacent bars that represent the classes or categories of a qualitative variable; the height of the bars corresponds to the number of observations in each class or category. Often constructed from a grouped frequency distribution, the histogram contains adjacent bars whose height represents the frequency of observations in a class interval; the feet of the bars are plotted at the true limits of each interval. A gap occurs between bars only if a zero frequency is recorded for a class interval. The frequency polygon contains points plotted at the midpoint of each class interval and connected by straight lines. The polygon is brought down to the x-axis by plotting a zero frequency at the midpoint of the interval immediately above and below those contained in the data.

Personal preference usually determines whether raw or relative frequency is plotted on the y-axis of the histogram or the frequency polygon. However, we *must* use relative frequency when we compare two or more sets of data which have different numbers of cases.

To avoid presenting distorted data, researchers must construct graphs and tables carefully. Otherwise, readers may be misled by the way data are presented. Rules of thumb are suggested for determining the number of class intervals in a grouped frequency distribution. A guideline is provided for constructing histograms and frequency polygons: special attention is given to establishing an appropriate relationship between the length of the x-axis and height of the y-axis. The shape of a distribution—whether it is symmetric or asymmetric—is a key factor in determining the choice of statistical tools to summarize quantitative data.

REFERENCES

Daniel W: *Biostatistics: A Foundation for Analysis in the Health Sciences,* 5th ed. Wiley, 1991.

Dawson-Saunders B, Trapp R: *Basic and Clinical Biostatistics,* 2nd ed. Appleton & Lange, 1994.

Gilliland B: Systemic sclerosis (Scleroderma). In: *Harrison's Principles of Internal Medicine,* 12th ed. Wilson J et al (editors). McGraw-Hill, 1991.

Greenberg R. *Medical Epidemiology.* Appleton & Lange, 1993.

Last JM (editor): *A Dictionary of Epidemiology.* Oxford University Press, 1983.

Lerner I, Kennedy B: The prevalence of questionable methods of cancer treatment in the United States. *CA* 1992;**42**:181.

Meyers H, Zepeda S: Alcohol and trauma: An endemic syndrome. *West J Med* 1990;**153**:149.

Minium E, King B, Bear G: *Statistical Reasoning in Psychology and Education,* 3rd ed. Wiley, 1993.

Stauffer J: Pulmonary diseases. In: *Current Medical Diagnosis & Treatment.* Schroeder S et al (editors). Appleton & Lange, 1988.

Varga J, Schumacher H, Jimenez S: Systemic sclerosis after augmentation mammoplasty with silicone implants. *Ann Intern Med* 1989;**111**:377.

Weinberger S, Drazen J: Disturbances of respiratory function. In: *Harrison's Principles of Internal Medicine,* 12th ed. Wilson J et al (editors). McGraw-Hill, 1991.

Self-study Questions

Part I: Definitions

Define each of the following terms.

Asymmetric distribution (skewed distribution)	Relative frequency distribution Risk factor

Bar diagram
Class intervals
Frequency polygon
Grouped frequency distribution
Grouping error
Histogram
Midpoint

Skewed distribution
Symmetric distribution
True limits (real limits)
Ungrouped frequency distribution
(ordered array)
Unordered array

Part II: Errors in Constructing a Grouped Frequency Distribution

Examine the Table 2–6 and identify errors, if any, in its construction.

Table 2–6. Total cholesterol (mg/dL) values of 150 men after 6 weeks on a fat-restricted diet.

Class Interval	Frequency
450–499	2
400–450	3
350–399	5
250–299	9
200–275	27
199–150	51
140–150	7
Total number (n)	150

Part III: Graphic Formats

Read each of the following descriptions and respond as indicated.

1. As part of a health-and-fitness screening program conducted in a large metropolitan area, weight (kg) and height measurements (m) were obtained from 3 groups of female adolescents, ages 15 to 17 years: African-American (n_{AA} = 279), Caucasian (n_C = 262), and Hispanic (n_H = 264). Body mass index was calculated (BMI = kg/m^2) and used to classify each participant as underweight, within normal range, obese, or morbidly obese.
   a. What information should be placed on the x-axis?
   b. What information should be placed on the y-axis?
   c. Which graph is appropriate to display these data?
2. Concerned by reports of an increase in mortality due to heart disease in adult women and men, an epidemiologist studied deaths per 100,000 adult women and men, respectively. Data were organized by sex (male/female) and year (1985 to 1994). The objectives were to compare on one set of axes men and women by year; men and women across years; men across years; and women across years with respect to heart disease deaths per 100,000 individuals.
   a. How is frequency defined in this clinical example?
   b. Which graph is appropriate to display this kind of information?
   c. Describe how the graph to display this type of information might be organized.
3. Oncologists examined the distribution of age at diagnosis (to the nearest whole year) of glioblastoma, a primary brain tumor, in 457 affected men and 323 affected women. They would like to compare the age-at-onset distribution in these two patient samples on the same set of axes to describe similarities and differences between affected men and women.
   a. Age at diagnosis is what kind of variable?
   b. What should be plotted on the y-axis?
   c. Which graph should be constructed in light of the information and objectives?

Table 2–7. Use of questionable treatment methods by selected cancer site.

Site	Number of Patients	Percentage of Patients in Which at Least One Questionable Method Was Used
Breast	889	9.2
Colon	643	8.2
Stomach	127	4.9
Pancreas	71	7.3
Lung	545	8.9
Cervix	321	6.5
Lymphomas	311	14.5
Leukemia	92	13.0
Spine/spinal cord	38	27.9
Brain and CNS	133	20.9
Ovary	117	16.0

Adapted with permission from Lerner I, Kennedy B: The prevalence of questionable methods of cancer treatment in the United States. *CA* 1992;**42**:181.

Part IV: Reading Tables

Examine the following tables and summarize your observations.

1. After conducting a national survey of therapies to treat cancer, the Committee on Questionable Methods of Cancer Management of the American Cancer Society identified therapies of questionable value by cancer site. Therapies defined as being of questionable value included scientifically unproven treatments, diet, nutritional supplements, psychic approaches, massages, and electrical stimulation. A portion of the data collected by the Committee is displayed in Table 2–7.
2. Consider that gastroenterologists obtained information on several thousand patients (n = 12,221) with a particular gastrointestinal disease and tabled age at diagnosis (years) and percentage of patients in each age group. Their data are displayed in Table 2–8. Their goal is to identify distributional patterns with respect to the age at which patients are diagnosed with this disease.
3. The school nurse in a midsized 4-year high school in a southern community is concerned by the apparent increase in the number of cases of mononucleosis in his school. Approximately 11% of students in each grade in the past several years developed mononucleosis in any given school year. The nurse reviewed health records of all students and counted

Table 2–8. Age at diagnosis of patients with a particular gastrointestinal disease (n = 12,221).

Age at Diagnosis (years)	Percentage Frequency
70+	0.5
65–69	0.4
60–64	0.3
55–59	0.3
50–54	0.8
45–49	2.0
40–44	3.0
35–39	12.0
30–34	27.7
25–29	8.2
20–24	9.8
15–19	29.0
10–14	5.5
5–9	1.5

Table 2–9. Number of new cases of mononucleosis in a school year in a 4-year high school in a southern community.

Grade	Students Enrolled	Number of New Cases	Percentage of Students Affected[a]
9	153	18	11.76
10	126	14	11.11
11	119	25	21.01
12	118	21	17.80

[a]Percentage = number of new cases in grade divided by number of students enrolled in the grade.

the number of new cases of mononucleosis by grade level during the 1992-1993 school year. His goal is to assess whether an increase has occurred in the number of new cases in each grade level relative to previous years. He organized his data in Table 2–9.

Part V: Reading a Graph

Study each of the following graphs and outline your observations.

1. In its national survey of therapies to treat cancer, the Committee on Questionable Methods of Cancer Management of the American Cancer Society identified therapies of questionable value by geographic site. Therapies defined as being of questionable value included scientifically unproven treatments, diet, nutritional supplements, psychic approaches, massages, and electrical stimulation. A portion of the data collected by the Committee is displayed in Figure 2–8.
2. Clinicians at a prominent medical center developed an experimental treatment for a rare childhood leukemia. Children with this disease who receive conventional chemotherapy survive only a short time following diagnosis. Affected children whose parents gave informed consent were assigned randomly to receive either the experimental or conventional treatment. Survival (months) following diagnosis is graphed in Figure 2–9.

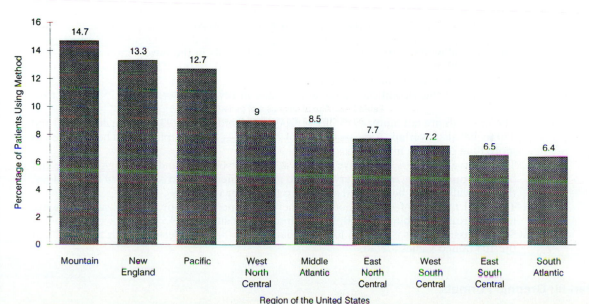

Figure 2–8. Use of questionable methods by Geographic Region. (Adapted with permission from Lerner I, Kennedy B: The prevalence of questionable methods of cancer treatment in the United States. *CA* 1992; **42**:181.)

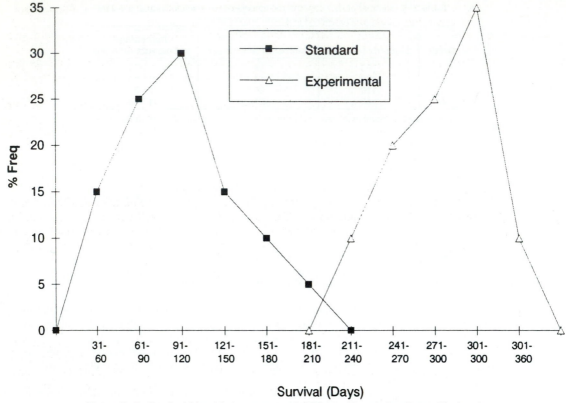

Figure 2–9. Survival (days) in two groups of children with a virulent form of leukemia.

Solutions

Part II: Errors in Constructing a Grouped Frequency Distribution

1. The interval width is not constant. The width is 11 units in the lowest interval (140–150: $150.5 - 139.5 = 11$ units) and 76 units in the interval 200 to 275 ($275.5 - 199.5 = 76$ units). In most other intervals, the width is 50 units.
2. The limits of the second class interval are listed in reverse order: 199 to 150 rather than 150 to 199.
3. The intervals are not mutually exclusive: 200 to 275 and 250 to 299 overlap; 400 to 450 and 450 to 499 also overlap. A measurement of 250 or 251, for example, would be classified in more than one class interval.
4. The intervals are not exhaustive. Observations between 300 and 398 (mg/dL) have not been captured in any of the intervals. If no measurements occurred between these values, the intervals should be included and a zero frequency recorded.
5. The total number of observations is either listed incorrectly or some observations are missing from the table; n = 150, but the frequencies sum to 104.
6. Seven class intervals is too few for these data. Note that two class intervals contain 78 of the 104 tallied values (75%).

Part III: Graphic Formats

1. a. The classes of body mass index should be placed on the x-axis: underweight, within normal range, obese, and morbidly obese.

    b. Relative frequency should appear on the y-axis because the number of females who were screened differs in each group.

    c. A bar diagram should be used because body mass index was treated as a qualitative variable.

2. a. The frequency of mortality due to heart disease is reported as the number of deaths per 100,000 adult women or men, depending on the group for whom information is reported.

    b. In light of the objectives and how the data were collected (by year and sex), a bar diagram should be used.

    c. The x-axis of the bar diagram should contain years. The y-axis should contain the number of deaths per 100,000 adults. Two rectangles should be constructed per year, one representing the number of deaths per 100,000 women and the other depicting the number of deaths per 100,000 men.

3. a. Age at diagnosis (to the nearest whole year) is quantitative.

    b. Relative frequency should be plotted on the y-axis because the number of affected men is different from the number of affected women (n_{MEN} = 457 versus n_{WOMEN} = 323).

    c. A percentage frequency polygon should be constructed. One polygon should be created for affected men; a second polygon should be constructed for affected women. Age at diagnosis should be placed on the x-axis. The polygon, rather than the histogram, will allow more rapid comparison between men and women.

Part IV: Reading Tables

1. Cancer sites are listed in Table 2–7 (column 1), along with the number of patients surveyed (column 2) and percentage of patients in which at least one treatment of questionable value was used (column 3). Because the number of patients differed for each cancer site, comparisons among sites must be based on a relative frequency; therefore, percentage frequencies were calculated.

    a. The use of questionable cancer treatment methods varied by site.

    b. The percentage of cancer patients for whom at least one questionable treatment was employed ranged from a high of 27.9% for patients with cancer of the spine or spinal cord to a low of 4.9% for patients with cancer of the stomach.

    c. The second largest percentage occurred for patients with brain cancer or cancer of the central nervous system (20.9%).

    d. Questionable methods were used in 13% or more of patients with lymphomas (14.5%), leukemia (13.0%), and ovarian cancer (16.0%).

    e. The percentage of questionable method use was fairly similar for patients with breast cancer (9.2%), lung cancer (8.9%), and colon cancer (8.2%); these percentages were only modestly higher than those for patients with cancer of the cervix (6.5%) and pancreas (7.3%).

2. Table 2–8 contains two columns of information; age at diagnosis (years) is grouped into 13 class intervals. Except for the open-ended top interval (70+ years), each interval is 5 units wide.

    a. A relatively small percentage of patients is diagnosed before age 15 (7% between the ages of 5 and 14 years).

    b. The largest percentage of patients (29%) is diagnosed between the ages of 15 and 19 years; the second largest percentage (27.7%) occurs between 30 and 34 years. Thus the distribution has two peak age classes in which patients are diagnosed. In fact, approximately 57% of affected patients are diagnosed either between the ages of 15 and 19 years or 30 and 34 years.

    c. Few patients, relatively speaking, are diagnosed after age 40 years. Approximately 7% of affected patients are diagnosed between the ages of 40 and 70+ years.

3. Table 2–9 consists of four columns of information; the first and last columns contain the information that may be of greatest interest to our school nurse.

    a. The percentage of affected students in grades 9 and 10 is fairly similar to the percentage in previous years (11.76% in grade 9, 11.11% in grade 10; 11% in previous years).

    b. The highest percentage of new cases of mononucleosis occurred in grade 11 (21.01%).

The percentage of affected students in grade 11 is almost double the percentage in grades 9 and 10 (1.79 times and 1.89 times greater, respectively) and almost double what occurred in previous years.
c. The percentage of new cases in grade 12 is slightly less than in grade 11 (17.8% versus 21.01%, respectively), but greater than in grades 9 and 10. The percentage of new cases in grade 12 is approximately 1.6 times greater than the percentage encountered in previous years.

Part V: Reading a Graph

1. Figure 2–8 contains the percentage of patients using questionable cancer treatment methods by geographic region.
   a. The use of questionable methods was greatest in the Mountain, New England, and Western (Pacific) states (14.7, 13.3, and 12.7%, respectively).
   b. The use of questionable methods occurred least often and was most similar in the East South Central (6.5%) and South Atlantic (6.4%) states.
   c. Among the remaining geographic regions, the use of questionable cancer treatment methods was noted in fewer than 10% of patients (West North Central, 9%; Middle Atlantic, 8.5%; East North Central, 7.7%; and West South Central, 7.2%).
2. Survival (days) is grouped into class intervals of 30 days and plotted for two groups of children in Figure 2–9.
   a. The distribution of survival is skewed positively for children who receive the standard treatment. The distribution of survival for children receiving the experimental treatment is skewed negatively.
   b. Affected children who received the standard treatment survived between 31 and 210 days. Affected children who received the experimental treatment survived between 211 and 360 days.
   c. The largest percentage of affected children receiving the standard treatment survive between 91 and 120 days (30%); the second largest percentage survived between 61 and 90 days (25%). In contrast, the largest percentage (35%) of children who received the experimental treatment survived 301 to 300 days; 25% survived between 271 and 300 days and 20% survived between 241 and 270 days.
   d. Five percent of patients who underwent standard treatment survived 181 to 210 days; none survived beyond 210 days. Ten percent of affected children who received the experimental treatment survived beyond 300 days; none survived beyond 360 days.

3

Summarizing Data: Statistical Indices for Quantitative Data

Clinical Example: Dietary Fat Control in Women

One hundred and fifty-six healthy women, ages 45 to 69 years, were enrolled in a study to evaluate the long-term effects of diet. Women in the intervention group followed a low-fat diet designed to reduce total dietary fat intake to 20% of baseline kilocalories (n_{INT} = 156). Women in the reference group (n_{REF} = 148) followed their normal diet with no dietary intervention. One year after the trial ended, the mean grams of saturated fat consumed by husbands of women in the intervention group was 19 g/day, with a standard deviation of 10.1 g/day. The mean grams of saturated fat consumed by husbands of women in the reference group was 23.9 g/day, with a standard deviation of 12.8 g/day. The investigators (Shattuck et al, 1992) conclude: "Our results suggest that a dietary intervention aimed at women can have an effect on their husbands and may be a low cost-effective approach to healthy dietary change for both women and men" (p 1244).

To appreciate the implications of the data summarized above, we must know what a mean and standard deviation are. How are these indices calculated? Can they be used with quantitative and qualitative data? Is the mean appropriate for skewed data? In this chapter, we address these and similar questions as they relate primarily to quantitative data. Measures appropriate for qualitative data (eg, proportions and rates) are covered in Chapter 4.

OBJECTIVES

When you complete this chapter, you should be able to:

- Define and describe the characteristics of the mean, median, mode, range, variance, standard deviation, and coefficient of variation.
- Discuss when to use the mean, median, mode, range, variance, standard deviation, and coefficient of variation.
- Calculate the median, mean, range, variance, standard deviation, and coefficient of variation.
- Identify the shape of a distribution from measures of central tendency.

Summarizing data and describing their salient characteristics are the goals of **descriptive statistics**. Two important characteristics of a distribution of *quantitative* observations are (1) the location of its central and (2) the spread or dispersion of observations about this center. A descriptive measure computed from a sample is a **statistic**; a descriptive index obtained from a population is a **parameter**. Statistics estimate parameters. We usually use Greek letters to designate parameters and Roman characters to represent statistics.

DESCRIBING THE CENTER OF A DISTRIBUTION

Quantitative indices that describe the center of a distribution are referred to as **measures of central tendency**. The mode, median, and mean are three common measures of central tendency.

Mode

Among all observations in an *ungrouped* frequency distribution, the **mode** is the value that occurs most often. For example, the mode of the systolic blood pressure readings in Table 2–1 in Chapter 2 is 140 mm Hg. A distribution may have more than one mode or no mode, if all values are different (Daniel, 1991, p 22). Examine Table 2–3 in Chapter 2 and note that three FEV_1 readings (79, 82, and 89) occur with equal frequency ($f = 5$). These readings also occur more often than any others. Because it has three modes, the distribution is said to be *trimodal*. A distribution with two modes is *bimodal;* a distribution with one mode is *unimodal*.

In a *grouped* frequency distribution, the mode is the midpoint of the class interval containing the largest number of observations. Review Table 2–5 in Chapter 2. The class interval of

85 to 92 contains the largest number of observations; the midpoint of this interval, 88.5, is the mode of these grouped data.

Unlike other measures of central tendency, the mode can be used with quantitative and qualitative data. For qualitative data, the mode is the category with the largest frequency. Consider Table 2–7, which appears in part IV of the exercises in Chapter 2. Observe that the cancers listed in Table 2–7 occur with differing frequency in the study population. For example, cancer of the spine/spinal cord occurs less often than colon cancer. Therefore, in determining the model category, we utilize percentage frequency. *Cancer of the spine/spinal cord* is the modal category. Approximately 28% of patients in this category have been subjected to at least one questionable treatment method.

Median

The **median,** sometimes designated *M, Md,* or *Mdn,* is the value that divides a distribution into two equal parts, so that the number of values equal to or greater than the median is equal to the number of values equal to or less than the median. The median is also referred to as the 50th percentile. A percentile is a point below which a specified percentage of observations occurs, when the observations are arranged in order of magnitude (Minium & Clarke, 1982, p 53). For example, the 50th percentile is that point below which 50% of the observations occur. Some statisticians use *M* to represent the mean (Hays, 1981, p 146); therefore, exercise care when interpreting a measure of central tendency designated by "*M*."

If the number of observations is *odd,* the median is the middle value when all observations are arranged in order of magnitude. Consider the following hemoglobin readings (g/dL) from 5 healthy adult females: 14.0, 15.5, 14.4, 13.0, and 16.0. To determine the median, arrange the readings in order from lowest to highest (or vice versa) and select the middle value: 13.0, 14.0, *14.4,* 15.5, and 16.0. The median is *14.4.*

If the number of observations is *even,* the median is the arithmetic average of the two middle values, when all observations are arranged in order of magnitude. Consider the following hematocrit readings (mL/dL) from a sample of 4 neonates between the ages of 1 and 13 days: 54.0, 60.2, 45.0, and 64.5. To determine the median, first arrange the observations from smallest to largest (or vice versa): 45.0, 54.0, 60.2, and 64.5. Next, identify the two middle values: 54.0 and 60.2. Finally, compute the arithmetic average of these two values (ie, add them together and divide by 2): (54.0 + 60.2)/2 = 57.1 Thus, the median is 57.1 mL/dL.

Now consider again the hematocrit readings obtained from a second sample of 4 neonates between the ages of 1 and 13 days. The readings from our second sample are 35.2, 54.0, 60.2, and 66.4. Note that the two middle readings are identical to those in our first sample. The median is (54.0 + 60.2)/2 = 57.1, which is identical to the value obtained earlier, even though the lowest and highest readings differ in the first and second sample. The median is determined by the number of observations below and above it; the median does not reflect how deviant these observations may be, however. Note also that when the number of observations is even, the value of median is not contained in the data.

Sokal and Rohlf illustrate how to compute the median from a grouped frequency distribution (1981, pp 45–46). Given the wide availability of personal computers and statistical software, researchers are advised to compute the median from raw data, even if the data will appear later in grouped form in a paper or journal article. Be sure to indicate clearly whether the median is computed from raw or grouped data.

Mean

The **mean,** known also as the **arithmetic mean** or **average,** is the sum of all observations divided by their number. The mean is the descriptive measure of central tendency equated most frequently with the term "average." Keep in mind, however, that the generic term "average" may refer to each of the three measures of central tendency. To minimize confusion, avoid using the term "average."

The arithmetic mean of a *sample* of X observations is represented by a capital letter X with a bar over it ($\overline{X}$) and is read as "X bar." The mean of a sample of Y observations is $\overline{Y}$. Recall that the sample mean is a statistic that estimates the population mean. For example, the mean of the systolic blood pressures in Table 2–1 is $(127 + 140 + 125 + \ldots + 139 + 140)/8 = 128.3750$, or 128.38 if rounded to two decimal places. The mean of the FEV_1 measurements in Table 2–3 is $(132 + 127 + 122 + \ldots + 29)/97 = 86.3608$, or 86.36 if rounded to two decimal places. The three dots, called ellipses, indicate that some values are not shown to conserve space. The formula for computing the mean of a sample of X observations is

$$\overline{X} = \sum_{i=1}^{n} X_i / n \qquad \qquad 3.1$$

The summation operator, represented by the upper-case Greek sigma, Σ, indicates addition. Note the lower case i attached to X as a subscript. The i is a place marker that indicates the observation number. X_1 is the first observation, X_2 is the second observation, X_3 is the third observation, and X_n is the nth or last observation. The subscript on the summation operator, $i = 1$, instructs us to begin our addition with the first observation. The superscript, n, on the summation operator directs us to continue summing observations until we have added the last, or n^{th}, value. Statisticians recommend determining the mean from raw rather than grouped data. Using raw data allows us to include every data value in our computation. When we calculate the mean from *grouped* data, we use the midpoint of each class interval and the corresponding frequency; we do not consider individual observations. Minium (1970, p 58) discusses how to compute the sample mean from grouped data.

The formula for computing the mean of a (finite) *population* of X observations is

$$\mu_X = \sum_{i=1}^{N} X_i / N \qquad \qquad 3.2$$

The mean of a (finite) population is represented by the lower-case Greek mu, μ. As noted earlier, some statisticians use M, the upper-case Greek mu, to designate the population mean. The subscript X in Formula 3.2 indicates a population of X observations; observe that N, rather than n, appears in the denominator and as the superscript on the summation operator. The upper-case N indicates population size; the lower case n denotes sample size. Summation begins with the first observation (as indicated by $i = 1$) and continues until all N values are added together. Actually, researchers are seldom able to compute the mean of a population, because most populations are too large to permit observation of all values. In many situations, data from thousands of patients are obtained and treated as if they constitute a population. The mean computed from such a collection of observations is then regarded as a parameter. In some contexts, however, population parameters can be determined, for example, with a rare disease like progeria. In 1992, only 10 progeria patients were known to live in the United States. Corresponding statistics for other countries are unavailable or unreliable (Progeria International Registry, W. Ted Brown, personal communication, January 25, 1993). Progeria, known also as premature aging, is characterized by accelerated atherosclerosis, alopecia, atrophy of subcutaneous fat, and skeletal hypoplasia (Friedman & Child, 1991, p 924). Few progeria patients live past their mid-teens.

PROPERTIES OF MEASURES OF CENTRAL TENDENCY

MODE

1. The mode is used in descriptive statistics, rarely in inferential statistics.

2. The mode is the most frequently occurring value in a set of observations. It is easy to obtain and can be determined by inspection. A set of data may have one mode, two or more modes, or no mode.

3. The mode is the only measure of central tendency that can be used to describe qualitative and quantitative data.

4. The mode is the least stable of the three measures of central tendency. That is, in repeated (random) sampling from a defined population, the value of the mode tends to vary more from sample to sample than does the value of the median or mean.

MEDIAN

1. The median is the value that divides a distribution into two equal halves, so that the number of observations above and below the median are equal. If the number of observations is odd, the median is the middle value when the observations are arranged in order of magnitude. When the number of observations is even, the median is the arithmetic average of the two middle values, when the data are arranged in order of magnitude.

2. A set of observations has only one median.

3. The median may be the preferred measure of central tendency for distributions that are strongly asymmetric (skewed negatively or positively). The median is used widely if the objective is to represent the bulk of the observations, without giving undue weight to a few extreme values (Minium & Clarke, 1982, p 60).

4. The median is subject to less sampling fluctuation than the mode; however, in many circumstances, the median demonstrates more sampling fluctuation than the mean.

MEAN

1. The mean is the arithmetic average of all observations. It is obtained by adding all values in a distribution and dividing by their number. The mean is used widely in descriptive and inferential statistics.

2. For a given set of data, the mean is unique—that is, only one mean exists.

3. The mean is the balance point of a distribution; the sum of all positive and negative deviations about the mean is zero: $\sum_{i=1}^{n}(X_i - \overline{X}) = 0$.

4. The mean is affected by the magnitude of every observation in a data set.

5. In many situations, the mean is the measure of central tendency with the best sampling stability. In some situations, however, the mean may not be the most suitable measure of central tendency, for example, when data are markedly skewed. In this case, extreme values can so distort the mean that its use is not appropriate (Daniel, 1991, p 21). When this occurs, the median may be more stable than the mean. In other contexts, the median may also be preferred over the mean. For example, heterogeneous populations that include healthy and severely diseased patients are often bimodal. In situations like these, the median is often more stable than the mean.

Statisticians sometimes use other types of means than the one just discussed. Interested readers may wish to consult Sokal and Rohlf (1981, pp 42–43) for a brief discussion of geometric and harmonic means, or Dawson-Saunders and Trapp (1994, pp 43–44) for a description of the geometric mean. Briefly, we compute the geometric mean when data have been transformed logarithmically or measured on a logarithmic scale (Dawson-Saunders & Trapp, 1994, p 44). We use the harmonic mean when observations have been transformed by taking the reciprocal of each value, or by measuring values on a reciprocal scale (Sokal & Rohlf, 1981, p 43).

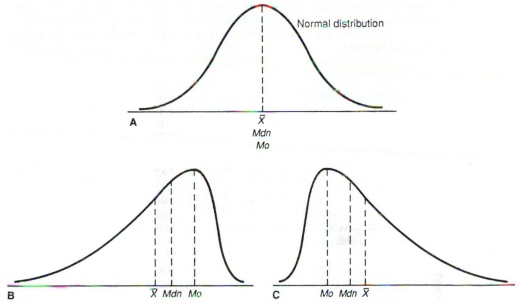

Figure 3–1. Relationship between the mean, median, and mode in bell-shaped, negatively skewed, and positively skewed distributions.

Shapes of Distributions and Measures of Central Tendency

Space limitations or cost may prevent us from displaying data in a table or graph in a journal article. Without access to a table or graph, it may not be easy for readers to determine the shape of a distribution, and therefore the extent to which the sampled population resembles the reader's patient base. An alternative is to provide two different measures of central tendency. If at least two of the three measures of central tendency appear in a report, readers can estimate the shape of a distribution (symmetric or asymmetric) and more thoroughly assess the generalizability of findings.

Three distributions are shown in Fig 3–1. Distribution A is symmetric and shaped like a bell. Bell-shaped distributions are often called **normal curves** or **Gaussian distributions**. (We discuss these distributions in Chapter 5.) In a bell-shaped curve, the mean, median, and mode are equal. Therefore, if the median and mean in a study are approximately equal, we can conclude that the observations in the study are distributed approximately like a bell-shaped curve.

Distribution B is skewed negatively. Because it is influenced by the extreme scores in the lower tail of the distribution, the mean is smaller numerically than the median and mode. The median is also smaller numerically than the mode. In this distribution, the mode is the largest of the three measures of central tendency: mean < median < mode.

In contrast, distribution C is skewed positively. The extreme observations in the upper tail "pull the mean toward them." Consequently, the mean is the largest numerically of the three measures of central tendency. In this case, the median occupies the middlemost numerical position; the mode is the smallest numerically: mean > median > mode.

DESCRIBING THE SCATTER OF OBSERVATIONS ABOUT THEIR CENTER

We have seen how measures of central tendency provide information about the location of the center of a set of observations. Other information, however, is necessary to describe the dispersion of observations about their center. Terms used synonymously with dispersion include variation, spread, variability, and scatter (Daniel, 1991, p 24). Indices used to describe dispersion or variation are called **measures of dispersion.** They include the range, variance, and standard deviation.

Range

The range is the difference between the smallest and largest observations (Daniel, 1991, p 24). The range of the systolic blood pressure readings in Table 2–1 in Chapter 2 is 38 (140 − 102 = 38). The range of the FEV_1 values in Table 2–3 is 103 (132 − 29 = 103).

Variance

In many studies, the mean is used to describe the location of the center of a distribution. Often researchers use a statistical measure, the variance, to describe the variation of observations about the mean. Variance is defined and calculated slightly differently for a sample versus a population. The variance of a *population* is the sum of squares of deviations of observations from the population mean, divided by the population size, N. The variance is represented symbolically by the square of the lower case Greek sigma (σ^2). The variance of a population of X observations is given in Formula 3.3. The X is attached as a subscript to σ^2 to indicate that we are calculating a the variance of a population of X observations.

$$\sigma^2_X = \frac{\sum_{i=1}^{N}(X_i - \mu_X)^2}{N}$$

3.3

Rather than determining each deviation from the mean and squaring it, it might seem appealing to disregard the squaring operation and use the simple sum of the deviations $\sum_{i=1}^{N}(X_i - \mu_X)$. This simple sum, however, equals zero, because the mean is the balance point of the distribution. The absolute value of the deviations $\sum_{i=1}^{N}|X_i - \mu_X|$ is not employed, because this quantity, although attractive conceptually, does not possess the desired qualities necessary for statistical inference (Dawson-Saunders & Trapp, 1994, p 45).

The variance of a *sample* of X observations appears in Formula 3.4. Observe that n replaces N and the denominator includes $n - 1$ rather than n. Note also that $\overline{X}$ replaces μ. The variance of a sample, represented by lower case s squared (s^2), is an estimate of the population variance.

$$s^2_X = \frac{\sum_{i=1}^{n}(X_i - \overline{X})^2}{n - 1}$$

3.4

In developing the best estimate of a population parameter, we want to compute a statistic which, when obtained from samples drawn repeatedly from the same population and averaged over all samples, equals the parameter (Sokal & Rohlf, 1981, p 52). A statistic possessing this property is an *unbiased estimator* of the population parameter. If n, rather than $n - 1$, is placed in the denominator of Formula 3.4, we obtain a *biased estimator*. Therefore, we use $n - 1$ in the denominator.

Return to the data on systolic blood pressure in Table 2–1, Chapter 2, for an illustration of the use of Formula 3.4. If the result is to be rounded to two decimal places, carry at least four

Box 3–1. Computation of the variance of systolic blood pressure readings (mm/Hg) of 8 women using formula 3.4.

X	$(X - \bar{X})$	$(X - \bar{X})^2$
140	140 − 128.3750 = 11.6250	135.1406
140	140 − 128.3750 = 11.6250	135.1406
139	139 − 128.3750 = 10.6250	112.8906
137	137 − 128.3750 = 8.6250	74.3906
127	127 − 128.3750 = −1.3750	1.8906
125	125 − 128.3750 = −3.3750	11.3906
117	117 − 128.3750 = −11.3750	129.3906
102	102 − 128.3750 = −26.3750	695.4606
$\Sigma X = 1027$	$\Sigma(X - \bar{X}) = 0.0000$	$\Sigma(X - \bar{X})^2 = 1295.6498$
		$\Sigma(X - \bar{X})^2 / (n - 1) = 185.0993$

in the calculation. To use Formula 3.4, organize the data as shown in Box 3–1 and compute the mean. (The mean, computed earlier, is 128.3750.) Next, obtain the deviation of each observation from its mean (column 2), square the deviation (column 3), add the squared deviations (bottom of column 3), and divide by $n - 1$ (bottom of column 3). To illustrate that the mean is the balance point of a distribution, the sum of the deviations appears at the bottom of column 2. The sample variance is 185.0993 or 185.10, rounded to two decimals. Unless a sample has only a few observations, Formula 3.4 is difficult to use. Therefore, we employ a modified version, Formula 3.5, with larger data sets. We arrive at Formula 3.5 by squaring the expression inside the parentheses of Formula 3.4, simplifying this result, distributing the summation operator, and simplifying the numerator. A demonstration of this mathematical procedure appears in Minium and associates (1993, p 104).

$$s^2_X = \frac{\sum_{i=1}^{n} X_i^2 - \dfrac{\left(\sum_{i=1}^{n} X_i\right)^2}{n}}{n - 1} \qquad 3.5$$

Examine Formula 3.5. The expression on the left of the numerator, $\sum_{i=1}^{n} X_i^2$, is the *sum-of-squares*. We obtain it by squaring each value and adding the squares together: $X_1^2 + X_2^2 + X_3^2 + \ldots + X_n^2$. The right portion of the numerator is the *square-of-the-sum*, $\left(\sum_{i=1}^{n} X_i\right)^2$. We compute it by adding together all values and then squaring the sum: $(X_1 + X_2 + X_3 + \ldots + X_n)^2$. This calculation appears in Box 3–2.

Box 3–2. Calculation of the variance of 8 systolic blood pressure readings using formula 3.5.

Description	Operation	Performance of Operation	Result of Operation
Compute the sum of all observations	$\sum_{i=1}^{n} X_i$	140 + 140 . . . + 102	1027
Compute the sum-of-squares	$\sum_{i=1}^{n} X_i^2$	$140^2 + 140^2 \ldots + 102^2$	133,137
Assemble the numerator	$\sum_{i=1}^{n} X_i^2 - \dfrac{\left(\sum_{i=1}^{n} X_i\right)^2}{n}$	$133{,}137 - (1027^2/8)$	1295.8750
Add the denominator and divide	$n - 1$	1295.8750/(8 − 1)	185.1250

For the sample of systolic blood pressure readings in Table 2–1, the variance is 185.1250. Note that the results in Box 3–1 (185.0993) and Box 3–2 (185.1250) differ slightly. This difference is due to rounding error introduced when deviations from the mean were created, squared, and summed in Box 3–1.

The variance, calculated with $n - 1$ in the denominator, expresses approximately the arithmetic average of squared deviations about the mean. If the variance equals zero, every observation is identical. As the spread about the mean increases, the squared deviations and the variance increase. Unfortunately, there is no rule-of-thumb to indicate what constitutes a "large" or "small" variance. An understanding of "large" and "small" comes with clinical experience.

Standard Deviation

The variance, used widely in statistical inference, is expressed in *squared units of measurement*. To express dispersion about the mean in the same units of measurement as the data, we use the square root of the variance, known as the **standard deviation.** Formula 3.6 is the standard deviation of a *population* (σ). Formula 3.7 represents the standard deviation of a sample of observations (s).

$$\sigma = \sqrt{\sigma^2} \qquad\qquad\qquad \textbf{3.6}$$

$$s = \sqrt{s^2} \qquad\qquad\qquad \textbf{3.7}$$

If we want to differentiate the standard deviation of total cholesterol values from the standard deviation of low-density lipoprotein measurements, for example, we attach different subscripts to s. We might identify total cholesterol values by TC and their standard deviation by s_{TC}; we might represent low-density lipoprotein values by LD and their standard deviation by s_{LD}.

Keep in mind that the standard deviation alone does not tell us whether the shape of a distribution is symmetric or asymmetric. For example, a "large" standard deviation does not indicate that a distribution is skewed. A "large" standard deviation only tells us that observations vary considerably about their mean. Fig 3–2 illustrates that the standard deviation alone cannot inform us about the shape of a distribution. Both distributions are bell shaped (symmetric) and have the same mean; the standard deviations differ, however. Distribution A (the tall, thin curve) exhibits less dispersion about its mean than distribution B.

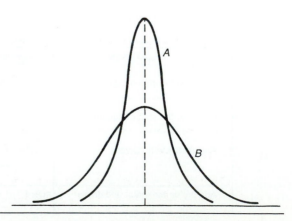

Figure 3–2. Two identically shaped distributions with equal means and unequal standard deviations.

Properties of the Range and Standard Deviation

RANGE

1. The range is the difference between the largest and smallest observation.

2. For *quantitative* data, the range often is reported with the mode. The range cannot be used with *qualitative* data.

3. With a grouped frequency distribution, the range is used to estimate the number of class intervals and interval width.

4. Because it is dependent on only two values, the range is more subject to sampling fluctuation than the variance and standard deviation.

5. The range is generally a function of sample size; the larger the sample size, the larger the range (Minium & Clarke, 1982, pp 75–76).

6. The range is used descriptively; it is used rarely in inferential procedures.

Standard Deviation

Because published reports often include the standard deviation, we describe its properties rather than those of the variance. The properties of the variance are essentially the same as those of the standard deviation, with the exception that the variance is expressed in *squared units of measurement*.

1. The standard deviation is the square root of the variance. The standard deviation is expressed in the same units of measurement as the observations of interest.

2. The standard deviation is the preferred measure of dispersion for *quantitative* data that are distributed relatively symmetrically. The standard deviation cannot be used with *qualitative* data.

3. The standard deviation, typically reported with the mean, is often used with the variance in advanced statistical work.

4. The calculation of the standard deviation is based on every observation in a distribution. Thus, the magnitude of the standard deviation is influenced by extreme (deviant) observations. For this reason, the standard deviation may not be the best measure of dispersion for markedly skewed distributions.

5. The standard deviation and variance typically possess the best sampling stability among measures of dispersion. If a distribution is markedly skewed, other measures of dispersion may be more appropriate; these are described briefly in "Measures of Dispersion and Shapes of Distributions" later in the chapter.

COMPARING VARIATION

Clinicians and investigators in the biomedical sciences examine many different variables and frequently attempt to identify relationships among them (eg, between dietary fat intake and the development of various cancers). Variables are measured on different scales, like blood

Table 3–1. Coefficient of variation for variables having different scales of measurement.

Variable	Mean ($\bar{X}$) and Standard Deviation (SD)		Coefficient of Variation (%)
Erythrocyte count (adult, males, millions/mm³)	$\bar{X}$	5.4	
	SD	0.9	16.67
Total serum–iron binding capacity (μg/dL)	$\bar{X}$	273.7	
	SD	59.6	21.78
Length of hospital stay (days) per surgical floor	$\bar{X}$	6.6	
	SD	0.9	13.64
Hematocrit (neonates, 1–13 days, mL/dL)	$\bar{X}$	54.0	
	SD	10.0	18.52

pressure (mm Hg), serum albumin (g/dL), total cholesterol (mg/dL), and erythrocyte count (millions/mm³). Clinicians often wish to compare distributions of variables, to determine the extent to which observations disperse about their center. When observations differ appreciably in their means or scales of measurement, however, it makes no sense to contrast standard deviations (Sokal & Rohlf, 1981, p 59). We then use the **coefficient of variation** to compare relative amounts of variation. The coefficient of variation (CV) is defined as the standard deviation, divided by the mean, and multiplied by 100% (Sokal & Rohlf, 1981, p 59):

$$CV = \left(\frac{s}{\bar{X}} \right) (100\%) \qquad\qquad 3.8$$

An example is provided in Table 3–1. Based on the information in this table, we conclude that relative variation is least for length of hospital stay and greatest for total serum–iron binding capacity.

Let us return to the clinical example at the beginning of the chapter and compare the relative variation in the dietary fat consumption of the husbands of women who participated in the trial. The mean and standard deviation, respectively, for the husbands of women in the intervention group is 19 and 10.1 g/day. The coefficient of variation is ([10.1/19] × 100%) = 53.16%. The comparable data for the husbands of women in the reference group is: ([12.8/23.9] × 100%) = 53.56%. Thus, the relative variation in these two groups is similar.

Dawson-Saunders & Trapp (1994, p 46) point out that the coefficient of variation is used frequently in laboratory testing and quality control procedures. For example, Potter and associates (1993) examined the effect of dietary soy fiber on human plasma lipid profiles. Blood samples were drawn from each participant in the study. To assess the reproducibility of the assay, staff in two different laboratories performed the same assay on each blood sample. The coefficient of variation for total cholesterol was 2.9%, for high-density lipoproteins 4.4%, and for total triglycerides 4.9% These values indicate good reproducibility, because the variation, as measured by the standard deviation, is quite small in relation to the mean (Dawson-Saunders & Trapp, 1994, p 46).

MEASURES OF DISPERSION AND SHAPES OF DISTRIBUTIONS

When a distribution of observations is relatively symmetric, the standard deviation and variance are the preferred measures of dispersion. When a distribution is markedly skewed (ie, when it contains some extremely deviant observations), the standard deviation and variance *may* be inappropriate. An investigator may use a mathematical transformation to try to create a relatively symmetric distribution and then work with the transformed data. Kirk (1982, p 84) provides an excellent discussion of different transformations, including square root and logarithmic transformations.

If a transformation cannot be used to produce a relatively symmetric distribution, the median may be the preferred measure of central tendency. In this case, the **semi-interquartile range** (Q) may be used as a measure of dispersion. The semi-interquartile range is half the distance between the 25th percentile (also called the first quartile or Q_1) and the 75th percentile (also called the third quartile or Q_3). Quartiles divide a distribution into four equal parts. The semi-interquartile range is

$$Q = \frac{Q_3 - Q_1}{2}$$

3.9

Less sensitive to deviant observations than the standard deviation and variance, the semi-interquartile range describes dispersion *in the central half of the distribution* (Sokal & Rohlf, 1981, p 49). The sampling stability of Q is acceptable, although often not as good as that of the variance. The usefulness of Q is limited to descriptive statistics. For more on the semi-interquartile range, readers are referred to Minium and Clarke (1982, pp 67–68, 74–75).

SELECTING THE MOST APPROPRIATE DESCRIPTIVE STATISTICS

The following factors contribute to selecting the most appropriate descriptive statistics: (1) whether a variable is quantitative or qualitative; and (2) the shape of the data, if quantitative. The count (frequency) and mode are the *only* descriptive statistics appropriate for use with nominal (ie, qualitative) data. Counts are used to indicate how many observations (eg, patients) fall into mutually exclusive categories. The mode is the category with the largest frequency; this category is referred to as the modal category. Although numbers may identify the categories of a qualitative variable, numerical operations are not performed on these identifiers.

Ordinal Data

A synonym for ordinal is *rank order*. For ordinal data, the most appropriate descriptive statistics are the count, mode, and median. Use of the mean and standard deviation for ordinal data is questionable, because the units on an ordinal scale are usually unequal. When investigators report the mean and standard deviation for ordinal data, we assume that the units on the scale are equal or approximately equal (Knapp & Miller, 1991, p 10).

Interval and Ratio Data

Interval and ratio variables are true quantitative variables for which all measures of central tendency and dispersion are appropriate. The choice of the measure of central tendency and dispersion, however, depends on the intended use of the statistics, and whether the data are relatively symmetric or asymmetric. The mode is used for simple description. If a distribution is relatively symmetric, the mean and standard deviation (or variance) are preferred. If a distribution is markedly skewed or if a few extremely deviant observations exist, the median and semi-interquartile range are often employed.

SUMMARY

We use measures of central tendency to describe the center of a distribution. The mode is the most frequently occurring value in a set of quantitative observations; for qualitative data, the category with the largest frequency is referred to as the modal category. The median and mean, unlike the mode, are used with quantitative data only. The median is the middle-most value in a distribution, such that half of the observations occur above and below it. The mean is the arithmetic average of a set of observations.

The mode is used primarily in descriptive statistics. Of the three measures of central tendency discussed in this chapter, the mode is the least stable. The median is subject to less sampling fluctuation than the mode. In many situations, however, the value of the median varies more from sample to sample than does the value of the mean. The mean is used widely in both descriptive and inferential statistics. Because the mean includes the value of every observation in a distribution, the magnitude of the mean is affected by extremely large or small values. Therefore, the median is often preferred for distributions that are markedly skewed, if the objective is to represent the bulk of the observations.

The amount of scatter of observations about their center is described by measures of dispersion, notably, the range, variance, and standard deviation. All three measures are used with quantitative data only. The difference between the largest and smallest observations is the range. It is the least stable measure of dispersion. In addition, the range is generally a function of sample size; the larger the sample, the larger the range. The variance, like the standard deviation, enjoys widespread use in descriptive and inferential statistics. The variance approximates the arithmetic average of the squared deviations about the mean. The standard deviation is the square root of the variance and is expressed in the same units of measurement as the variable itself. The standard deviation is typically reported with the mean. Like the mean, the magnitudes of the standard deviation (and variance) are influenced by extremely deviant observations. As a result, it may not be the best measure of dispersion for markedly skewed distributions. In this case, another measure, known as the semi-interquartile range, may be preferred.

Because many variables are measured on scales having different metrics (eg, grams, mg/dL, mm Hg), we cannot directly compare standard deviations to describe whether a set of observations is more or less variable than another. We use the coefficient of variation for this purpose. It is defined as the standard deviation, divided by the mean, and multiplied by 100%. The larger the coefficient of variation, the greater the relative variation about the mean. In addition, the coefficient of variation is a useful measure for describing the reproducibility of a quatitative clinical assay.

Several factors are considered when selecting the most appropriate descriptive statistics, in particular (1) whether a variable is qualitative or quantitative; and (2) the shape of the distribution, if the data are quantitative. The count and mode are the only descriptive statistics appropriate for qualitative data. The count, mode, and median may be used with ordinal (rank-order) data. Using the mean and standard deviation with ordinal data is questionable, because the units of an ordinal scale are usually unequal. All of the descriptive statistics described in this chapter can be used to characterize interval and ratio data. The choice of the measure of central tendency and dispersion depends on the intended use of the statistics and whether the data are bell-shaped or markedly skewed.

REFERENCES

Daniel W: *Biostatistics: A Foundation for Analysis in the Health Sciences,* 5th ed. Wiley, 1991.
Dawson-Saunders B, Trapp R: *Basic and Clinical Biostatistics,* 2nd ed. Appleton & Lange, 1994.
Hays W: *Statistics,* 3rd ed. Holt, Rinehart & Winston, 1981.
Kirk R: *Experimental Design: Procedures for the Behavioral Sciences,* 2nd ed. Brooks/Cole, 1982.
Knapp R, Miller MC III: *Clinical Epidemiology and Biostatistics.* Williams & Wilkins, 1991.
Minium E: *Statistical Reasoning in Psychology and Education.* Wiley, 1970.
Minium E, Clarke R: *Elements of Statistical Reasoning.* Wiley, 1982.
Minium E, King B, Bear G: *Statistical Reasoning in Psychology and Education,* 3rd ed. Wiley, 1993.

Potter SM, et al: Depression of plasma cholesterol in mildly hypercholesterolemic men by consumption of baked products containing soy protein. *Am J Clin Nutrition* 1993; 501.

Shattuck A, White E, Kristal A: How women's adopted low-fat diets affect their husbands. *Am J Public Health* 1992;82:1244.

Sokal R, Rohlf F: *Biometry,* 2nd ed. W. H. Freeman, 1981.

Self-study Questions

1. Define the mode, median, and mean. Describe the properties of each.
2. Define the range, variance, and standard deviation. Describe the properties of each.
3. Define the coefficient of variation. Describe when it is useful.
4. Differentiate between *statistics* and *parameters*.
5. Identify which measures of central tendency and dispersion, if any, are appropriate for use with nominal, ordinal, interval, and ratio variables.
    a. Describe how the choice of the most appropriate measure of central tendency and dispersion is affected by the symmetry, or lack of it, of a distribution of observations measured on an interval or ratio scale.
    b. With ordinal data, the mean and standard deviation usually are not used. If these measures appear in a report with ordinal data, what can we assume about the ordinal scale of measurement?
6. Describe the relationship between the *numerical magnitude* of measures of central tendency for observations that are distributed symmetrically, skewed negatively, and skewed positively.
7. If you would like to practice calculating a mean and standard deviation, turn back to the pulmonary function data in Chapter 2, Table 2–3. Calculate the sum and sum-of-squares. Assemble the calculated quantities to determine the mean and standard deviation. (Answers: $n = 97$, $\Sigma X = 8377$, $\Sigma X^2 = 761{,}087$, $\overline{X} = 83.3608$, $s = 19.8017$.)

Summarizing Data: Indices to Describe Health Status

4

Clinical Example 1: Meningococcal Meningitis

At the health center of a large university, a 21-year-old female student presents with cough, headache, vomiting, sore throat, fever, chills, and muscle pains. She also has a petechial rash on her axillae, flanks, wrists, and ankles. A lumbar puncture reveals a purulent cerebrospinal fluid, with elevated pressure, increased protein, and decreased glucose content. Other laboratory findings include prolonged prothrombin time, partial thromboplastin time, and a depressed platelet count.

In this hypothetical example based on actual clinical experiences, several questions must be addressed before an appropriate treatment plan can be developed. Based on the available information, how *likely* is it that the patient has meningococcal meningitis? Is further testing required to confirm a diagnosis? If the patient has meningococcal meningitis, how *likely* is it that she will develop shock, myocarditis, cranial nerve damage, nephritis, or other problems? If the patient is treated with aqueous penicillin G, how *likely* is it that she will have an allergic reaction that requires the use of a different drug? How *likely* is it that individuals who have had recent contact with her will develop meningococcal meningitis? Should these individuals be traced and treated with rifampin?

Clinical Example 2: Exposure to Environmental Tobacco Smoke

> Exposure to environmental tobacco smoke is studied to determine if this exposure increased the *risk* of death from heart disease. The investigator finds that male never-smokers living with a current or former smoker have an approximately 9.6% *chance* of dying of ischemic heart disease by age 74, compared with a 7.4% *chance* for male never-smokers living with a nonsmoker. The corresponding life-time *risks* for women are 6.1% and 4.9%" (Steenland, 1992, p 94).

In this second example, what is meant by the statement that "exposure to environmental tobacco smoke is studied to determine if this exposure increases the *risk* of death from heart disease?" What does it mean to say that "male never-smokers living with a current or former smoker have an approximately 9.6% *chance* of dying of ischemic heart disease by age 74?"

Clinical Example 1 focuses primarily on an individual patient. Clinical Example 2 generalizes to male and female never-smokers. Although different, the scenarios share a common element: the frequency of health outcomes, estimated by their likeliness or chance of occurrence under particular circumstances. Many outcomes (eg, platelet count) are quantitative. Other outcomes, however, are qualitative. In this chapter, we present indices used to describe the frequency of *qualitative* outcomes; these indices are employed to characterize the health status of populations and subgroups of individuals. For example, we can describe disease status (diseased/not diseased), survival (survived/did not survive), remission (in remission/ disease active), recurrence (disease recurred/disease not detectable), prognosis (poor/good), and other similar outcomes. Measures that describe health status, such as births and deaths, are called **vital statistics** (Dawson-Saunders & Trapp, 1994, p 42).

COMMON MEASURES OF HEALTH STATUS

Count

A **count** is the number of events or individuals that satisfy specified criteria. This definition of count is synonymous with our definition of frequency. For example, Roscoe and associates indicate that "Colorectal cancer was the second leading cause of cancer deaths in the United States in 1989, accounting for an estimated 30,000 deaths or 11% of all cancer deaths" (1992, p 759). In this example, 30,000 is the *count* of the number of persons who died from colorectal cancer in the United States in 1989.

Ratio

A **ratio** contains a numerator (A) that represents the count of the number of events that meet a specified criterion and a denominator (B) that represents the count of the number of events that satisfy a *different* criterion:

$$\text{Ratio} = \frac{A}{B} \qquad\qquad 4.1$$

Common examples of a ratio are:

$$\text{Sex Ratio} = \frac{\text{Number of Liveborn Males}}{\text{Number of Liveborn Females}}$$

$$\text{Fetal Mortality Ratio} = \frac{\text{Fetal Deaths in Year}}{\text{Live Births in Year}} \times 1000$$

Note that we include a multiplier (1000) in the fetal mortality ratio. The multiplier is a **base** used to produce a number that quantifies fetal mortality *per 1000 live births* in a specified year. In biostatistics, the following bases are often used with ratios and other measures: 1000, 10,000, and 100,000.

Proportion

Like a ratio, a **proportion** contains a numerator and denominator. The denominator of a proportion is defined differently, however. In a proportion, the numerator is the count of the number of persons or events that satisfy specified criteria; the denominator is the *maximum* number of individuals or events that could satisfy the numerator criteria. Thus, a proportion is a part divided by a whole. Observe that the numerator in a proportion is subsumed by the denominator:

$$\text{Proportion} = \frac{A}{A + B}. \qquad\qquad 4.2$$

In their study of the link between the dietary habits of husbands and wives, Shattuck and associates (1992, p 1246) classified participants into four age categories: 30 to 49, 50 to 59, 60 to 69, and 70 years and above. In the reference (no dietary intervention) group, 73 of 148 women are between the ages of 50 and 59 years. Therefore, the proportion of women in this age group is 73/148 = 0.4932. If we write the denominator in a slightly different way to indicate the number of women in each of these four age groups, we can see more clearly that the numerator is part of the denominator:

$$73/(4 + 73 + 59 + 12) = 0.4932.$$

In 1987, 2,123,323 deaths from all causes were recorded in the United States (Boring et al, 1991, p 24). Of these fatalities, 760,353 are attributed to diseases of the heart. The proportion of deaths attributed to heart disease in 1987 is (760,353)/(2,123,323) = 0.3581. Thus, in 1987, approximately one third of all deaths in the United States are attributable to diseases of the heart.

Percentage

A **percentage** is a proportion multiplied by 100%:

$$\text{Percentage} = \frac{A}{A + B} (100\%). \qquad\qquad 4.3$$

The percentage of all deaths attributed to diseases of the heart in 1987 is 35.81%. In the study on dietary habits, 49.32% of women in the reference group are between the ages of 50 and 59 years.

Rate

According to Mausner and Kramer (1985, p 43), "The rate is the basic measure of disease occurrence because it is the measure that most clearly expresses probability or risk of disease in a defined population over a specified period of time." In general terms, *risk* is the chance of occurrence of some untoward event (Fletcher et al, 1988, p 91). Many epidemiologists define **rate** as a measure that expresses rapidity, intensity, velocity, or force of some event; an example would be the occurrence of new cases of disease in a specified time period. The numerator of a rate is the number of events or individuals satisfying specified criteria. The denominator is the number of *units of exposure* examined in counting the numerator (Greenberg, 1993, p 133).

A unit of exposure is defined ordinarily as the passage of an individual through a certain experience or situation. A common unit of exposure is a *person-year*, which is a year lived by one person. Another common unit of exposure is pack-years of smoking. In a pack-year, one individual smokes a pack of cigarettes every day for one year. Midyear population sometimes appears in the denominator as an estimate of person-years lived by members of a population during a certain year. We use midyear population when available, because it is more stable than population estimates taken at the beginning and end of a year. A rate is:

$$\text{Rate} = \frac{\text{Number of Events Satisfying Specified Criteria}}{\text{Number of Units of Exposure Examined in Counting Numerator}} \text{ (Base).} \qquad \textbf{4.4}$$

Distinctions are made between crude and specific rates. A **crude rate** is a summary statistic that ignores the heterogeneity of the population under investigation. An example of a crude rate is birth rate—also referred to as the *crude birth rate* because it relates to the population in general, without specific reference to homogeneous groupings.

$$\text{Crude Birth Rate} = \frac{\text{Births in Specified Year}}{\text{Midyear Population in Specified Year}} \text{ (1000).}$$

Note that the crude birth rate is reported per 1000 population. Midyear population appears in the denominator as an estimate of the person-years lived by the population's members during the year.

In contrast, **specific rates** break down the population into homogeneous groups or strata, depending upon one or more demographic or other factors thought to be related to the outcome of interest. Reported for each homogeneous grouping, specific rates allow us to understand the influence of individual factors: for example, between 1984 and 1988, the age–race specific, cumulative *incidence* (number of new cases) for prostrate cancer in Caucasian men, ages 85 years or older, was approximately 1100 per 100,000 (*MMWR*, June 12, 1992, p 403). During this period, the age–race specific, cumulative incidence "rate" was approximately 350 per 100,000 Caucasian men, ages 65 to 69 years (*MMWR*, June 12, 1992, p 403). Here is another example of an age-specific birth rate:

$$\text{Age-specific Birth Rate} = \frac{\text{Births to Women of a Given Age in a Specific Year}}{\text{Midyear Population of Women of That Age}}.$$

Adjusting Rates

Suppose we wish to compare the crude rates for death due to heart disease in 1940 and 1990. We can compare two or more rates only if the populations from which they are developed are similar in all characteristics that affect the rate. Thus, the rates due to heart disease deaths will be confounded by age, because the distribution of individuals according to age has changed from 1940 to 1990: a greater relative number of individuals lived to older age in the 1990 population than in the 1940 population. This difference in age structure allows for the possibility that a greater number of persons developed and died of heart disease in the 1990 population. Consequently, in order to make valid comparisons, the crude rates must be adjusted to account for age differences in the two populations (Greenberg, 1993, p 37). The process of adjustment, referred to by some epidemiologists as *standardization,* produces a single summary rate that takes into account differences between the populations of interest (in the example just given, differences in the relative frequency of individuals of different ages). Thus, when comparing rates adjusted for a specific factor, remaining differences between the populations cannot be attributed to confounding by that factor (Hennekens & Buring, 1987, p 70). Procedures for adjusting rates are beyond the scope of this chapter. Interested individuals may wish to consult Hennekens and Buring (1987) or Dawson-Saunders & Trapp (1994).

A Comment About Rates

The term "rate" is often used to characterize demographic and epidemiologic measures that are either true rates, proportions, or ratios (Hennekens & Buring 1987, p 56). Consequently, individuals who read the literature must pay special attention to how a rate is defined. In particular, we must have a clear definition of the denominator to interpret the rate correctly. For example, if the denominator contains units of exposure, such as person-years exposed to asbestos, then the "rate" is a true rate. For a true rate, we discuss the number of new cases of disease per person-time of observation (eg, 3.5 cases per person-year). In contrast, if the denominator contains a count of the number of individuals exposed to asbestos during a specified time period, then the "rate" is actually a proportion. In this case, we focus on the proportion of the at-risk population that developed disease during the time frame of interest (eg, 5 cases per 100 individuals).

MEASURES OF PREVALENCE AND INCIDENCE

Measures of prevalence and incidence occur frequently in the medical and epidemiological literature to describe the commonness of health outcomes, such as the prevalence of existing cases of disease at a specific point in time.

Prevalence

Prevalence is the *proportion* of individuals in a population who have a specified clinical characteristic, such as a disease, at a *specific point in time.* Prevalence is often called a rate, even though it is a proportion (Hennekens & Buring, 1987, p 57). Prevalence is defined as

$$\text{Prevalence} = \frac{\text{Cases of a Specific Disease at Time } t}{\text{Population at Time } t} \text{ (Base).} \qquad 4.5$$

Note the inclusion of the base in Formula 4.5. Prevalence is often reported per 1000 or 100,000 persons, although some researchers omit the base in their calculation (Greenberg, 1993, p 15). For example, investigators conducted a population-based, HIV (human immunodeficiency virus) serosurvey among women delivering infants in Georgia during 1991; the researchers found that the prevalencee of HIV infection was 1.6 per 1000 women in Atlanta, 1.8 in health districts in smaller cities, and 0.9 in rural areas (*MMWR*, November 20, 1992, p 876).

Prevalence (1) provides an estimate of the chance that an individual in the population will be ill at a point in time and (2) reflects the status of disease in a population at a point in time (Hennekens & Buring, 1987, p 57). Prevalence is determined from a *cross-sectional study:* a defined population is surveyed at a point in time, the number of diseased individuals is determined, and the relationship between concurrent disease and the presence or absence of risk factors is evaluated (Fletcher et al, 1988, p 74; Greenberg, 1993, p 131).

Incidence

Cumulative incidence and **incidence density** are measures of incidence that relate the development of new cases of disease in a defined population over a specified period of time (Greenberg, 1993, p 16; Hennekens & Buring, 1987, p 57). These two measures have identical numerators; their denominators differ, however. Both measures are derived from a cohort study in which a population free of the event or disease of interest is followed over time with "periodic examinations to determine occurrences of the event" (Fletcher et al, 1988, p 80).

CUMULATIVE INCIDENCE (CI)

Cumulative incidence is the number of new cases of disease that accumulate during a specified time period (eg, 1 year), divided by the number of persons in the population at risk. Individuals who are newly diagnosed with a disease are referred to as *incident cases*. Cumulative incidence (CI) is defined as

$$CI = \frac{\text{Number of New Cases of Disease During a Defined Time Period}}{\text{Total Population at Risk}} . \qquad 4.6$$

The population-at-risk (the population susceptible to the disease or event) is counted in the denominator (Fletcher et al, 1988, p 82). Cumulative incidence is a proportion, even though it is sometimes called a rate. Hennekens and Buring (1987, pp 57–58) note that "cumulative incidence provides an estimate of the probability, or risk, that an individual will develop a disease during a specified period of time." Thus, some epidemiologists use risk as a synonym for cumulative incidence (Greenberg, 1993, p 17). When calculating cumulative incidence, we assume that the population-at-risk is available throughout the specified observation period.

Thun and colleagues (1992) prospectively evaluated the relationship of diet and other factors (eg, physical activity and family history) on the development of fatal colon cancer. From September 1, 1982 through August 31, 1988, the investigators followed 1,185,124 individuals and recorded 2757 deaths due to colon cancer. We define the observed individuals as the total population-at-risk, and the 2757 deaths as the number of deaths due to colon cancer during the observation period. In this case, the cumulative incidence of fatal colon cancer is 0.0023 or 0.23%. Approximately 233 cases of fatal colon cancer occurred per 100,000 persons. These data suggest that approximately 0.2 of 1% of an at-risk population, currently free of disease, will develop fatal colon cancer in the next 6 years. The probability that a member of this population will develop this fatal disease in the specified time-frame is 0.0023.

INCIDENCE DENSITY (ID)

Incidence density (ID), also referred to as incidence rate (IR), is the number of new cases of disease during a defined period of time, divided by total person-time of observation or at risk (Hennekens & Buring, 1987, p 58). Incidence density is a true rate, rather than a proportion.

$$ID = \frac{\text{Number of New Cases of Disease During a Defined Time Period}}{\text{Total Person Time of Observation}} \qquad 4.7$$

The denominator is the sum of the amount of time each individual is observed while *free of disease* (Hennekens & Buring, 1987, p 58). Consider a hypothetical example in which 3000 new cases of disease occur during 4,000,000 person-years of observation. The incidence density is 0.0075 or 75 cases per 100,000 person years.

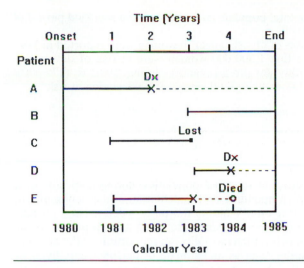

Figure 4–1. Depiction of a hypothetical study of 5 patients.

EXAMPLE CALCULATION OF RISK AND INCIDENCE DENSITY

A hypothetical study of 5 patients is depicted in Fig 4–1 to illustrate the calculation of risk and incidence density. The study began in 1980 and concluded in 1985. Although patients entered the study at different times, they were all disease-free at enrollment. The solid line indicates disease-free observation; the "X" marks the diagnosis of disease ("Dx"); the dashed line marks the amount of time the patient was observed after disease development. Note that all patients were observed for at least 1 year.

In particular, patient A was observed for 2 years before he developed disease; he was followed until 1985 when the study ended. Patient B entered the study in 1983 and was observed until 1985; she remained disease free during this 2-year period. Patient C, who enrolled in 1981, was followed until 1983 when he was lost to follow-up. He remained disease-free during the 2-year observation period. Patient D developed disease within 1 year of entering the study in 1983; she was followed until 1985. Patient E, who enrolled in the study in 1981, was observed for 2 years before she developed disease (1983); she died 1 year later.

To compute cumulative incidence, we must recognize that all patients were observed for at least 1 year. The 1-year cumulative incidence, or 1-year risk, of disease is the number of new cases occurring within 1 year divided by the total number of patients observed for 1 year: $\frac{1}{5} = 0.20$ or 20%. Thus, 20% of patients developed disease within 1 year of entry into the study. To determine the incidence density, first count the number of new cases of disease (3). Second, obtain the person-time. Person-time is based on the amount of time a patient is eligible to develop disease. Patient A contributes 2 person-years; patient B, 2 person-years; patient C, 2 person-years; D, 1 person year; and E, 2 person-years. The total person-time is 9 person-years. Third, divide the number of new cases by total person-time. The incidence density is (3 new cases/9 person-years) = 0.33 cases per person-year.

COMMON MEASURES OF PREVALENCE AND INCIDENCE

Morbidity

Morbidity is "any departure, subjective or objective, from a state of physiological or psychological well being" (Last, 1983, p 64). A common measure of incidence, morbidity is a proportion that is sometimes referred to as a rate. **Morbidity** is the number of nonfatal cases of newly reported disease, divided by the total population-at-risk during a specified period of time (Hennekens & Buring, 1987, p 61).

Consider that 175,000 new nonfatal cases of breast cancer in women were reported in 1991 (Boring et al, 1991, p 28). Suppose also that 1,500,000 women were at risk of developing breast cancer during this year. Morbidity for breast cancer during 1991 is (175,000)/(1,500,000) = 0.1167, or approximately 117 new nonfatal cases per 1000 women at risk.

Mortality

Mortality expresses the incidence of death in a specified population during a specific time period (Hennekens & Buring, 1987, p 62). Depending on the definition of the denominator, mortality can be either a proportion or a true rate. Whether mortality is defined as a proportion or a true rate, the numerator is the number of persons who die in a given period. If the denominator is the size of the population-at-risk, then mortality is a proportion. If the denominator, however, contains units of exposure—such as an estimate of persons-years lived by members of the population during a specified time—mortality is a true rate. Mortality may be stated as *crude mortality,* which reflects deaths due to all causes, or *cause-specific mortality,* which reflects deaths due to a specific disease or event. For example, in 1987 in the United States, there were 2,213,323 deaths due to all causes (Boring et al, 1991, p 24). If we assume a midyear population of 260,000,000 and use this to estimate person-years lived by members of the population during 1987, the crude mortality rate is 0.00851278, or approximately 851 deaths per 100,000 person years. There were 69,225 deaths due to pneumonia and influenza in 1987 (Squires et al, 1991, p 24). If we use 260,000,000 again as an estimate of person-years lived by the population during 1987, we can compute the cause-specific mortality due to pneumonia and influenza in 1987 as (69,225 deaths)/(260,000,000) = 0.00026625, or approximately 27 cases per 100,000 person-years. In these examples, it is difficult to differentiate cumulative incidence from incidence density (incidence rate), because the "total population at risk" (the denominator of cumulative incidence) can be represented by midyear population; but midyear population can also be used as a surrogate for person-years of observation (the denominator for incidence density). In the examples just cited, cumulative incidence and incidence density are the same. This is frequently not the case, however.

Other Measures of Prevalence and Incidence

Hennekens and Buring (1987, p 62) note that there are several other common measures of incidence and prevalence, including case-fatality rate (incidence), attack rate (incidence), disease rate at autopsy (prevalence), and birth defect rate (prevalence). For example, case fatality is the "propensity of disease to cause the death of affected persons" (Greenberg, 1993, p 19). Case fatality (CF) is computed as the number of deaths divided by the number of patients diagnosed with disease. Let us return for a moment to our hypothetical example in Fig 4–1. Note that patients D and E die within 1 year of diagnosis. The 1-year case fatality for this disease is ⅔ = 0.6667 or 67%. Thus, approximately 67% of patients diagnosed with this disease die within 1 year of diagnosis. Those interested in reading more about other measures or prevalence and incidence may wish to consult Greenberg (1993) or Hennekens and Buring (1987).

USING MEASURES OF PREVALENCE AND INCIDENCE

Measures of prevalence and incidence have many uses, including exploring the development of disease, predicting the future, estimating risk, and describing prognosis.

Exploring the Development of Disease

In exploring the development of disease, clinicians are interested in the antecedent conditions or risk factors that contribute to disease occurrence. Cohort investigations, which yield measures of incidence, "provide the clearest evidence concerning the development of the disease in relation to antecedent exposures" (Hennekens & Buring, 1987, p 66). Therefore, cohort investigations are used frequently to study disease etiology. It is tempting, however, to use measures of prevalence to explore disease development, because prevalence is based on *existing* cases of disease and appropriate sample sizes can be obtained fairly readily. Nevertheless, epidemiologists argue against using existing cases of disease because prevalent cases are affected by two sets of factors: (1) etiologic factors, which affect the development or occurrence of disease, and (2) prognostic factors, which affect the course of disease after its development (Hennekens & Buring, 1987, p 66). As a result, differences between cases and controls may be due to events that occur after disease development, that is, to prognostic factors. Thus, we risk confounding our studies of disease development if we use measures of prevalence to characterize etiology.

Predicting the Future

Measures of incidence characterize the force or rate at which new cases of disease develop in an at-risk population during a specified period. Thus, incidence is useful for predicting the likelihood that members of an at-risk population will develop disease (Fletcher et al, 1988, p 88; Greenberg, 1993, p 17). In contrast, prevalence reflects *existing* cases of disease (Greenberg, 1993, p 16), but gives no information about the chance of *future* development of the disease (Fletcher et al, 1988, p 88). Rather, prevalence provides information about the chance that an individual with certain demographic and clinical characteristics currently has the disease. Thus, prevalence helps clinicians make decisions about ordering diagnostic tests, interpreting test results, and planning treatment (Fletcher et al, 1988, p 88).

Assessing Risk and Making Comparisons

In general terms, *risk* refers to the chance that some untoward event will occur (Fletcher et al, 1988, p 91). In a more restricted sense, risk is the chance that disease-free persons who are exposed to certain factors, or who possess certain clinical or demographic characteristics, will develop disease (Fletcher et al, 1988, p 91). As we noted previously, some epidemiologists equate risk and cumulative incidence (Greenberg, 1993, p 17). Risk is assessed easily if data are organized in a 2 × 2 table, in which individuals are cross-classified on the presence or absence of disease and the presence or absence of exposure or some other factor. Table 4–1 is an example of a 2 × 2 table. Disease status (diseased/not diseased) appears along the top and exposure status (exposed/not exposed) appears on the left margin of the table. Letters are used as follows:

A	Number of exposed persons who are diseased
B	Number of exposed persons who are not diseased
C	Number of not exposed persons who are diseased
D	Number of not exposed persons who are not diseased
A + D	Total number of diseased persons
B + D	Total number of not diseased persons
A + B	Total number of exposed persons
D + D	Total number of not exposed persons

Table 4–1. Layout of a two-by-two table for developing estimates of risk.

Exposure Status	Diseased	Not Diseased	Total
Exposed	A	B	A + B
Not exposed	C	D	C + D
TOTAL	A + C	B + D	A + B + C + D

The totals (A + B, C + D, A + C, and B + D) are *marginal totals:* A + C represents the number of diseased persons, without regard to their exposure status; A + B indicates the number of exposed persons without regard to their disease status.

RISK DIFFERENCE

Risk difference (RD), also known as *attributable risk (AR)*, is the difference between the cumulative incidences in the exposed and unexposed group. Recall that measures of incidence derive from cohort studies. Attributable risk represents the excess of disease in the exposed group. Thus, it provides information about the absolute effect of the exposure or excess risk of disease in individuals who are exposed, compared to persons who are not exposed (Hennekens & Buring, 1987, p 87). Allow *CI* to represent cumulative incidence; attributable risk is

$$RD = CI_{EXPOSED} - CI_{NONEXPOSED} \qquad \textbf{4.8a}$$

$$= \frac{A}{(A + B)} - \frac{C}{(C + D)} \qquad \textbf{4.8b}$$

Let us consider the RD within the context of a hypothetical case based on actual studies. Suppose a prospective cohort study is undertaken to chart the development of colon cancer in two groups, one thought to be at risk for disease development because of dietary habits, and the other not at risk for cancer. Assume also that members of the two groups are as similar as possible on important demographic and clinical characteristics, thus minimizing the possibility of confounding and reducing the chance that results will be erroneously attributed to the variables of interest. Data from a 5-year study of colon cancer development appear in Table 4–2. The cumulative incidence of colon cancer development is 535/1500 = 0.3567 in the at-risk group and 533/5700 = 0.1612 in the group without risk. The attributable risk is RD = 0.3567 − 0.0935 = 0.2632 or approximately 0.26. The risk of colon cancer is increased by 0.26 in individuals whose dietary habits place them at risk. Thus, in at-risk patients the excess occurrence of colon cancer that is attributable to dietary habits is approximately 260 per 1000. If we are willing to assume a causal association between these two variables, the risk difference provides the clinician with valuable information about the role of diet in colon cancer development. If no association exists between dietary habits and colon cancer development, the RD will equal zero.

Table 4–2. Five-year prospective study of colon cancer development.

Dietary Group	Colon Cancer	Colon Cancer Free	Total
At risk	535	965	1500
Not at risk	533	5167	5700
TOTAL	1068	6132	7200

ATTRIBUTABLE RISK PERCENT

The **attributable risk percent (AR%)** is an estimate of the proportion of disease in exposed individuals that is attributable to the exposure. It also represents the percentage of disease in the exposed group that could be eliminated by removing the exposure (Hennekens & Buring,

1987, pp 87–88). Like the risk difference, attributable risk percent is developed from cohort investigations. Attributable risk percent is defined as:

$$AR\% = \frac{RD}{CI_{EXPOSED}} \times 100. \qquad 4.9$$

In our hypothetical colon cancer example, AR% equals $[0.2632/(535/1500)] \times 100 = 73.79$. If a causal link exists between dietary habits and colon cancer, we can assume that dietary habits account for approximately 74% of colon cancer in patients whose dietary habits place them at-risk. Thus, if we could modify these dietary habits, we could eliminate approximately 74% of the colon cancer in this at-risk group.

RELATIVE RISK

Relative risk (RR), known also as the risk ratio, is the cumulative incidence of disease in exposed persons, divided by the cumulative incidence of disease in unexposed individuals (Greenberg, 1993, p 91):

$$RR = \frac{A / (A + B)}{C / (C + D)}. \qquad 4.10$$

Relative risk addresses the question: "How many times more likely are *exposed* persons to become diseased than *nonexposed* persons?" (Fletcher et al, 1988, p 102). Greenberg (1993, p 91) points out that if exposed and unexposed persons have the same risk of experiencing some outcome, the relative risk will equal 1.0, which suggests that exposure is unrelated to the outcome. If the relative risk is greater than 1.0, the risk of disease development is greater in exposed than unexposed individuals. If the relative risk is less than 1.0, however, exposure affords some degree of protection to exposed individuals, compared to their unexposed counterparts.

The RR computed from the data in Table 4–2 for our colon cancer study is

$$RR = \frac{535 / (535 + 965)}{533 / (533 + 5167)} = \frac{535 / 1500}{533 / 5700} = 3.81.$$

Persons in the at-risk group are approximately *3.8 times more likely* than to develop colon cancer than their not-at-risk counterparts. Greenberg (1993, p 91) indicates that a relative risk of this magnitude signals the existence of a moderate to strong relationship between exposure and disease development.

ODDS RATIO

The **odds ratio (OR)** is developed from a case-control study in which participants are selected on the basis of their known disease status. The odds ratio is used by some epidemiologists to estimate relative risk (Greenberg, 1993, p 104; Hennekens & Buring, 1987, p 79). In a case-control study, cases (persons with disease) and controls (disease-free individuals) are selected and the proportion exposed in each group is compared (Hennekens & Buring, 1987, p 22). In a similar way, the OR compares the odds that cases have been exposed to a particular factor or event to the odds that controls also have been exposed.

$$\text{Odds that a } case \text{ is exposed} \quad = \frac{A / (A + C)}{C / (A + C)} \qquad 4.11a$$

$$\text{Odds that a } control \text{ is exposed} = \frac{B / (B + D)}{D / (B + D)} \qquad 4.11b$$

Table 4–3. Cross-sectional study of individuals with or without chronic cough in an industry in which sulfur dioxide is used routinely.

Exposure Group	Chronic Cough	No Chronic Cough	Total
Exposed to SO_2	100	350	450
Not exposed to SO_2	8	108	116
TOTAL	108	458	566

We obtain the odds ratio by forming the ratio of the two odds given in Formula 4.11a and 4.11b, and simplifying the numerator and denominator:

$$OR = \frac{a(d)}{b(c)} \qquad \qquad 4.12$$

We see from Formula 4.12 that the odds-ratio is the cross-product of the diagonals in a 2×2 table. For this reason, it is sometimes called the cross-product ratio.

Consider that a case-control study is done in an industry in which sulfur dioxide (SO_2) is used regularly (Table 4–3). Male workers who present with chronic cough and those without chronic cough are examined relative to their SO_2 exposure. Assume that no confounding exists (due to age, cigarette smoking habits, race, or length of workplace exposure to SO_2). In this hypothetical example, the odds ratio is $(100 \times 108)/(8 \times 350)$, which equals 3.86. This OR indicates that male workers with chronic cough are approximately four times more likely to have been exposed to SO_2 than their counterparts who do not cough chronically.

Describing Prognosis

"*Prognosis* is a prediction of the *future course of disease following its onset*" (Fletcher et al, 1988, p 106, italics added). Risk, in contrast, focuses on factors that affect the chance of *developing disease*. The literature abounds with numerous prognostic "rates," many of which are proportions rather than true rates. Fletcher and associates (1988) describe several common "rates" used to describe prognosis (p 111). For example, the 5-year survival rate is the proportion or percentage of patients surviving 5 years from some point in their disease, such as time of diagnosis. Remission rate is the proportion or percentage of patients who enter a period in which their disease is quiescent or undetectable. Recurrence rate is the proportion of percentage of patients whose disease returns, after having been in remission. A description of prognostic rates and issues affecting their interpretation is presented by Fletcher and associates (1988, pp 110–113).

SUMMARY

In this chapter, we discuss measures often used to describe the health status of individuals in groups, including the count to identify simple frequency, measures of incidence to characterize the development of new disease, and measures of risk to address the chance that disease may develop. The term "rate" is used to identify various expressions, including ratios, proportions, and true rates. Thus, care must be exercised when interpreting rates. In particular, a clear and specific definition of the denominator of a rate is necessary for correct interpretation.

Measures of prevalence and incidence occur frequently in the medical literature. Prevalence is the proportion of individuals in a population who have a specified clinical characteristic, such as disease, at a specific point in time. Cumulative incidence and incidence density relate the development of new cases of disease in a defined population over a particular period of time, such as 1 year. Cumulative incidence is the number of new cases that accumulate during a specified period of time, divided by the size of the population-at-risk. Incidence density is the number of new cases of disease during a defined period of time, divided by the total person-time or at-risk observation. Cumulative incidence is a proportion; incidence density is a true rate.

Morbidity and mortality are common measures of prevalence and incidence. Morbidity is "Any departure, subjective or objective, from a state of physiological or psychological well being" (Last, 1983, p 64). Morbidity is the number of nonfatal cases of newly reported disease, divided by the total population-at-risk during a specified period of time. Mortality, in contrast to morbidity, expresses the incidence of death in a specified population during a specific time period.

Measures of prevalence and incidence are used to (1) explore disease development, (2) predict the future, and (3) assess risk and make comparisons. Cohort investigations and the measures of incidence developed from them provide the clearest information about the association between disease and antecedent exposures. Measures of incidence are also useful for predicting the future, that is, the likelihood that members of an at-risk population will develop disease.

Several different measures are used to assess risk and compare groups. The risk difference, which is determined from cohort investigations, is the difference between the cumulative incidences in the exposed and unexposed groups. It provides information about the excess of disease in exposed, compared to unexposed, individuals. Attributable risk percent estimates the proportion of disease in exposed individuals that is attributable to the exposure. Like the risk difference, the attributable risk percent is developed from cohort investigations. Relative risk, also developed from cohort investigations, answers the following question: "How many times more likely are exposed individuals to develop disease compared to unexposed persons?" If the relative risk is greater than 1.0, the risk of disease development is greater in exposed than unexposed individuals. Determined from a case-control study, the odds ratio compares the odds that cases have been exposed to a particular factor or event to the odds that controls have also been exposed.

Measures that describe prognosis stand in contrast to measures of risk. Risk provides information about the chance of developing disease. Prognosis predicts the future course of disease following its onset. Five-year survival, remission, and recurrence are common measures of prognosis.

REFERENCES

Boring C, Squires T, Tong T: Cancer statistics, 1991. *CA* 1991;**41**:19.

Centers for Disease Control: HIV infection and AIDS, Georgia, 1991. *MMWR* 1992;**41**:876.

Centers for Disease Control: Trends in prostate cancer, United States, 1980–1988. *MMWR* 1992;**41**:401.

Dawson-Saunders B, Trapp R: *Basic and Clinical Biostatistics,* 2nd ed. Appleton & Lange, 1994.

Fletcher R, Fletcher S, Wagner E: *Clinical Epidemiology: The Essentials,* 2nd ed. Williams & Wilkins, 1988.

Greenberg R: *Medical Epidemiology.* Appleton & Lange, 1993.

Hennekens C, Buring J: *Epidemiology in Medicine.* Little Brown, 1987.

Last J: *A Dictionary of Epidemiology.* Oxford University Press, 1983.

Roscoe R, et al: Colon and stomach cancer mortality among automotive wood model makers. *J Occupational Med* 1992;**34**:759.

Shattuck A, White E, Kristal A: How women's adopted low-fat diets affect their husbands. *Am J Public Health* 1992;**82**:1244.

Steenland K: Passive smoking and the risk of heart disease. *JAMA* 1992;**267**:94.

Thun M, et al: Risk factors for fatal colon cancer in a large prospective study. *JNCI* 1992;**84**:1491.

Self-study Questions

Part I: Thought Questions

1. Describe briefly the information provided by measures of health status.
2. Compare and contrast a *ratio, proportion,* and (true) *rate.*
3. Explain briefly the purpose behind *adjusting* (or standardizing) rates.
4. Identify the similarities and differences between measures of *prevalence* and *incidence.*
5. Describe the similarities and differences between *cumulative incidence* and *incidence density.*
6. Differentiate between measures of *morbidity* and *mortality.*
7. Identify and describe common *uses* of measures of prevalence and incidence.
8. Define *risk difference, attributable risk percent, relative risk,* and *odds-ratio;* make sure your definition includes the type of study from which each is obtained.
9. Specify the difference between *risk* and *prognosis.*
10. Describe the meaning of the following statement: "In a study of over 100,000 women, investigators found that women who smoke 25 or more cigarettes per day have nearly twice the risk of developing diabetes than women who smoke between 1 and 14 cigarettes per day."

Part II: Computation of Risk

Use the following clinical scenario to respond to Questions 1 to 4. A clinical trial was done with patients who (1) had suffered at least two recurrences of duodenal ulcers, (2) were currently in remission, and (3) tested positive for the presence of *H. pylori,* a bacterium commonly found in the human duodenum. Participants were divided randomly into two groups. One group received a frequently used ulcer medication; the other group received the same ulcer medication plus an appropriate antibiotic. Patients were followed for 1 year; a simple determination was made for each patient—whether an ulcer recurred (yes/no) during the 12-month observation period. The data appear in Table 4–4.

1. Is calculation of the *odds ratio* or *relative risk* more appropriate for these data? Why?
2. Calculate the cumulative incidence of ulcer recurrence in each group of patients.
3. Compute the relative risk of ulcer recurrence.
4. The investigators who conducted this study indicated that the combined therapy of ulcer medication and antibiotics virtually eliminated the risk of recurrence. Do you agree or disagree with this statement? Why?

Table 4–4. Ulcer recurrence in patients treated with a common ulcer medication and those treated with the same medication plus an antibiotic.

Treatment	Recurrence During Observation Period		Total
	Yes	No	
Ulcer medication plus antibiotic	9	99	108
Ulcer medication only	89	15	104
TOTAL	98	114	212

Solutions

1. *Relative risk;* a *cohort* design was used in which patients were followed over time. An odds ratio is computed from a cross-sectional study in which measures of prevalence are presented.

2. *Ulcer medication and antibiotics:* CI = 9/108 = 0.083. The ulcer recurred in approximately 8% of patients during the follow-up period. *Ulcer medication only:* CI = 89/104 = 0.0858. The ulcer recurred during follow-up in approximately 86% of patients treated with ulcer medication only.
3. RR = (9/108)/(89/104) = 0.0974. In this study, patients treated with ulcer medication and antibiotics were approximately one tenth as likely to suffer a recurrence, compared to patients treated only with ulcer medication.
4. *Agree,* because the relative risk of recurrence is negligible for patients receiving the combined therapy. We must be cautious, however, about generalizing these results to all ulcer patients, because it has not been demonstrated that patients with other types of ulcers will respond similarly.

Quantifying Uncertainty—Defining the Basic Rules of Probability

5

Clinical Example 1: Hypertension

After a thorough history, physical examination, and appropriate diagnostic tests, a patient is diagnosed with hypertension. The available clinical information suggests that drug management is warranted. The treating physician prescribes Inderal. How likely is it that this beta blocker will control the patient's hypertension? How likely is it that the patient will experience sleep disturbance or develop increased plasma triglyceride levels after several weeks of drug therapy?

Clinical Example 2: Myocardial Infarction

A man experiences an acute myocardial infarction while dining with his family. What is the chance that he will die within the first hour after the infarction?

Clinical Example 3: Lupus Versus Rheumatoid Arthritis

A woman, age 33 years, presents with fever, anorexia, malaise, and weight loss. She reports that her joints are tender. She also indicates that she develops skin rashes in areas exposed to sunlight. Examination by an ophthalmologist reveals cotton-wool spots on the retina (cytoid bodies). Serologic studies indicate the presence of antinuclear antibodies with high titer to native DNA. In addition, her hemoglobin level and white blood cell count are depressed. Is this patient more likely to have systemic lupus erythematosus or rheumatoid arthritis?

When clinicians interpret test results, establish a diagnosis, predict clinical outcomes, or summarize research, some degree of uncertainty always exists. This degree of uncertainty can be quantified through probability theory. In this chapter, we define basic probability concepts and discuss the fundamental rules of probability. These concepts and rules underlie diagnostic testing, medical decision making, and statistical inference.

OBJECTIVES

When you complete this chapter, you should be able to:

- Define basic probability concepts, such as independent events, mutually exclusive events, and conditional probability.
- Read a table and determine the probability of specified events.
- Compute the probability of specified events.
- Understand the relationship between probability and relative frequency.
- Translate probability calculations.

DEFINING BASIC CONCEPTS

In this section, we minimize the use of calculations. The fundamental rules of probability are illustrated in Table 5–1, which contains data from the first 1000 children admitted to a clinic for retarded children. Note that the data are cross-classified according to diagnostic classification and level of retardation. Diagnostic classification, labeled A, appears in rows A_1, A_2, and so on. Observe that 160 children have Down's syndrome (A_2). The level of retardation, designated B, appears in columns B_1, B_2, and so on. Note that 44 children are profoundly retarded (B_1). Each child can be placed in only one diagnostic classification. Likewise, each child can be categorized as having only one level of retardation. The row totals represent the number of children in each diagnostic classification, without regard to level of retardation. The column totals indicate the number of children with a specified level of retardation, without regard to diagnostic classification. The sum of the row totals equals 1000; the sum of the column totals equals 1000.

Table 5–1. Level of retardation and diagnostic classification of the first 1000 patients admitted to a clinic for retarded children.

A: Diagnostic Classification	B: Level of Retardation						Total
	B_1 Profound	B_2 Severe	B_3 Moderate	B_4 Mild	B_5 Borderline	B_6 Not Retarded	
A_1 Encephalopathies	38	57	114	103	55	33	400
A_2 Down's syndrome	4	34	88	27	5	2	160
A_3 Congenital cerebral defect	2	6	6	6	0	10	30
A_4 Mental retardation of unknown cause	0	9	36	62	35	0	142
A_5 Other	0	8	16	8	75	161	268
TOTAL	44	114	260	206	170	206	1000

Adapted with permission of publisher from Daniel W: *Biostatistics: A Foundation for Analysis in the Health Sciences,* 5th ed. Wiley, 1991, p 64.

Probability

Daniel (1991, p 45) defines probability in the following way: "If some process is repeated a large number of times, *n*, and if some resulting event with the characteristic, *E*, occurs *m* times, the relative frequency of occurrence of *E*, *m/n*, will be approximately equal to the probability of *E*." If we use **pr** to represent probability, the probability of *E* is:

$$pr(E) = \frac{m}{n}.$$

5.1

We now consider the five elements of the definition just described. The probability of an event (eg, the development of tuberculosis):

Is estimated by *relative frequency.*
Results from a *process* that is *repeated a large number of times.*
Requires the ability to *count the number of times the event occurs.*
Requires the ability to *count the number of repetitions* (*n*, the maximum number of times the event *could* occur).
Depends upon the *number of repetitions; as n increases,* the *relative frequency approximates the probability of the event.*

We illustrate the last point with the following hypothetical example. Consider that the probability that a woman will develop a new case of breast cancer in the next year is 0.1250, or approximately 125 new cases per 1000 women. Suppose we observe 100 women and record 10 new cases of breast cancer in a 1-year period. The relative frequency of new disease is 10/100 or 0.10. If we increase the number of women observed to 1000 and count 110 new cases, the corresponding relative frequency is 110/1000 = 0.11. If we follow 100,000 women for 1 year and chart 12,500 new cases, the relative frequency of new disease is 12,500/100,000 = 0.1250. Thus, as the number of women observed *increases,* the difference between the probability and an estimate based on relative frequency *decreases.* Moreover, for a large number of observations, the relative frequency approximates the probability quite well.

EXAMPLE OF PROBABILITY

The probability of randomly selecting a Down's syndrome child from the 1000 patients whose data appear in Table 5–1 is $pr(A_2) = 160/1000 = 0.16$. The probability of selecting a child who is profoundly retarded is $pr(B_1) = 44/1000 = 0.044$.

Set

A **set** is a collection of distinct objects, such as a sample of patients (Daniel, 1991, p 47). A set is sometimes called a sample space (Hays, 1981, p 10). The 1000 children in Table 5–1 constitute our set.

Element

The distinct objects that constitute a set are **elements** or members of the set (Daniel, 1991, p 47). Each individual patient in our sample is an element or a member of the set.

Event

An **event** is a group or collection of elements. Capital letters are used to identify an event. Numerical subscripts are used, when necessary, to distinguish one event from another. For example, the event of being severely retarded (B_2) contains 114 children (with each child being an element). The probability of this event is $pr(B_2) = 114/1000 = 0.1140$. The event of having a congenital cerebral defect is A_3. The probability of this event is $pr(A_3) = 30/1000 = 0.03$.

Mutually Exclusive Events

Two events, A and B, are **mutually exclusive** if they cannot occur at the same time. For example, mild retardation (B_4) and no retardation (B_6) are mutually exclusive because they cannot occur at the same time in the same child.

Union (Or)

The union of two events (eg, A_3 or B_4) contains all the elements belonging *either* to event A_3 *or* event B_4 *or both* events A_3 and B_4. The union of A_3 or B_4 is written as

$$pr(A_3 \text{ or } B_4).$$

Intersection (And)

The intersection of two events (eg, B_1 and A_1) contains all children who have both encephalopathies and profound retardation. The intersection of events, A_1 and B_1, is designated as $pr(B_1 \text{ and } A_1)$ and referred to as a joint probability.

Independent Events

Two events are **independent** if the probability of one does not affect the probability of the other, or vice versa. If the probability of occurrence of one event increases or decreases the probability of the other event, the two events are dependent. In our example, if the probability of moderate retardation (B_3) does not increase or decrease with the presence or absence of Down's syndrome (A_2), the events are independent. The concept of conditional probability is central to determining if events are independent.

Conditional Probability (Given the Occurrence of)

The **conditional probability** of event A *given the occurrence of* B is $pr(A|B)$. The vertical line is read as *"given;"* $pr(A|B)$ is read as the probability of A *given* B.

Let us return to Clinical Example 2 at the beginning of the chapter. If a man experiences an acute myocardial infarction, what is the probability that he will die within the first hour after the infarction? According to Massie and Sokolow (1993), among patients with an acute infarction, approximately 20% die within the first hour (p 300). We can represent this conditional probability as

$$pr(\textit{Death Within First Hour}|\textit{Acute MI}) = 0.20.$$

Thus, the conditional probability of death within the first hour, *given* the occurrence of an acute infarction, is approximately 0.20; that is, 20% of patients die within the first hour, given an acute infarction.

CONDITIONAL VERSUS UNCONDITIONAL PROBABILITY

Unconditional probability is synonymous with the conventional probability statement. For example, the probability of encephalopathies from Table 5–1 is

$$pr(A_1) = \frac{400}{1000} = 0.40.$$

This probability is *unconditional* because it is computed without knowing whether another event occurs. Note that the denominator of an unconditional probability is the total number of patients observed.

In contrast, conditional probabilities focus on the occurrence of an event, *given* that another outcome has occurred. For example, what is the (conditional) probability that an infant will be severely retarded if he or she is born with Down's syndrome—$pr(B_2|A_2)$? In calculating this probability, we restrict our denominator to a subset of the total sample (children born with Down's syndrome); we then consider those who have severe retardation. Calculation of conditional probability is illustrated later in this chapter.

CONDITIONAL PROBABILITY VERSUS JOINT PROBABILITY

Conditional probability (A given B) and joint probability (both A and B) are often confused. The joint probabilty represents the simultaneous occurrence (or intersection) of two events (the probability that a child will have Down's syndrome and mild retardation). Conditional probability, in contrast, addresses this question: Given that one event has already occurred, what is the probability that the other event will occur? In our hypothetical example, we ask this question: Given that an infant is born with Down's syndrome, what is the probability that he or she will be mildly retarded?

TWO IMPORTANT PRINCIPLES OF PROBABILITY

Principle 1

The probability of an event is a nonnegative number between 0 and 1.0:

$$0 \le pr(A) \le 1.0. \qquad \textbf{5.2}$$

A probability of zero indicates absolute certainty that an event will not occur; a probability of 1.0 reflects absolute certainty that an event will occur. A value of 0.50 indicates that the probability that the event will occur is the same as the probability that it will not occur.

Principle 2

The sum of the probabilities of all possible events is 1.0:

$$pr(A_1 + A_2 + A_3 \ldots + A_n) = 1.0. \qquad \textbf{5.3}$$

Stated somewhat more statistically, the sum of the probabilities of all mutually exclusive, events ($A_1, A_2, \ldots, A_n$) equals 1.0 (Hodges & Lehman, 1970, p 17). This property of *exhaustiveness* requires that the "observer of a probabilistic process must allow for all possible events, and when all are taken together, their total probability is 1" (Daniel, 1991, p 46).

Example

For the diagnostic classification variable in Table 5–1, the sum of the probability of all mutually exclusive events defining is 1.0:

$$pr(A_1 + A_2 + A_3 + A_4 + A_5) = \left(\frac{400}{1000} + \frac{160}{1000} + \frac{30}{1000} + \frac{142}{1000} + \frac{268}{1000} \right) = 1.0.$$

RULES FOR COMBINING PROBABILITIES

What is the Probability of Event A *or* Event B?

The **addition rule** of probability allows us to add probabilities to answer the question: What is the probability of event A *or* event B? Before we simply add probabilities together, however, we must determine whether the events are mutually exclusive (they cannot occur together at the same time).

Addition Rule for Mutually Exclusive Events

$$pr(A \text{ or } B) = pr(A) + pr(B) \qquad \text{5.4}$$

The probability of mutually exclusive events A *or* B is the sum of their respective probabilities.

DIAGRAM OF A OR B FOR MUTUALLY EXCLUSIVE EVENTS

The union of two events is depicted in Diagram A of Fig 5–1. Allow the rectangle to represent the entire set. The two circle-like objects represent two different events that are *mutually exclusive*. Because mutually exclusive events cannot occur simultaneously, no overlap exists between these events; they share no common elements. Therefore, the probability of A or B is the sum of their individual probabilities.

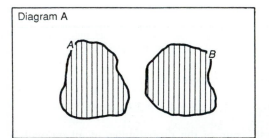
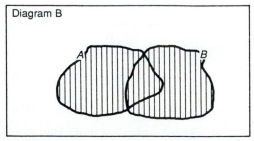

Figure 5–1. Union of two events. Diagram A contains mutually exclusive events. The events in diagram B are *not* mutually exclusive. Their union is the *entire* vertical lined area.

CALCULATION

What is the probability of moderate retardation (B_3) or mild retardation (B_4)? These two events are mutually exclusive because a child cannot be both moderately or mildly retarded. Therefore, the probability of B_3 or B_4 is

$$pr(B_3 \text{ or } B_4) = pr(B_3) + pr(B_4) = \frac{260}{1000} + \frac{206}{1000} = \frac{466}{1000} = 0.466.$$

From these 1000 youngsters, the probability of selecting a child at random who has moderate retardation or borderline retardation is 0.466. In terms of relative frequency, slightly less than half of the children in this sample are moderately retarded or borderline retarded (466 in 1000).

The probability of selecting a child at random who is classified as having encephalopathies (A_1) or a congenital cerebral defect (A_3) is

$$pr(A_1 \text{ or } A_3) = pr(A_1) + pr(A_3) = \frac{400}{1000} + \frac{30}{1000} = \frac{430}{1000} = 0.43.$$

Addition Rule for Events That Are Not Mutually Exclusive

$$pr(A \text{ or } B) = pr(A) + pr(B) - pr(A \text{ and } B) \qquad \text{5.5}$$

For events that are *not* mutually exclusive, we modify the addition rule to reflect that pr (A and B) *is added twice in the calculation*. Note that $pr(A \text{ and } B)$ does not appear in Formula 5.4 (the addition rule for mutually exclusive events). Because no overlap exists between mutually exclusive events, $pr(A \text{ and } B)$ equals 0 and, therefore, does not affect the calculation of $pr(A$ or $B)$.

DIAGRAM OF A OR B FOR EVENTS THAT ARE NOT MUTUALLY EXCLUSIVE

Diagram B in Fig 5–1 depicts a sample space with two events that are not mutually exclusive. The union consists of all elements that are in *either* A or B or *both* A and B. The union of these two events is given by the entire shaded area encompassed by both circle-like objects.

CALCULATION

What is the probability of mental retardation of unknown cause (A_4) or severe retardation (B_2)? To calculate $pr(A_4 \text{ or } B_2)$ from Formula 5.5, we must know or calculate the probability of A_4 and B_2, $pr(A_4 \text{ and } B_2)$. To obtain $pr(A_4 \text{ and } B_2)$, however, we must determine if A_4 and B_2 are independent. Determining independence of events is discussed below.

To compute $pr(A_4 \text{ or } B_2)$, we first read $pr(A_4 \text{ and } B_2)$ from Table 5–1. Reading from the table at the intersection of row 4 and column 2, we find that 9 children in 1000 have mental retardation of unknown cause *and* severe retardation. Therefore, $pr(A_4 \text{ and } B_2) = 9/1000$. We can confirm our result as follows:

$$pr(A_4 \text{ or } B_2) = pr(A_4) + pr(B_2) - pr(A_4 \text{ and } B_2)$$

$$= \frac{142}{1000} + \frac{114}{1000} - \frac{9}{1000} = \frac{247}{1000} = 0.247$$

Examine Table 5–1 and note that 9 is included in the column total of 114 (B_2, the number of children having severe retardation) *and* the row total of 142 (A_4, the number with mental retardation of unknown cause). Therefore, *we must subtract the 9 because it is been included twice in our calculation.* For our sample, the probability of randomly selecting a child who has mental retardation of unknown cause *or* severe retardation is 0.247.

Next, we discuss the concept of independence because it is central to calculating the probability of A_4 *and* B_2.

Conditional Probability Revisited

Conditional probabilities focus on the chance that one event will occur, given that another event has already occurred. The concept of independence of events is illustrated through the use of conditional probability.

Conditional Probability for Independent Events

If events are independent, the probability of A is unaffected by the occurrence of B. Therefore, the conditional probability of A, given that B has occurred, is the probability of A:

$$pr(A|B) = pr(A).$$
                                                                                              5.6

CONDITIONAL PROBABILITY FOR EVENTS THAT ARE NOT INDEPENDENT

The conditional probability of A, given B, equals the joint probability divided by the probability of B:

$$pr(A|B) = \frac{pr(A \text{ and } B)}{pr(B)},$$
                                                                                              5.7

where $pr(B) \neq 0$.

Computation Assuming Nonindependence

Given that a child is born with Down's syndrome (A_2), what is the probability that he or she will be borderline retarded (B_5)—$pr(B_5|A_2)$? Based on extensive clinical observation and research, we know that a child born with Down's syndrome is likely to have some degree of mental retardation; therefore, it is appropriate to assume that these two events are not independent. The conditional probability of borderline retardation given Down syndrome is

$$pr(B_5|A_2) = \frac{pr(B_5 \text{ and } A_2)}{pr(A_2)} = \frac{(5 / 1000)}{(160 / 1000)} = 0.0313$$

Among children born with Down's syndrome, the probability is approximately 0.03 that a child will be classified as borderline retarded. Thus, approximately 3% of Down's syndrome babies will be borderline retarded.

Given that an infant is born with Down's syndrome (A_2), what is the probability that he or she will be severely (B_2) or moderately retarded (B_3)? To answer this question, we extend the addition rule and combine it with Formula 5.7. We recognize first that severe and moderate retardation are mutually exclusive events, because both cannot occur simultaneously in the same child. We represent the probability of interest as

$$pr(B_2|A_2 \text{ or } B_3|A_2) = pr(B_2|A_2) + pr(B_3|A_2)$$

$$= \frac{pr(B_2 \text{ and } A_2)}{pr(A_2)} + \frac{pr(B_3 \text{ and } A_2)}{pr(A_2)}$$

$$= \frac{(34 / 1000)}{(160 / 1000)} + \frac{(88 / 1000)}{(160 / 1000)} = 0.7625$$

Thus, given that an infant is born with Down syndrome, the probability is approximately 0.76 that he or she will be severely or moderately retarded. In terms of percentage frequency, given that a child is born with Down syndrome, 122 of 160 such children, or approximately 76% in our sample, are severely or moderately retarded.

WHAT IS THE PROBABILITY OF A *AND* B?

We use the **multiplication rule** to determine joint probability (intersection), the probability that A *and* B will occur—$pr(A \text{ and } B)$. The probability of A and B is represented by the intersection of these two events, which is diagrammed in Fig 5–2. The intersection consists only of the overlapping, cross-hatched area. To compute the probability of both A and B, we must ask whether the events are independent.

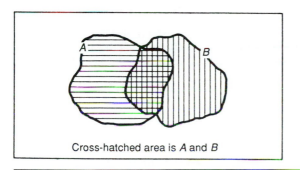

Cross-hatched area is *A* and *B*

Figure 5–2. Intersection of two events, A and B. The cross-hatched (overlapping) area represents the intersection.

Multiplication Rule for Independent Events

If events are independent, the probability that A and B occur jointly is the product of their individual probabilities:

$$pr(A \text{ and } B) = pr(A)pr(B) \tag{5.8}$$

Multiplication Rule for Events That Are Not Independent

If events are not independent, the joint probability of A and B is equal to the conditional probability of A, given the occurrence of B, divided by the probability of B—assuming that the probability of B is not zero:

$$pr(A \text{ and } B) = pr(A|B)pr(B) \tag{5.9a}$$

where $pr(B) \neq 0$.

This formula is obtained by multiplying both sides of Formula 5.7 (conditional probability for events that are not independent) by $pr(B)$. The "and" in the expression $pr(A$ and $B)$ does not signify the order of events; thus, $pr(A$ and $B)$ equals $pr(B$ and $A)$. Therefore, the multiplication rule also can be written as

$$pr(B \text{ and } A) = pr(B|A)pr(A) \qquad \textbf{5.9b}$$

where $pr(A) \neq 0$.

COMPUTATION

What is the probability of Mental Retardation of Unknown Cause and Severe Retardation— $pr(A_4$ and $B_2)$?

To compute this joint probability, we must first know whether the events are independent. Sometimes, we know events are independent based on extensive clinical observation or research. When the relationship between events remains unknown, we follow these steps:

1. From Table 5–1, obtain $pr(A_4$ and $B_2)$: $pr(A_4$ and $B_2) = 9/1000 = 0.009$.

2. Use Formula 5.8 to compute $pr(A_4$ and $B_2) = pr(A_4)pr(B_2)$. Check to determine if the result equals the value obtained in step 1. If it does, *the events are independent.* In this case, $pr(A_4$ and $B_2) = pr(A_4)pr(B_2) = C142/1000) \times (114/1000) = 0.0162.-0.009$. Therefore, these events are not independent. We cannot use Formula 5.8 to obtain the joint probability; instead, we use Formula 5.9 for events that are not independent.

3. Use Formula 5.9 to calculate the conditional probability of mental retardation of unknown case and severe retardation: $pr(A_4$ and $B_2) = pr(B_2|A_4)pr(A_4) = (9/142) \times (142/1000) = 9/1000 = 0.009$. Note that this probability is identical to the value we read from Table 5–1.

Complement

Consider that two events, A and B, are mutually exclusive. By definition, B occurs only when A is *not* present. Event B is the **complement** of A:

$$pr(B) = pr(\text{Not } A) = 1 - pr(A). \qquad \textbf{5.10}$$

Examples of complementary events include disease status (diseased/disease free), remission (disease not detectable/disease active), 5-year survival (yes/no), and mortality (yes/no). Consider the hypothetical case in Clinical Example 3 at the beginning of the chapter. If the probability of disease (D^+) is 0.95, the probability of being disease-free (D^-) is

$$pr(D^-) = 1 - pr(D^+) = 1 - 0.95 = 0.05.$$

We can state this in terms of relative percentage frequency: approximately 5% of patients who present with these symptoms are disease-free.

SUMMARY

Researchers rely on the rules of probability to predict future outcomes, develop diagnoses, interpret diagnostic tests, and formulate clinical decisions. In this chapter, fundamental rules of probability are presented and illustrated with data from Table 5–1; these rules are summarized in Table 5–2.

Table 5–2. Summary of fundamental rules of probability.

Concept	Rule
Probability (estimated as relative frequency)	$\dfrac{\text{Number of Times an Event Occurs}}{\text{Maximum Number of Times It Could Occur}}$
	Addition rule for mutually exclusive events
	$pr(A \text{ or } B) = pr(A) + pr(B)$
Addition rule for events that are not mutually exclusive	$pr(A \text{ or } B) = pr(A) + pr(B) - pr(A \text{ and } B)$
Conditional probability for independent events	$pr(A|B) = pr(A)$
Conditional probability for events that are not independent	$pr(A|B) = \dfrac{pr(A \text{ and } B)}{pr(B)}$, where $pr(B) \neq 0$
Multiplication rule for independent events	$pr(A \text{ and } B) = pr(A)pr(B)$
Multiplication rule for events that are not independent	$pr(A \text{ and } B) = pr(A|B)pr(B)$
Complement of two mutually exclusive events	$pr(B) = pr(\text{Not } A) = 1 - pr(A)$

Probability is defined as a relative frequency that assumes values between 0.00 and +1.00. A probability of zero indicates absolute certainty that an event will not occur; a probability of +1.00 reflects absolute certainty that an event will occur. Two events, A and B, are mutually exclusive if they cannot occur at the same time. Two events are independent if the probability of one does not affect the probability of the other or vice versa.

The addition rule is used to compute the probability of A or B, also known as the union—pr(A or B). For example, what is the probability that a patient has ulcerative colitis or Crohn's disease? To compute this probability, we must take into account whether or not the events are mutually exclusive. The multiplication rule is employed to determine the probability of A and B, also referred to as the joint probability—pr(A and B). For example, what is the probability that a patient has a body temperature of 103 °F and meningitis. To calculate this probability, we must consider whether or not the events are independent. If events are not independent, conditional probability plays a role in determining the joint probability of A and B. The conditional probability of an event, given the occurrence of another event, is pr(A|B). For example, what is the probability that a patient is having an acute myocardial infarction, given that he has aching chest pain that radiates to the left arm? We will revisit this important concept of conditional probability in Chapter 7.

REFERENCES

Daniel W: *Biostatistics: A Foundation for Analysis in the Health Sciences,* 5th ed. Wiley, 1991.
Hays W. *Statistics,* 3rd ed. Holt, Rinehart, & Winston, 1981.
Hodges J, Lehman E: *Basic Concepts of Probability and Statistics,* 2nd ed. Holden-Day, 1970.
Massie B, Sokolow M: Cardiovascular disease. In: *Current Medical Diagnosis and Treatment.* Tierney L Jr, et al (editors). Appleton & Lange, 1993.

Self-study Questions

Part I: Thought Questions

1. Define *probability, mutually exclusive events,* and *independent events.* Provide an example of each.
2. Describe the difference between *unconditional* and *conditional* probability.
3. Translate the following statement into its symbolic equivalent: Approximately 1 in 70 women will develop ovarian cancer in their lifetime.
4. Allow *ANA* to represent antinuclear antibodies, *SLE* to designate systematic lupus erythematosus, and + to denote the presence of an event. Translate the following symbolic representation: $pr(ANA^+|SLE^+) = 0.99$.

Part II: Angioplasty and Subsequent Death

A multicenter study was conducted to assess the occurrence of death following angioplasty to reopen occluded coronary arteries. The study involved 4030 patients undergoing angioplasty. Among the 3000 men in the study, 7 died in the hospital following the procedure. Among the 1030 women in the study, 27 died in the hospital following the procedure.

1. What is the probability that a patient selected at random will be male?
2. What is the probability that a patient selected at random will be female?
3. What is the probability of death following angioplasty?
4. What is the probability of death following angioplasty, given that the patient is male?
5. What is the probability of death following angioplasty, given that the patient is female?

Suggestions for calculating the above probabilities: First, define the events as described below. Second, array the data in a two-by-two table, with the rows defining sex (M/F) and the columns defining outcome (death/survival).

D^+ Death following angioplasty to reopen occluded coronary arteries
D^- Survival following angioplasty to reopen occluded coronary arteries
M   Patient is male
F   Patient is female

Part III: Additional Probability Calculation Exercises

Refer to Table 5–1. Determine or calculate the following:

1. How many children in the sample
   a. Have Down's syndrome?
   b. Have moderate retardation?
   c. Have no retardation or borderline retardation?
   d. Have moderate retardation and encephalopathies?
2. What is the probability that a randomly selected child will
   a. Have a congenital cerebral defect?
   b. Be identified as having no retardation?
   c. Be profoundly retarded?
3. What is the probability of selecting a child at random who will
   a. Have a congenital cerebral defect or mental retardation of unknown cause?
   b. Have profound or severe retardation?
   c. Be classified diagnostically as having encephalopathies or Down's syndrome or a congenital cerebral defect or mental retardation of unknown cause?
   d. Will have retardation that is profound or severe or moderate?
   e. Will have Down's syndrome or no retardation?
4. What is the probability that a child selected randomly will have Down's syndrome and profound retardation?
   a. Read the probability directly from the table.
   b. Calculate the probability; assume first that the events are independent.
   c. Calculate the probability; assume that the events are not independent.
   d. Compare the results in A, B, and C. Comment on your calculations.

Solutions

Part I: Thought Questions

1. *Probability:* Relative frequency. *Mutually exclusive events:* Events that cannot occur at the same time. *Independent events:* The occurrence of one event in no way affects the occurrence of the other.

2. Conditional probabilities represent the probability of occurrence of one event, given that another event has occurred. Unconditional probabilities address the occurrence of an event, without regard to the presence or absence of another event.
3. "Approximately 1 in 70 women will develop ovarian cancer in their lifetime." If we recall that probability is a relative frequency, we can translate this statement as follows: The probability that a woman will develop ovarian cancer in her lifetime is approximately (1/70) or 0.0143.
4. Translate: $pr(ANA^+|SLE^+) = 0.99$. Ninety-nine percent of patients who have systemic lupus erythematosus test positive for antinuclear antibodies.

Part II: Angioplasty

The following two-by-two layout is used in all calculations.

Angioplasty and Mortality Postprocedure

Sex of Patient	Postprocedure Outcome		Total
	Death (D$^+$)	Survival (D$^-$)	
Male	7	2993	3000
Female	27	1003	1030
TOTAL	34	3996	4030

1. What is the probability that a patient selected at random will be male?

$$pr(M) = \frac{3000}{4030} = 0.7444$$

2. What is the probability that a patient selected at random will be female?

$$pr(F) = \frac{1030}{4030} = 0.2556$$

3. What is the probability of death following angioplasty?

$$pr(D^+) = \frac{34}{4030} = 0.0084$$

4. What is the probability of death following angioplasty given the patient is male?

$$pr(D^+|M) = \frac{pr(D^+ \text{ and } M)}{pr(M)} = \frac{(7 / 4030)}{(3000 / 4030)} = 0.0023$$

5. What is the probability of death following angioplasty given the patient is female?

$$pr(D^+|F) = \frac{pr(D^+ \text{ and } F)}{pr(F)} = \frac{(27 / 4030)}{(1030 / 4030)} = 0.0262$$

Note that the probability of death following angioplasty is nearly 10 times greater if the patient is female. As an aside, let us calculate relative risk based on the cumulative incidence of death in each group:

$$RR = \frac{CI_{Death\ for\ Females}}{CI_{Death\ for\ Males}} = \frac{(27 / 1030)}{(7 / 3000)} = 11.2344$$

Based on the calculation of relative risk, we find that women have approximately an 11 times greater risk of death following the procedure, compared to their male counterparts.

Part III: Additional Calculation from Table 5–1

1. How many children in the sample
   a. Have Down's syndrome? $A_2 = 160$.
   b. Have moderate retardation? $B_3 = 260$.
   c. Have no retardation or borderline retardation? B_6 or $B_5 = 206 + 170 = 376$.
   d. Have moderate retardation and encephalopathies? A_1 and $B_3 = 114$.
2. What is the probability that a randomly selected child will
   a. Have a congenital cerebral defect? $pr(A_3) = \dfrac{30}{1000} = 0.03$.

   b. Be identified as having no retardation? $pr(B_6) = \dfrac{206}{1000} = 0.206$.

   c. Be profoundly retarded? $pr(B_1) = \dfrac{44}{1000} = 0.044$.

3. What is the probability of selecting a child at random who will
   a. Have a congenital cerebral defect or mental retardation of unknown cause? (Use the addition rule because the two events are mutually exclusive.)

   $$pr(A_3 \text{ or } A_4) = pr(A_3) + pr(A_4) = \frac{30}{1000} + \frac{142}{1000} = 0.1720$$

   b. Have profound or severe retardation? (Use the addition rule because the two events are mutually exclusive.)

   $$pr(B_1 \text{ or } B_2) = pr(B_1) + pr(B_2) = \frac{44}{1000} + \frac{114}{1000} = 0.1580$$

   c. Be classified diagnostically as having encephalopathies or Down's syndrome or a congenital cerebral defect or mental retardation of unknown cause?

   $$pr(A_1 \text{ or } A_2 \text{ or } A_3 \text{ or } A_4) = pr(A_1) + pr(A_2) + pr(A_3) + pr(A_4)$$

   $$= \frac{400}{1000} + \frac{160}{1000} + \frac{30}{1000} + \frac{142}{1000}$$

   $$= 0.7320$$

   We could also use the following approach, because the sum of all mutually exclusive events must equal 1.0:

   $$pr(A_1 \text{ or } A_2 \text{ or } A_3 \text{ or } A_4) = 1 - pr(A_5) = 1 - \frac{268}{1000} = 0.7230$$

   d. Will have profound or severe or moderate retardation?

   $$pr(B_1 \text{ or } B_2 \text{ or } B_3) = pr(B_1) + pr(B_2) + pr(B_3)$$

   $$= \frac{44}{1000} + \frac{114}{1000} + \frac{260}{1000} = 0.4180$$

   e. Will have Down's syndrome or no retardation? (Modify the addition rule because Down's syndrome and no retardation are *not* mutually exclusive. Therefore, subtract the intersection to avoid "double counting" it.)

   $$pr(A_2 \text{ or } B_6) = pr(A_2) + pr(B_6) - pr(A_2 \text{ and } B_6)$$

   $$= \frac{160}{1000} + \frac{206}{1000} - \frac{2}{1000} = 0.3640$$

4. What is the probability that a child selected randomly will have Down's syndrome and profound retardation? $pr(A_2 \text{ and } B_1)$
   a. Read the probability directly from the table. The numerator of the probability represents the intersection of the second row and the first column (4 children). Divide by 1000 (the total number of children in the sample). The probability is 0.004.
   b. Calculate the probability; assume first that the events are independent. Use the multiplication rule for independent events.

$$pr(A_2 \text{ and } B_1) = pr(A_2)pr(B_1) = \frac{160}{1000} \times \frac{44}{1000} = 0.0070$$

   c. Calculate the probability; assume that the events are not independent. Modify the multiplication rule for events that are not independent.

$$pr(A_2 \text{ and } B_1) = pr(A_2|B_1)pr(B_1) = \frac{4}{44} \times \frac{44}{1000} = 0.004$$

   d. Compare the results in a, b, and c. Comment on your calculations. If the events are independent, the probability determined from Table 5–1 (0.004) equals the value computed in part b (0.0070). By determining that these probabilities are unequal, we find that the events are not independent. This observation is confirmed in part c above.

Describing Distributions of Quantitative Measurements—The Normal Probability Distribution

6

Clinical Example: Hypertension

During a routine physical examination, a 47-year-old Caucasian male presents with an arterial blood pressure of 170/120 mm Hg. He smokes 1 to 1½ packs of cigarettes per day, as he has done for approximately 25 years. His paternal great grandfather died of a heart attack at age 47 and his paternal grandfather suffered a fatal stroke at age 53. His 72-year-old father has had three strokes within the past 5 years. The patient's weight is within the normal range for his height, age, and frame. All other physical findings are unremarkable. Laboratory results from routinely ordered blood chemistries are pending.

Is this patient hypertensive? How is hypertension defined? Is hypertension a significant health problem? What are the implications if we use different cutoff values to define hypertension with respect to the proportion of the population identified as hypertensive or requiring additional screening? In this chapter, we explore a mathematical model, known as the normal curve or Gaussian distribution, that allows us to answer these and similar questions.

OBJECTIVES

When you complete this chapter, you should be able to:

- Define the properties of a normal curve.
- Discuss the uses of the standard normal curve.
- Use the standard normal curve to compute the probability of outcomes and to translate that probability into a relative frequency.
- Explain how increasing or decreasing a clinical laboratory cutoff value affects the proportion of individuals identified as *within the range of normal* or *outside the range of normal.*

HYPERTENSION SCREENING

Massie and Sokolow (1993) explain that "Hypertension is an important treatable cause of cardiovascular disease; untreated, it increases the incidence of early demise, stroke, coronary events, heart failure, and renal failure." The researchers also point out that approximately one half of the hypertensive population is "aware they have the condition, and only half of those who are aware of it have their pressure normalized by treatment" (p 352). According to the 1988 report of the Joint National Committee on the Detection, Evaluation, and Treatment of High Blood Pressure, the diagnosis of hypertension in adults occurs when the average diastolic blood pressure is 90 mm Hg or greater (p 1024). The Committee provided the guidelines given in Table 6–1 for the classification of arterial blood pressure in adults aged 18 years and older.

Blood pressure readings from large-scale community screening programs are usually distributed like symmetric, bell-shaped curves. The results of such a program are described by the Hypertension Detection and Follow-up Program Cooperative Group (1977). By employing well-established statistical principles, we can address the question raised in the opening paragraph of this chapter: What are the implications if we use different cutoff values to define hypertension with respect to the proportion of the population identified as hypertensive or requiring additional screening?

In this chapter, we discuss the bell-shaped distribution as a mathematical model. We define the characteristics of the bell-shaped distribution and illustrate its use within the context of hypothetical examples based on actual research in hypertension. Of course, the usefulness of the bell-shaped distribution extends well beyond blood pressure screening. The bell-shaped distribution plays a central role in statistical inference, in which findings from a sample are generalized to a target population. Many variables in medicine are measured quantitatively; in very large groups of individuals, these variables often follow a bell-shaped distribution. If a quantitative diagnostic test result falls above or below a specified **cutoff value,** patients may be

Table 6–1. Classification of arterial diastolic blood pressure (mm Hg) in adults, 18 years and older.

Diastolic Blood Pressure (mm Hg)	Blood Pressure Classification
Less than 85	Normal
85–89	High normal
90–104	Mild hypertension
105–114	Moderate hypertension
Greater than or equal to 115	Severe hypertension

Used with permission from 1988 Report of the Joint National Committee on the Detection, Evaluation, and Treatment of High Blood Pressure. *Arch Intern Med* 1988;**148**:1023.

Insert verti

categorized as having normal or abnormal readings or being diseased or disease-free. Cutoff values, presented in **tables of reference values,** represent statistical data for 95% of the population (Wallach, 1992, p 7). Wallach (1992) and Rodriguez (1991) provide tables of reference values for many clinical laboratory tests.

THE BELL-SHAPED DISTRIBUTION

The bell-shaped distribution is known also as the **normal curve, normal probability distribution,** or **Gaussian distribution** after Carl Friedrich Gauss, who made significant contributions in the beginning of the 19th century to its development (Minium et al, 1993, p 111). Colton (1974, p 82) notes that " 'Normal' is perhaps not the most appropriate label for this distribution [because] the statistical meaning of the term differs from the medical meaning of 'normal.' " Because the Gaussian distribution is usually referred to as the "normal curve," we use this designation.

The normal curve is a mathematical *abstraction* or *model*; it is a probability distribution (sometimes referred to as a probability density function), that describes an infinite number of observations measured continuously (Daniel, 1991, pp 86–87). The normal curve is specified by the following mathematical rule (Hays, 1981, p 205):

$$f(x) = \frac{1}{\sqrt{2\pi}\sigma}e^{-(X-\mu)^2/2\sigma^2} \quad for -\infty < X < \infty. \qquad \textbf{6.1}$$

Pi (π) equals 3.14159 and e is 2.71828; X is a random variable that can assume values between negative ($-\infty$) and positive (∞) infinity. A random variable is one for which different values occur because of chance factors, such as biologic variation within and between patients. The density function depends only on the values of μ and σ for a given X, because these two parameters are the only components of the function that vary (Hays, 1981, p 205). The graph generated by the mathematical rule (Formula 6.1) produces the familiar bell-shaped curve shown in Figure 6.1. The x-axis (abscissa) contains the values of the random variable; the y-axis (ordinate) contains relative frequency, denoted as $f(x)$.

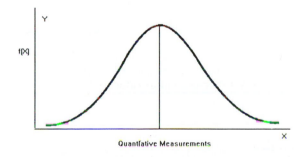

Figure 6–1. Normal curve with quantitative measurements on the x-axis and relative frequency, given by the density function, $f(x)$, on the y-axis.

Because the parameter μ can assume any finite number and σ can assume any finite positive number, the normal curve is a *family of distributions* as displayed in Figure 6–2 (Hays, 1981, p 205). Normal curves may have equal means but different standard deviations (Figure 6–2a), unequal means and unequal standard deviations (Figure 6–2b), or different means but equal standard deviations (Figure 6–2c). Each curve, however, is generated by the same mathematical function (Formula 6.1).

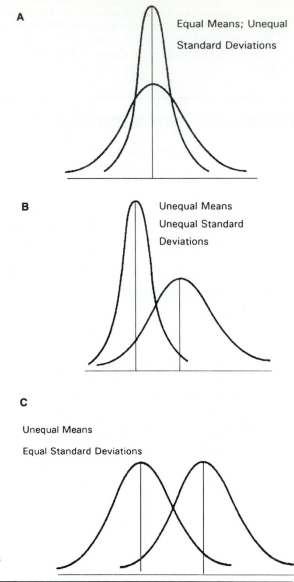

A

Equal Means; Unequal

Standard Deviations

B

Unequal Means

Unequal Standard

Deviations

C

Unequal Means

Equal Standard Deviations

Figure 6–2. The normal curve as a family of distributions
with different means and standard deviations.

Characteristics of the Normal Curve

The normal curve has the following characteristics:

1. The normal curve is a *theoretical probability distribution* representing an infinite number of observations measured continuously. Although it is a mathematical abstraction, the normal curve often provides a suitable description of the distribution that results from a large number of observations.

2. The normal curve is a *family of distributions,* with each distribution determined by two parameters, μ and σ. A change in the value of the mean (**μ**) shifts the center of the distribution along the x-axis. For example, the two normal curves in Figure 6–2c have different means but the same standard deviation. A change in the value of the standard deviation (**σ**) affects the degree to which observations spread out about the mean. Note that the standard deviation

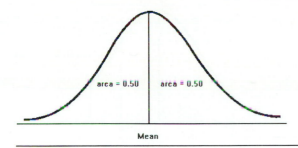

Figure 6–3. Normal curve showing that the total area of one square unit is divided equally to the right and left of the mean.

of the curve on the left in Figure 6–2b is smaller than the standard deviation of the distribution on the right. The left-hand distribution is more peaked than the one on the right; conversely, the right-handed distribution is flatter (more spread out) than the one on the left.

3. The normal curve is *symmetric* about its mean, μ, and *bell-shaped*. The left-hand portion of the distribution is the mirror image of the right-hand portion.

4. The normal curve is *asymptotic* to the x-axis. The curve descends rapidly to the x-axis, but never touches it.

5. The normal curve is *unimodal*. It has a single center located at the middle of the distribution. Because the curve is symmetric, bell-shaped, and unimodal, the mean, median, and mode are equal.

6. The total area under the curve above the x-axis equals one square unit. Recall that the normal curve is a probability distribution (Property 1). Thus, Property 6 derives from one of the important principles of probability—the sum of the probabilities (relative frequencies) of all possible events (all possible values of X) equals 1.0 (Principle 2, Chapter 5). Because the normal curve is symmetric, bell-shaped, and unimodal, 50% of the area under the curve resides to the left of a perpendicular erected at the mean and 50% resides to the right. This is illustrated in Figure 6–3.

7. If perpendiculars are erected at a distance of one standard deviation above and one standard deviation below the mean, approximately 68% of the total area is captured between these perpendiculars, the x-axis, and the curve. If perpendiculars are constructed at a distance of approximately two standard deviations above and below the mean, approximately 95% of the total area is enclosed. If perpendiculars are set at a distance of approximately three standard deviations to the left and right of the mean, approximately 99.7% of the total area is included. The approximate areas are shown in Figure 6–4.

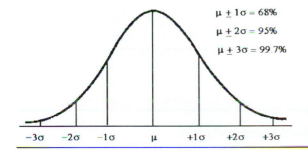

$\mu \pm 1\sigma = 68\%$

$\mu \pm 2\sigma = 95\%$

$\mu \pm 3\sigma = 99.7\%$

Figure 6–4. Approximate percentage of observations between the mean and specified points above and below the mean.

STANDARD NORMAL CURVE

We use the normal curve for many purposes; one purpose is to obtain the relative frequency (probability) of observations between any two points, *a* and *b*. The relative frequency of

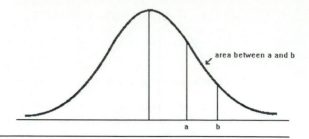

Figure 6–5. Area between two points, *a* and *b*.

observations between points *a* and *b* on the x-axis is given by the area bounded by the x-axis, the curve, and perpendiculars erected on the x-axis at the two points of interest. This is illustrated in Fig 6–5. The probability of an observation occurring between these two points is determined by integrating Formula 6.1 between *a* and *b,* where $(-\infty)$ is assigned the value *a* and (∞) is given the value *b:*

$$\int_b^a \frac{1}{\sqrt{2\pi}\,\sigma} e^{-(X-\mu)^2/2\sigma^2} \qquad\qquad 6.2$$

We focus on the area between two points to determine probabilities because the probability of any specific observation is zero. This is true because the area above any single point on the x-axis area is zero.

For a given set of X observations, it would be extraordinarily time consuming to apply Formula 6.2 to integrate the function for different values of *a* and *b* and for every curve defined by a different mean and standard deviation. Fortunately, tables provide the results of all such integrations. One particular member of the family of normal distributions interests us because the table of areas under the curve has been constructed for this specific curve. This curve is the **standard normal curve** (known also as the **unit normal curve**).

The standard normal curve has a mean of zero ($\mu = 0$) and standard deviation of one ($\sigma = 1$). To use tables of the standard normal curve, we must perform a simple linear transformation, called a *z*-**transformation,** for observations coming from distributions that have a mean and standard deviation other than 0 and 1, respectively. The *z*-transformation appears in Formula 6.3:

$$z = \frac{X - \mu}{\sigma}. \qquad\qquad 6.3$$

This transformation produces a **standard normal deviate,** which we compute by subtracting the mean of a set of observations from X, the specific observation of interest, and dividing the difference by the standard deviation. A standard normal deviate "expresses the deviations from the mean in standard deviation units" (Dawson-Saunders & Trapp, 1994, p 78). for example, a standard normal deviate of 1.0 ($z = 1.0$) indicates that an observation is one standard deviation above the mean. A value of -2.5 ($z = -2.5$) reveals that an observation is 2.5 standard deviations below the mean. Note that the sign attached to the value of z signals direction—above ($+$) or below ($-$) the mean.

Summary of Characteristics of the Standard Normal Curve

Central to many applications in diagnostic testing, descriptive statistics, and inferential statistics, the standard normal curve has the following characteristics:

1. The mean of any set of *z*-values (standard normal deviates) is zero. If $X = \mu$, the standard normal deviate equals zero:

$$z = \frac{\mu - \mu}{\sigma} = \frac{0}{\sigma} = 0.$$

2. The standard deviation of any set of z-values (standard normal deviates) is 1.0. The standard deviation is used as the unit of measurement in Formula 6.3 and, therefore, the standard deviation of a set of z-values is 1.0.

3. A distribution of z-values (standard normal deviates) possesses the same shape as the set of observations from which they are derived.

One common mistake in using standard normal deviates is to assume that their distribution is normal even if the shape of the distribution of original observations is not. Keep in mind that the z-transformation is a *linear* procedure, which does not change the relative (proportional) distance between and among original observations. Thus, if a distribution of original observations is skewed negatively, the distribution of standard normal deviates will also be skewed negatively.

Using the Standard Normal Curve—Hypertension Screening

Consider that blood pressure readings are obtained from nearly 200,000 participants in a large-scale community blood pressure screening program (similar to the one described by the Hypertension Detection and Follow-up Program Cooperative Group, 1977), and that these measurements follow a normal (Gaussian) distribution. The mean is 85 mm Hg, with a standard deviation of 13 mm Hg. Suppose also that in keeping with the recommendation of the 1988 Report of the Joint National Committee on Detection, Evaluation, and Treatment of High Blood Pressure, we screen for hypertension based on arterial diastolic blood pressure. We recommend that a physician be consulted if an individual has an arterial diastolic blood pressure equal to or greater than 90 mm Hg.

Clinical Example 1

What proportion of individuals in our screening program have a diastolic blood pressure $X \geq 90$ mm Hg? To answer the question, follow these steps:

1. Compute the standard normal deviate associated with a measurement of 90:

$$z = \frac{X - \mu}{\sigma} = \frac{90 - 85}{13} = 0.3846 = 0.38$$

The diastolic blood pressure of 90 mm Hg is approximately 0.38 standard deviations above the mean of 85.

2. Turn to Table A–1 in the appendix of statistical tables. Locate the z-value of 0.38. Read across to the column labeled "one-tailed area." This column contains the area beyond a z-value of 0.38. The area equals 0.3520. Figure 6–6 shows the area; the shaded portion in the upper tail of the standard normal curve corresponds to the area beyond a z-value of 0.38. Approximately 35% of the individuals in our sample have a diastolic blood pressure $\geq$ 90 mm Hg. If we randomly select a study participant, the probability is 0.35 that this individual has a diastolic pressure of 90 mm Hg or greater.

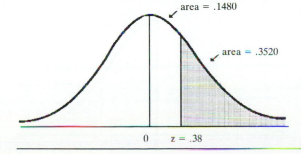

area = .1480

area = .3520

0   z = .38

Figure 6–6. Area beyond a z-value of 0.38 that corresponds to a diastolic-blood-pressure of 90 mm Hg or greater.

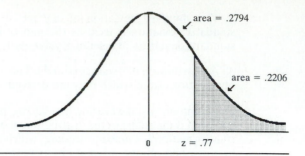

Figure 6–7. Area beyond a z-value of 0.77 that corresponds to a diastolic blood pressure of 95 mm Hg or greater.

3. To convert the area, which represents a proportion to a relative frequency, multiply the area by the total number in the sample (200,000). In the screening sample, 70,400 will be asked to consult a physician because their diastolic blood pressure is 90 mm Hg or greater (0.3520 × 200,000 = 70,400).

Clinical Example 2

What proportion of adults in our screening program have a diastolic blood pressure of 95 mm Hg or greater?

1. Compute the standard normal deviate for X = 95.

$$z = \frac{95 - 85}{13} = 0.7692 = 0.77$$

2. Consult Table A–1 and identify the area beyond a z-value of 0.77. The area from the one-tailed column is 0.2206. Approximately 22% of the participants in our program have diastolic blood pressures ≥ 95 mm Hg. Figure 6–7 depicts the area above a z-value of 0.77.

3. To translate this area to a relative frequency, multiply the area by the number participating in the program: 0.2206 × 200,000 = 44,120.

Thus, 44,120 individuals have a diastolic blood pressure ≥ 95 mm Hg, a value in the mildly hypertensive range (defined as 90 to 114 mm Hg).

Clinical Example 3

What proportion of our sample has a diastolic blood pressure of 100 mm Hg or above?

1. Obtain the standard normal deviate corresponding to a measurement of 100:

$$z = \frac{100 - 85}{13} = 1.1538 = 1.15.$$

2. Identify the one-tailed area from Table A–1. The area beyond a standard normal deviate of 1.15 is 0.1251, as shown in Figure 6–8.

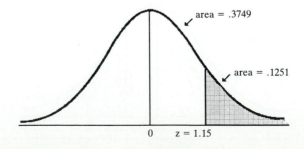

Figure 6–8. Area beyond z-value of 1.15 that corresponds to a diastolic blood pressure of 100 mm Hg or greater.

3. Translate the area into a relative frequency: $0.1251 \times 200{,}000 = 25{,}020$.

Thus, slightly more than 25,000 individuals in our sample have an arterial diastolic blood pressure ≥ 100 mg Hg.

Clinical Example 4

What proportion of individuals have diastolic blood pressures in the mildly hypertensive range of 90 to 104 mm Hg?

1. Compute the z-value corresponding to a value of 90 (note: we computed it already in the first example).

$$z = \frac{90 - 85}{13} = 0.3846 = 0.38$$

2. Obtain the z-value for X = 104 mm Hg.

$$z = \frac{104 - 85}{13} = 1.4615 = 1.46$$

3. Determine the area between a z-value of 0.38 and a z-value of 1.46. The area is 0.2799.

There are several ways to obtain this area. First, we determine that the area between a z-value of zero and a z-value of 0.38 is 0.1480 (column labeled "Area Between Mean and z"). Next, we identify the one-tailed area beyond the $z = 1.46$; this area is 0.0721. Third, we add these two areas: $0.1480 + 0.0721 = 0.2201$. This is the area *not captured* between the z-values of 0.38 and 1.46. Finally, we subtract 0.2201 from 0.50 to determine the area between the z-values of interest: $0.50 - 0.2201 = 0.2799$. Figure 6–9 illustrates the areas involved in these computations.

An alternative approach proceeds as follows. We specify the area corresponding to a z-value of 0.38 and above (the area corresponding to X $\geq$ 90 mm Hg); this area is 0.3520. Second, we obtain the area associated with a z-value of 1.46 (the area corresponding to X $\geq$ 104); this area is 0.0721. Third, because we are interested in the area *between* two z-values, we subtract 0.0721 from 0.3520: $0.3520 - 0.0721 = 0.2799$. These areas can be seen in Figure 6–9. Note that all these areas add to 0.50—the total area to the right of the mean.

4. Approximately 28% of the individuals in our screening program have an arterial diastolic blood pressure between 90 and 104 mm Hg. Thus, 55,980 individuals have a diastolic measurement in this range.

Clinical Example 5

What proportion of the sample has an arterial diastolic blood pressure between 105 and 114 mm Hg (the moderately hypertensive category)?

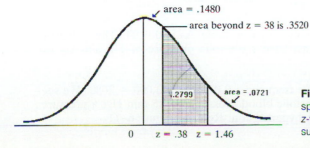

Figure 6–9. Area between a z-value of 0.38 that corresponds to a diastolic blood pressure of 90 mm Hg and a z-value of 1.46 that corresponds to a diastolic blood pressure of 104 mm Hg.

1. Determine the z-value for X = 105.

$$z = \frac{105 - 85}{13} = 1.5385 = 1.54$$

2. Identify the one-tailed area for z = 1.54: 0.0618.

3. Calculate the z-value corresponding to a measurement of 114.

$$z = \frac{114 - 85}{13} = 2.2308 = 2.23$$

4. Look-up the area associated with a z-value of 2.23 or greater: 0.0129.

5. Subtract 0.0129 from 0.0618 to obtain the area between the two z-values of interest: 0.0618 − 0.0129 = 0.0489.

Alternatively, obtain the area between the mean and z = 1.54 (for X = 105); use the column labeled "area between mean and z" to locate this area: 0.4382. Subtract 0.4382 and 0.0129 (one-tailed area for z = 2.23) from 0.50: 0.50 − 0.4382 − 0.0129 = 0.0489. The areas just discussed are illustrated in Figure 6–10.

6. Convert the area into a relative frequency: 0.0489 × 200,000 = 9780.

In our sample, approximately 9800 individuals have arterial diastolic blood pressures between 105 and 114 mm Hg (the moderately hypertensive range).

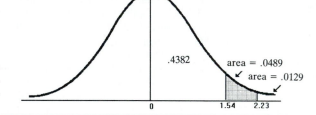

Figure 6–10. Area between a z-value of 1.54 that corresponds to a diastolic blood pressure of 105 mm Hg and z-value of 2.23 that corresponds to a diastolic blood pressure of 114 mm Hg.

Clinical Example 6

If we use a cutoff of 115 mm Hg to define severe hypertension, what proportion of our sample will be categorized as severely hypertensive, based on one measurement?

1. Calculate the standard normal deviate that corresponds to a measurement of 115:

$$z = \frac{115 - 85}{13} = 2.3077 = 2.31$$

2. Locate the appropriate one-tailed area in Table A–1: 0.0104. Thus, slightly more than 1% of our participants have a diastolic pressure of 115 mm Hg or greater.

3. Translate the area to a relative frequency: 0.0104 × 200,000 = 2080. We see that 2080 participants have a diastolic blood pressure ≥ 115 mm Hg, a pressure considered in the range of severe hypertension. Refer to Figure 6–11.

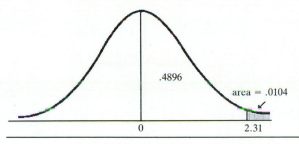

.4896

area = .0104

0   2.31

Figure 6–11. Area beyond z-value of 2.31 that corre-sponds to a diastolic blood pressure of 115 mm Hg or greater.

Clinical Example 7

Within what central limits do 95% of the diastolic blood pressure measurements occur? In this example, we work from the area to determine the value of z, then compute the diastolic pressures that bound the 95% limits.

1. Because the normal curve is symmetric, the area representing the 95% central limits is divided equally about the mean, 47.5% occurs between the z-value to be determined and the mean on the left- and right-hand side of the curve. Observe that 2.5% of the total area occurs in each tail.

2. Refer to the body of Table A–1, using either column two or three. If you use column two, look for an area of 0.475. You can also consult column three and find the z-value associated with the area of 0.025; this z-value is 1.96. Because the curve is symmetric, $z = \pm 1.96$.

3. Use the formula for a standard normal deviate (Formula 6.3), substitute the known z-value and solve for the 95% central limits. Express the answer in mm Hg.

$$z = \frac{X - \mu}{\sigma}$$

$$\pm 1.96 = \frac{X - \mu}{\sigma}$$

$$X = \mu \pm 1.96\sigma$$

4. Calculate the upper limit:

$$X_{Upper} = \mu + 1.96\sigma$$

$$= 85 + (1.96)(13)$$

$$= 110.48 = 111 \; mm \; Hg$$

5. Calculate the lower limit:

$$X_{Lower} = \mu - 1.96\sigma$$

$$= 85 - (1.96)(13)$$

$$= 59.52 = 60 \; mm \; Hg$$

Thus, 95% of participants in the community screening program have blood pres-sure values between 60 and 111 mm Hg. Figures 6–12 and 6–13 illustrate the results of our calculations.

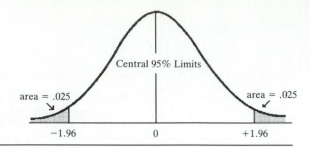

Figure 6–12. Central 95% limits on the standard normal curve, z-values correspond to ± 1.96.

The above examples illustrate three important concepts:

1. Examples 1 to 7 demonstrate how we can use the normal curve to answer a variety of questions about quantitative data that approximate a normal distribution. Many variables in medicine, when obtained from large groups of individuals, are described adequately by the normal curve.

2. Many quantitative diagnostic tests are developed so that the range of normal captures the central 95% of a nondiseased population (calculation principles illustrated in Example 7).

3. The percentage of a population regarded as being diseased or having abnormal test results varies substantially with the cutoff value, also referred to as a referent or critical value (Ingelfinger et al, 1987, p 94). If we use a cutoff value of 90 mm Hg in our hypertension screening program, 38% of the screenees will have a diastolic blood pressure that may require additional screening or treatment for hypertension (Example 1). If we use a cutoff value of 115 mm Hg, however, only 1.05% of our screening sample will have an arterial diastolic blood pressure that requires follow up or therapy.

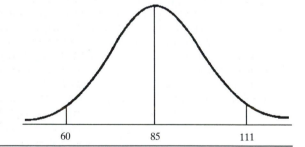

Figure 6–13. Distribution of diastolic blood pressure with a mean of 85 mm Hg and 95% of the measurements occurring between values of 60 mm Hg and 111 mm Hg.

SUMMARY

We would regard the 47-year-old Caucasian male in the opening clinical example as severely hypertensive, if his average diastolic blood pressure is found to be 115 mm Hg or greater. According to guidelines developed in the 1988 Report of the Joint National Committee on Detection, Evaluation, and Treatment of High Blood Pressure, this patient's family history, smoking history, and blood pressure require that he consult a physician. An important model in clinical biostatistics, the normal curve enjoys varied uses, ranging from developing limits of normal for many quantitative diagnostic tests to drawing inferences about treatment effectiveness from a segment of an appropriate target population.

The normal curve is a theoretical probability distribution representing an infinite number of observations measured continuously. The normal curve is a family of distributions, with each distribution determined by its mean and standard deviation. The normal curve is a bell-shaped, symmetric, unimodal, and asymptotic. The total area under the curve is one square unit.

Perhaps the most widely used member of the family of normal curves, the standard normal curve allows us to relate the position of an observation with respect to its mean. We describe the position by calculating a z-value, which expresses deviations from the mean in standard deviation units. For example, $z = 1.0$ indicates that the observation is one standard deviation above the mean. These z-values allow us to use the table of the standard normal curve to determine the area between two observations; this area represents relative frequency, that is, probability. For example, 68% of the area in a normal curve occurs between $z = -1.0$ and $z = +1.0$. Thus, in a normal distribution, we expect 68% of the observations to fall between these two points. Similarly, we expect approximately 95% of observations to occur between $\mu \pm 2\sigma$ and approximately 99.7% of values to fall between $\mu \pm 3\sigma$. Therefore, if we randomly select an individual from a normally distributed distribution, the probability is 0.68 that his or her observation is within one standard deviation above and below the mean.

By using the standard normal curve, we can understand quickly the effect of changing the cutoff value that differentiates normal from abnormally high or low quantitative test results. The 95% central limits are used by many clinical laboratories to distinguish between values "within the normal range" from those that are outside this range. Thus, even in a population that is healthy, we expect 5% of its members to have test results that are identified as being outside the range of normal (assuming, of course, that the distribution of test results is bell shaped).

REFERENCES

Colton T: *Statistics in Medicine*. Little, Brown, 1974.

Daniel W: (1991). *Biostatistics: A Foundation for Analysis in the Health Sciences*, 5th ed. Wiley, 1991.

Dawson-Saunders B, Trapp R: *Basic and Clinical Biostatistics*, 2nd ed. Appleton & Lange, 1993.

Hays W: *Statistics*, 3rd ed. Holt, Rinehart & Winston, 1981.

Hypertension Detection and Follow-up Program Cooperative Group: The hypertension detection and follow-up program: A progress report. *Circ Res* 1977;**40**(suppl 1):106.

Ingelfinger J, Mosteller F, Thibodeau L, Ware J: *Biostatistics in Clinical Medicine*, 2nd ed. Macmillan, 1987.

Massie B, Sokolow M: Systemic hypertension. In: *Current Medical Diagnosis & Treatment*. Tierney L Jr, et al (editors). Appleton & Lange, 1993.

Minium E, King B, Bear G: *Statistical Reasoning in Psychology and Education*, 3rd ed. Wiley, 1993.

1988 Report of the Joint National Committee on the Detection, Evaluation, and Treatment of High Blood Pressure. *Arch Intern Med* 1988;**148**:1023.

Rodriguez A: *Medi-Data: Normal Reference Library and Function Test Values*, 2nd ed. Rodram Corporacion, 1991.

Wallach J: Interpretation of Diagnostic Tests: A Synopsis of Laboratory Medicine, 5th ed. Little, Brown, 1992.

Self-study Questions

Part I: Thought Problems

1. List the characteristics of the normal curve.
2. Identify the characteristics of the standard normal curve.
3. Discuss the implications of changing the cutoff value for quantitative diagnostic tests.

Part II: Thought Problems About Cholesterol Screening

Clinicians examined total cholesterol levels of 2000 school children, grades 1 to 8, in a large metropolitan area. Cholesterol was measured quantitatively. The range was found to be 140 to 300 mg/dL, with approxiamtely 10% of the values between 140 and 160 mg/dL, 60% between 220 and 260 mg/dL, and 15% above 261 mg/dL.

1. Comment on the appropriateness of using the mean to characterize the central tendency of these observations.
2. Comment on the appropriateness of calculating standard normal deviates and referencing them to tables of the normal curve, in order to determine the proportion of observations that occur between cholesterol measurements.

Part III: Computations for Blood Pressure Screening

For each of the following problems, use the systolic blood pressure data from the community screening program described in this chapter. Assume normally distributed observations, $\mu = 85$, and $\sigma = 13$.

1. What proportion of participants have a diastolic blood pressure of 70 mm Hg or greater?
2. What proportion of individuals have a diastolic blood pressure of 70 mm Hg or less?
3. Within what central limits do 99% of the diastolic measurements occur?

Part IV: Computations for Total Cholesterol

Total cholesterol is measured in a large number of adults and found to be distributed normally, with a mean of 150 mg/dL and standard deviation of 15 mg/dL.

1. What proportion of adults has a total cholesterol measurement of 160 mg/dL or greater?
2. What proportion of participants has a total cholesterol value of 135 mg/dL or greater?
3. What proportion of individuals has a total cholesterol reading between 160 and 175 mg/dL?
4. Within what central limits do 95% of the total cholesterol measurements occur?
5. Within what central limits do 99% of the total cholesterol readings occur?

Solutions

Part II: Cholesterol Screening

The total cholesterol levels of these children are negatively skewed, with a greater percentage of observations in the upper tail of the distribution. Therefore, the median rather than the mean is the preferred measure of central tendency (question 1). Because the distribution is skewed, it is inappropriate to compute standard normal deviates and reference them to tables of the normal curve. In tables of the normal curve, areas are translated into proportions or percentages with the assumption that observations are distributed normally.

Part III: Diastolic Blood Pressure

1. $z = \dfrac{70 - 85}{13} = -1.15$. The area between -1.15 and the mean of zero is 0.3749. This area is added to 0.50, the total area to the right of the mean. Thus, the total area is 0.8749. The proportion of individuals with a diastolic blood pressure ≥ 70 mm Hg is 0.8749.
2. The one-tailed area to the left of the z-value of -1.15 equals 0.1251. Therefore, the proportion of individuals with a diastolic blood pressure ≤ 70 mm Hg is 0.1251. We could

have obtained this value by subtracting 0.3759, the area between the z-value of -1.15 and the mean of zero, from 0.50, the total area to the left of the mean.

3. The two-tailed area is 0.01. Consult Table A–1 to identify the z-value that corresponds to this two-tailed area: $z = \pm 2.57$, approximately. Use this value to solve for the upper and lower limits within which 99% of the measurements occur.

$$z = \frac{X - \mu}{\sigma}$$

$$X = \mu \pm z\sigma$$

$$X_{Lower} = 85 - 2.57(13) = 51.59 = 52$$

$$X_{Upper} = 85 + 2.57(13) = 118.41 = 119$$

Part IV: Total Cholesterol

1. $z = \dfrac{160 - 150}{15} = 0.6667 = 0.67$. The one-tailed area to the right of 0.67 is 0.2514. Therefore, the proportion of individuals who have a total cholesterol reading $\geq$ 160 mg/dL is 0.2514.

2. $z = \dfrac{135 - 150}{15} = -1.00$. The area between a z-value of -1.00 and the mean of zero is 0.3413. The area to the right of the mean is 0.50. Therefore, the proportion of participants who have a total cholesterol $\geq$ 135 mg/dL is 0.8413 ($0.3413 + 0.50 = 0.8413$).

3. Calculate the two z-values first:

$$z = \frac{160 - 150}{15} = 0.6667 = 0.67$$

$$z = \frac{175 - 150}{15} = 1.6667 = 1.67$$

The one-tailed area beyond a z-value of 0.67 is 0.2514. The area beyond a z-value of 1.67 is 0.0475. Subtract 0.0475 from 0.2514 to obtain the area between the two z-values: $0.2514 - 0.0475 = 0.2039$. You can also identify the area between the mean of zero and the z-value of 0.67 (0.2486), add it to the area to the right of a z-value of 1.67 (0.0475), and subtract the sum from 0.50 ($0.50 - 0.2486 + 0.0475 = 0.2039$). The proportion of readings between 160 and 175 mg/dL is 0.2039.

4. The central 95% limits are computed as: $X = 150 \pm 1.96(15) = 120.60, 179.40$. The two-tailed area of 0.05 is used to locate $z;$ the z-value is ± 1.96. If the total cholesterol values are rounded off, 95% of the measurements are captured between 121 and 180 mg/dL.

5. Calculation of the central 99% limits proceeds identically. The two-tailed area is 0.01. Consult Table A–1 to identify the corresponding z-value: $z = \pm 2.57$, approximately. Compute the 99% central limits, as follows: $X = 150 \pm 2.57(15) = 111.45, 188.55$. Approximately 99% of adults in our sample have measurements between approximately 112 and 189 mg/dL.

7   Interpreting Clinical Laboratory Tests

Clinical Example: Screening for Hepatocellular Carcinoma

> Sera from 2225 men are screened for alpha$_1$-fetoprotein (AFP). One hundred seven men have primary hepatocellular carcinoma; 2118 have other diseases. Raised serum AFP levels ($\geq$ 200 ng/mL) are detected in 129 patients. Among the 107 patients with hepatocellular carcinoma, 90 men have increased serum AFP levels (Kohn & Weaver, 1974). Is serum AFP a *sensitive* and *specific* serologic marker of hepatocellular carcinoma?

Answering the question about the value of AFP as a serologic marker of hepatocellular carcinoma requires that we move beyond the simple query of "Is this test result normal?" (Galen & Gambino, 1975, p 2). The value of a test or procedure depends on several factors, including the quantitative characteristics of the test and the degree to which test results reduce uncertainty about diagnostic hypotheses and questions. The purpose of this chapter is to introduce fundamental concepts central to interpreting clinical laboratory tests. Because test interpretation is complex, it is impossible to address all relevant issues in this chapter. Readers who would like a more in-depth treatment of this topic may want to consult books by Galen and Gambino (1975) and Kraemer (1992).

OBJECTIVES

When you complete this chapter, you should be able to:

- Discuss the fundamental rules of probability that describe performance characteristics of clinical laboratory tests.
- Discuss the clinical and statistical factors that determine the choice of laboratory tests.
- Define and discuss the performance characteristics of clinical laboratory tests.
- Differentiate between sensitivity and specificity and predictive values.
- Identify the factors that influence predictive values.

IDENTIFYING THE PURPOSES OF CLINICAL LABORATORY TESTS

The generic term "clinical laboratory tests" refers to blood chemistries and procedures such as x-rays and CT scans. Tests are ordered for two basic purposes: screening and patient management.

Screening

The goal of screening is "to detect diseases whose morbidity and mortality can be reduced by early detection and treatment" (Griner et al, 1981, p 559). Additionally, treatment must exist to change the natural course of the disease (Griner et al, 1981, p 559). If not treated, the disease typically leads to significant morbidity or mortality. Tests used to screen patients should be abnormal in almost all patients with disease. Conversely, when the test result is normal, the clinician should be confident that the patient is disease free.

Patient Management

Patient management is the second major purpose for which tests are ordered. Tests may be repeated frequently for several reasons:

1. The clinician may want to monitor a disease by asking questions such as these: Has the disease progressed? Is the patient stable? Is the disease in remission?

2. The clinician may wish to identify and reverse complications of treatment (eg, treatment-induced anemia or drug toxicity).

3. The clinician may want to ensure a therapeutic level of one or more drugs.

4. The clinician may repeat one or more tests because the results will help to describe prognosis.

5. If an unexpected result occurs, the clinician may repeat a test to verify the result. "The reproducibility of the test is the most important characteristic" when it is used to manage patients (Griner et al, 1981, p 559).

Various factors help to determine the optimal frequency for monitoring patients with repeat tests, including an in-depth awareness of physiology; knowledge of the natural course of the disease; awareness of the range of tests used to monitor the disease's history; and understanding of nonmedical factors that may affect a result, such as the time of day a test is performed and whether the patient fasted before the test (Griner et al, 1981, p 559). We now consider the general performance characteristics of tests used to screen and diagnose disease.

DEFINING TEST PERFORMANCE CHARACTERISTICS

The following symbols are used throughout the rest of this chapter to designate disease status and test result.

Symbols
D+   Patient has the disease
D−   Patient is disease-free
T+   Test result is positive
T−   Test result is negative

TEST PERFORMANCE CHARACTERISTICS

The performance characteristics of a test include its sensitivity, specificity, false positives, false negatives, and predictive values. Performance characteristics are sometimes called test operating characteristics.

SENSITIVITY (Positivity in Disease)

Sensitivity is the conditional probability that a diseased patient has a positive test result, that is, $pr(T+|D+)$. When a diseased patient (D+) tests positive (T+), a *true positive* outcome has occurred.

SPECIFICITY (Negativity in Health)

Specificity is the conditional probability that a disease-free patient has a negative test result, that is, $pr(T-|D-)$. When a disease-free patient (D−) has a negative test result (T−), a *true negative* outcome has occurred.

FALSE NEGATIVE

A false negative is the conditional probability that a diseased patient has a negative test result, that is, $pr(T-|D+)$. A false negative is the complement of sensitivity:

$$\text{False Negative} = (1 - \text{Sensitivity}) \text{ and}$$

$$pr(T+|D+) + pr(T-|D+) = 1.0$$

FALSE POSITIVE

A false positive is the conditional probability that a disease-free patient has a positive test result, that is, $pr(T+|D-)$. A false positive is the complement of specificity:

$$\text{False Positive} = (1 - \text{Specificity}) \text{ and}$$

$$pr(T-|D-) + pr(T+|D-) = 1.0$$

FALSE POSITIVES AND FALSE NEGATIVES REFERRED TO AS RATES

Some clinicians, epidemiologists, and statisticians refer to the proportion of false positive and negative results as a "rate." This term should be avoided because it does not satisfy the definition of a true rate: the denominator of a true rate contains units of exposure (eg, person-years), as discussed in Chapter 4. The relative frequency of false-negative outcomes, when calculated correctly, is a *proportion*.

POSITIVE PREDICTIVE VALUE (PPV or PV+)

The positive predictive value is the conditional probability that a patient with a positive test result is a true positive: $pr(D+|T+)$.

NEGATIVE PREDICTIVE VALUE (NPV or PV−)

The negative predictive value is the conditional probability that a patient with a negative test result is a true negative: $pr(D-|T-)$.

CUTOFF POINT

A **cutoff point** for test results measured on a numerical continuum is an arbitrarily selected value that separates positive (abnormal) from negative (normal) results (Griner et al, 1981, p 557). A cutoff point is referred to by some clinicians as a *reference* or *referent value, cut point,* or *positivity criterion*. For example, if we follow the 1988 recommendation of the Joint National Committee on the Detection, Evaluation, and Treatment of High Blood Pressure to identify severe hypertension, we define the cutoff point for diastolic blood pressure as 115 mm Hg or greater.

DIFFERENTIATING POSITIVE FROM NEGATIVE RESULTS—OR DEFINING NORMALITY

Laboratory tests are either qualitative or quantitative. **Qualitative tests** categorize patients as diseased or disease free, according to the presence or absence of the clinical sign or symptom. For example, a patient may have a chest x-ray to confirm or rule out pneumonia; or a softball player may have an x-ray to determine if she fractured her leg when she slid into second base. The results help to prove or disprove a clinical condition.

Quantitative tests yield results on a *numerical continuum* and classify patients as having a positive or negative result, based on an arbitrarily selected cutoff point. Often, distributions of results from quantitative tests approximate a Gaussian distribution. Statistical properties of the distribution are used to define cutoff points and to differentiate positive from negative results (Fletcher et al, 1988, p 33). This involves defining a *range of values* within which results are considered negative (normal), and outside of which results are considered positive (abnormal). The limits of normal for most quantitative tests are set arbitrarily, based on the Gaussian model, as the range captured by the mean *plus and minus two standard deviations* (Griner et al, 1981, p 568). These limits are determined from measurements taken from a large number of individuals, known as a **reference population.**

In developing many tests, we assume that the reference population is disease free. In many situations, however, the reference population is drawn from the general population, which includes diseased individuals. When the general population is sampled, we assume that the sample is large enough to minimize the impact of diseased individuals (Griner et al, 1981, p 568). Even if all members of the reference population are disease free, however, approximately 5% will have test results at the extreme upper and lower end of the distribution of results, if the Gaussian model applies. Thus, even though they are disease free, some individuals may be identified as having positive (abnormal) results. The effect of varying the cutoff point on the proportion of individuals identified as diseased or disease free, and the subsequent impact on sensitivity and specificity, is discussed in "Sensitivity Versus Specificity" later in the chapter.

Note that we speak of the sampled individuals as a population, even though, according to the definition presented in Chapter 1, this collection of individuals is called a sample. In referring to this collection as a population, we assume that the sample is representative of the target population of interest and is large enough to be treated, for all practical purposes, as a population.

The way we define the reference population determines how we evaluate and interpret test results. We define the reference population in terms of inclusion criteria, exclusion criteria, and clinical characteristics. Conclusions drawn from the reference population should not be generalized beyond that population (Kraemer, 1992, p 32). For example, suppose a test is developed to detect nodular involvement in men suspected of having prostrate cancer. The conclusions drawn about the value of the test as a marker of nodular involvement apply only to men suspected of having prostate cancer, and not to men in the general population.

DEFINING THE PERFORMANCE CHARACTERISTICS OF A TEST

We can easily calculate the performance characteristics of a test if results are arrayed in a 2×2 table. In Table 7–1, the cells represent one of four possible outcomes: true positive, false positive, true negative, or false negative. Each cell is lettered a, b, c, or d. The margins represent cell totals. For example, the marginal total a + b represents the sum of the number of results in cell a plus the frequency in cell b. The *rows* of the 2×2 table depict test results, classified either as positive (T+) or negative (T−). The *columns* indicate disease state, identified either as present (D+) or absent (D−). Assessment of disase state is based on a **gold standard,** which is the best available test or procedure to diagnose the disease of interest. The gold standard may be a simple, relatively inexpensive test, such as a throat culture for group A β-hemolytic streptococcus (Fletcher et al, 1988, p 44). Often, however, the gold standard is a more expensive, more invasive test or procedure that poses some risk to the patient, such as tissue biopsies or radiologic contrast procedures (Fletcher et al, 1988, p 44).

Table 7–1. Two-by-two table for determining test performance characteristics.

	Disease State		
Test Result	Present (D+)	Absent (D−)	Total
Positive (T+)	*a* True Positive	*b* False Positive	*a* + *b*
Negative (T−)	*c* False Negative	*d* True Negative	*c* + *d*
TOTAL	*a* + *c*	*b* + *d*	*a* + *b* + *c* + *d* = N

As medicine and technology advance, a gold standard may be replaced by a new, improved test or procedure (Kraemer, 1992, p 7).

The cells and margins of the 2 × 2 table are defined in Table 7–2. For example, we see that cell a in a 2 × 2 table is the number of true positive outcomes. If the number of true positives is divided by the total number of patients tested, we obtain a relative frequency. This relative frequency is a probability that represents the intersection of two outcomes that are not mutually exclusive:

$$pr(T+ \text{ and } D+) = \frac{\text{Number of True Positives}}{\text{Total Number Tested}} = \frac{a}{a+b+c+d} = \frac{a}{N}.$$

Thus, the probability that an individual selected at random from the reference population will be diseased *and* test positive is $pr(T+ \text{ and } D+)$, which equals (a/N). Cells b, c, and d and the marginal totals are defined similarly.

Examine the (a + c) marginal total in Tables 7–1 and 7–2; this total corresponds to the number of individuals known to have disease, based on the gold standard. When we divide (a + c) by the total number of persons tested [(a + c)/N], we obtain the probability of disease $pr(D+)$. Note that this probability represents disease prevalence. Similarly, the probability that an individual is disease free is $pr(D−) = [(b + d)/N]$. These two probabilities are unconditional probabilities or *prior* or *pretest* probabilities, because they are obtained prior to (not based on) laboratory test results.

We use the four cells and the marginal totals to define test performance characteristics. Formula 5.7 is used to determine the formula for each test characteristic. Formula 5.7 applies

Table 7–2. Definition of the cells and margins of the 2 × 2 table.

Cell	Definition	Represented as a Proportion of Those Tested	Proportion Represented Algebraically	Translated into a Probability Equivalent
a	Number of true-positive outcomes	$\dfrac{\text{Number of True Positives}}{\text{Total Number of Patients Tested}}$	$\dfrac{a}{a+b+c+d} = \dfrac{a}{N}$	$pr\,(T+ \text{ and } D+)$
b	Number of false-positive outcomes	$\dfrac{\text{Number of False Positives}}{\text{Total Number of Patients Tested}}$	$\dfrac{b}{a+b+c+d} = \dfrac{b}{N}$	$pr(T+ \text{ and } D−)$
c	Number of false-negative outcomes	$\dfrac{\text{Number of False Negatives}}{\text{Total Number of Patients Tested}}$	$\dfrac{c}{a+b+c+d} = \dfrac{c}{N}$	$pr(T− \text{ and } D+)$
d	Number of true-negative outcomes	$\dfrac{\text{Number of True Negatives}}{\text{Total Number of Patients Tested}}$	$\dfrac{d}{a+b+c+d} = \dfrac{d}{N}$	$pr(T− \text{ and } D−)$
Margins				
a + b	Number of patients who tested positive	$\dfrac{\text{Number of Positive Tests}}{\text{Total Number of Patients Tested}}$	$\dfrac{a+b}{a+b+c+d} = \dfrac{a+b}{N}$	$pr(T+)$
c + d	Number of patients who tested negative	$\dfrac{\text{Number of Negative Tests}}{\text{Total Number of Patients Tested}}$	$\dfrac{c+d}{a+b+c+d} = \dfrac{c+d}{N}$	$pr(T−)$
a + c	Number of diseased patients	$\dfrac{\text{Number of Diseased Patients}}{\text{Total Number of Patients Tested}}$	$\dfrac{a+c}{a+b+c+d} = \dfrac{a+c}{N}$	$pr(D+)$
b + d	Number of disease-free patients	$\dfrac{\text{Number of Disease = free Patients}}{\text{Total Number of Patients Tested}}$	$\dfrac{b+d}{a+b+c+d} = \dfrac{b+d}{N}$	$pr(D−)$

Table 7–3. Definition of performance characteristics of clinical laboratory tests.

Characteristic	Definition	Conditional Probability	Translated into Probability Formula	Translated According to the Cells and Margins of the 2 × 2 table
Sensitivity	Probability that test will be positive, given the patient is diseased	$pr(T+ \mid D+)$	$\dfrac{pr(T+ \text{ and } D+)}{pr(D+)}$	$\dfrac{a/N}{(a+c)/N} = \dfrac{a}{a+c}$
Specificity	Probability that the test will be negative, given the patient is disease free	$pr(T- \mid D-)$	$\dfrac{pr(T- \text{ and } D-)}{pr(D-)}$	$\dfrac{d/N}{(b+d)/N} = \dfrac{d}{b+d}$
False negative = (1 − sensitivity)	Probability that a test will be negative, given the patient is diseased	$pr(T- \mid D+)$	$\dfrac{pr(T- \text{ and } D+)}{pr(D+)}$	$\dfrac{c/N}{(a+c)/N} = \dfrac{c}{a+c}$
False positive = (1 − specificity)	Probability that a test will be positive, given the patient is disease free	$pr(T+ \mid D-)$	$\dfrac{pr(T+ \text{ and } D-)}{pr(D-)}$	$\dfrac{b/N}{(b+d)/N} = \dfrac{b}{b+d}$
Positive predictive value	Probability that a patient is diseased, given a positive test	$pr(D+ \mid T+)$	$\dfrac{pr(T+ \text{ and } D+)}{pr(T+)}$	$\dfrac{a/N}{(a+b)/N} = \dfrac{a}{a+b}$
Negative predictive value	Probability that a patient is disease free, given a negative test	$pr(D- \mid T-)$	$\dfrac{pr(T- \text{ and } D-)}{pr(T-)}$	$\dfrac{d/N}{(c+d)/N} = \dfrac{d}{c+d}$

to conditional probability for events that are not independent (refer to Chapter 5). A summary of test performance characteristics appears in Table 7–3.

The **sensitivity** of a test is the conditional probability that a test will be positive if the patient is diseased. This *conditional* probability is

$$pr(T+|D+) = \frac{pr(T+ \text{ and } D+)}{pr(D+)} = \frac{a/N}{(a+c)/N} = \frac{a}{a+c}. \qquad 7.1$$

Sensitivity is computed from the number of true positive results (cell a), divided by the total number of diseased patients (marginal total a + c). Note that the total number of diseased patients (D+) includes those who are true positives and those who are false negatives.

Specificity is the conditional probability that a negative test result will occur if the patient is disease free:

$$pr(T-|D-) = \frac{pr(T- \text{ and } D-)}{pr(D-)} = \frac{d/N}{(b+d)/N} = \frac{d}{b+d}. \qquad 7.2$$

Specificity is the frequency of true negative results (cell d), divided by the total number of disease-free patients (marginal total, b + d). The number of disease-free patients (D−) includes those who are false positives and those who are true negatives.

The complement of sensitivity is the proportion of false negatives:

$$pr(T-|D+)= \frac{pr(T- \text{ and } D+)}{pr(D+)} = \frac{c/N}{(a+c)/N} = \frac{c}{a+c}. \qquad 7.3$$

This proportion is derived from the number of false-negative results, divided by the number of diseased patients. Keep in mind that false negatives equal (1 − sensitivity).

The complement of specificity is the proportion of false positives, which equals (1 − specificity) or

$$pr(T+|D-) = \frac{pr(T+ \text{ and } D-)}{pr(D-)} = \frac{b/N}{(b+d)/N} = \frac{b}{b+d}. \qquad 7.4$$

This proportion is determined from the number of false positives, divided by the number of disease-free patients.

The positive and negative predictive values of the test appear in the last two rows of Table 7–3. The **positive predictive value** addresses the question: Given a positive test result, what is the probability that the patient is diseased? The positive predictive value is

$$pr(D+|T+) = \frac{pr(T+ \text{ and } D+)}{pr(T+)} = \frac{a}{a + b}. \qquad 7.5$$

This probability is also called a *posterior* or *posttest* probability.

The **negative predictive value** answers the question: Given a negative test result, what is the probability that a patient is disease free? Like the positive predictive value, the negative predictive value is conditioned on knowledge of the test result. The negative predictive value is

$$pr(D-|T-) = \frac{pr(T- \text{ and } D-)}{pr(T-)} = \frac{d}{c + d}. \qquad 7.6$$

Sensitivity, Specificity, and Predictive Values: A Source of Confusion

The difference between the positive predictive value and sensitivity, and the difference between the negative predictive value and specificity, confuse many people. Examine the conditional probability for each of these four characteristics. Note that the numerator of sensitivity and the positive predictive value are identical. The numerator of specificity and negative predictive value are the same. Observe, however, that *sensitivity and specificity are conditioned on knowledge of the disease state* of the patient. In contrast, *predictive values are conditioned on knowledge of the test result*. This difference is reflected in the denominator of the performance characteristic. For example, the denominator of sensitivity contains the probability of disease; the denominator of the positive predictive value contains the probability of a positive test result. Thus, predictive values answer different questions than sensitivity and specificity.

CALCULATING PERFORMANCE CHARACTERISTICS

Screening for Hepatocellular Carcinoma

We use the clinical example at the beginning of the chapter to illustrate how to calculate the performance characteristics of alpha$_1$-fetoprotein (AFP) as a serologic marker of hepatocellular carcinoma (Kohn & Weaver, 1974, p 334). According to Kohn and Weaver (1974, p 334), "AFP detection and assay correctly performed and interpreted is a valuable, sensitive, and specific serological marker of hepatocellular carcinoma." A serum AFP level ≥ 200 ng/mL is the cutoff point that separates positive from negative results. Is the serum AFP a sensitive and specific serologic marker of hepatocellular carcinoma? To answer this question, we create a 2 × 2 table based on the data presented in the clinical example. Table 7–4 contains these data. We use subtraction and addition to fill in the cells and margins of the table:

1. Note that 2225 men are screened. The marginal totals must add to 2225.

2. Among these 2225 men, 129 have serum AFP levels ≥ 200 ng/mL. Therefore, 129 men have positive results (T+); this number corresponds to the (a + b) marginal total.

Table 7–4. Alpha$_1$-fetoprotein and hepatocellular carcinoma.

Test Result	Hepatocellular Carcinoma		Total
	Present (D+)	Absent (D−)	
Positive (T+)	a 90	b 39	a + b 129
Negative (T−)	c 17	d 2079	c + d 2096
TOTAL	a + c 107	b + d 2118	2225

3. To obtain the number of negative results (T−), subtract 129 from 2225: (2225 − 129 = 2096). This number is the (c + d) marginal total.

4. Observe that 107 men are known to have disease (D+). Enter 107 as the (a + c) marginal total.

5. Determine the number of disease-free men (D−) by subtracting the number who are diseased from the total number tested: (2225 − 107 = 2118). Use this number (2118) as the (b + d) marginal total.

6. Among the 107 men known to have cancer, 90 have raised serum AFP levels. Ninety, which corresponds to the intersection of T+ and D+, is the number of diseased men who have a positive test result. Enter 90 in cell a.

7. Subtract 90 (cell a) from 129 (the number of positive test results; marginal total a + b) to obtain cell b. Cell b is the number of disease-free men who have a positive result (cell b = 129 − 90 = 39).

8. Subtract the cell a value (90) from the number of men who have disease (marginal total a + c) to compute the cell c value: (107 − 90 = 17).

9. Use either the value in cell b or c to determine the value of cell d (the number of men who are disease-free and test negative). If you use the cell b value, subtract 39 from the b + d marginal total: 2118 − 39 = 2079. If you use the count in cell c, subtract the frequency in cell c (17) from the c + d marginal (2096): 2096 − 17 = 2079.

10. Finally, verify that the cell values add to the appropriate marginal totals and the marginal totals add to the total number of men tested.

Now use the data in the 2 × 2 table to calculate the performance characteristics of AFP. Calculations appear in Box 7–1. The sensitivity of serum-AFP levels is 0.8411. If a patient has hepatocellular cancer, the probability is approximately 0.84 that he will have a raised serum AFP level. If we translate this conditional probability to a relative frequency by multiplying by 100%, we observe that approximately 84% of men with disease test positive. The specificity is 0.9816. Given that a patient is free of liver cancer, the probability that he will have a

Box 7–1. Performance characteristics of serum AFP levels as a serologic marker of hepatocellular carcinoma.

Test Characteristic	Basic Definition	Definition Using Lettered Cells of the 2 × 2 Table	Computation
Sensitivity	$pr(T+\mid D+)$	a / (a + c)	90 / 107 = 0.8411
Specificity	$pr(T-\mid D-)$	d / (b + d)	2079 / 2118 = 0.9816
False negative	$pr(T-\mid D+)$	c / (a + c)	17 / 107 = 0.1589
False positive	$pr(T+\mid D-)$	b / (b + d)	39 / 2118 = 0.0184
Positive predictive value	$pr(D+\mid T+)$	a / (a + b)	90 / 129 = 0.6977
Negative predictive value	$pr(D-\mid T-)$	d / (c + d)	2079 / 2096 = 0.9919

normal serum AFP level is approximately 0.98. Thus, among men who are free of liver cancer, approximately 98% will have serum AFP levels below the cutoff point of 200 ng/mL. Relative to the percentage of false-negative outcomes, 15.89% of the diseased men will be incorrectly identified as disease free. In terms of the relative frequency of false positives, among patients who are free of liver cancer, 1.8% will test positive. The positive predictive value indicates that among patients who test positive (have raised serum AFP levels), approximately 70% have hepatocellular carcinoma. Based on the negative predictive value among men who test negative, approximately 99% are free of hepatocellular carcinoma.

USES OF SENSITIVE AND SPECIFIC TESTS

In determining whether to select a test with maximum sensitivity or specificity, the clinician is guided by two considerations: (1) the reason for ordering the test (eg, to rule out a disease) and (2) the characteristics of the suspected disease.

Uses of Sensitive Tests

A sensitive test is usually positive in the presence of disease. A sensitive test should be selected when "there is an important penalty for missing a disease" (Fletcher et al, 1988, p 47). A sensitive test should be used when the clinician has evidence, based perhaps on patient history or physical examination, that a serious but treatable condition exists (eg, a sexually transmitted disease, tuberculosis, Hodgkin's lymphoma, dissecting thoracic aneurysm, malignant melanoma).

In addition, highly sensitive tests are useful to screen for disease. For example, numerous screening programs exist to detect hypertension, a serious disease with greater morbidity and mortality if untreated (Littenberg et al, 1990, p 192). Diagnosis and early treatment for hypertension significantly reduce morbidity and mortality from stroke and vascular diseases (Hypertension and Detection and Follow-up Program, 1977; Littenberg et al, 1990).

Highly sensitive tests are helpful in screening for relatively rare diseases, such as phenyl ketonuria (PKU), which is estimated to occur in 1 in 10,000 individuals (Behrman & Kliegman, 1990, p 138). PKU is a serious disease that causes mental retardation if not diagnosed and treated in newborns. A highly sensitive, simple, inexpensive blood test is used to diagnose PKU (Behrman & Kliegman, 1990, p 138; Hennekens & Buring, 1987, p 330). If treatment is begun shortly after birth in a PKU-diagnosed infant, mental retardation can be prevented. Although PKU is rare, many states require that each newborn be tested for the disease.

Highly sensitive tests are also useful during the early phases of a diagnostic workup, when the objective is to reduce the number of diagnostic possibilities. The goal, then, is to *rule out* disease by establishing that certain diseases are unlikely. For example, Fletcher and associates (1988, p 48) point out that a clinician might select a tuberculin skin test "early in the evaluation of lung infiltrates because this test is usually positive in people with active tuberculosis." Because a highly sensitive test has few false negatives, a clinician can confidently exclude a disease when a negative test result occurs (Griner et al, 1981, p 561). Therefore, *a highly sensitive test is most helpful when the result is negative* (Fletcher et al, 1988, p 48).

Uses of Specific Tests

A specific test is usually negative in a disease-free patient. A highly specific test is rarely positive in the absence of disease. As a result, the number of false-positive results is small (Fletcher et al, 1988, p 48). A test with high specificity is selected when other data, such as physical findings, suggest the presence of a serious disease that cannot be treated effectively or cured (eg, multiple sclerosis, Alzheimer's disease, or amyotrophic lateral sclerosis). A test with high specificity is also selected when knowledge that a disease is *absent* has significant psychologic or public health value (Galen & Gambino, 1975, p 50). In selecting a test with high specificity, the clinician seeks to confirm or *rule in* disease (Griner et al, 1981, p 561). Consequently, *a specific test is most helpful when the result is positive.*

SENSITIVITY VERSUS SPECIFICITY

In the ideal clinical world, the physician orders tests that are both highly sensitive and specific. Few tests, however, are highly sensitive and specific. Trade-offs between these two characteristics usually occur. For quantitative tests, trade-offs are associated with the cutoff point that differentiates abnormal from normal results. Lowering a cutoff point to make it less stringent can increase sensitivity. In this case, more individuals with disease will test positive; specificity, however, may decrease because more disease-free individuals may also test positive. Increasing the cutoff point and making the test more stringent decreases sensitivity, because a greater proportion of diseased individuals will test negative. Specificity, however, may increase because a greater proportion of disease-free individuals may also test negative. Take a moment to review the hypertension screening example in Chapter 6. The proportion of individuals referred for additional testing changes in direct relation to changes in the cutoff point to identify hypertension.

An example provided by the Public Health Service (Table 7–5) illustrates how altering the cutoff point affects sensitivity and specificity. Results from the Somogyi-Nelson blood test to screen for diabetes 2 hours after eating appear in the table. Clinicians screened 70 patients with diabetes and 510 diabetes-free individuals. Note that as the cutoff point increases (becomes more stringent), sensitivity decreases and specificity increases. Observe also that as sensitivity decreases, the number of false negatives increases. As specificity increases, however, the number of false positives decreases. For example, if a cutoff point of 70 mg/100 mL is used to screen for diabetes, sensitivity is high, with 98.6% of diabetics having a positive test result. Thus, nearly all diabetics are identified correctly; only 1.4% are missed. Note, however, that specificity is extremely low, with 8.8% of diabetes-free individuals having a negative test result. The percentage of false positives is large, 91.2%. Therefore, if a cutoff point of 70 mg/100 mL is used, the test will be sensitive but nonspecific.

The complex tradeoffs between sensitivity and specificity require that we consider (1) the

Table 7–5. Specificity and sensitivity of Somogyi-Nelson blood test for diabetes at different cutoff points, two hours after eating.

Cutoff Point (mg/100 mL)	Sensitivity (%) $pr(T+|D+)$	False Negatives (%) $pr(T-|D+)$	Specificity (%) $pr(T-|D-)$	False Positives (%) $pr(T+|D-)$
70	98.6	1.4	8.8	91.2
80	97.1	2.9	25.5	74.5
90	94.3	5.7	47.6	52.4
100	88.6	11.4	69.8	30.2
110	85.7	14.3	84.1	15.9
120	71.4	28.6	92.5	7.5
130	64.3	35.7	96.9	3.1
140	57.1	42.9	99.4	0.6
150	50.0	50.0	99.6	0.4
160	47.1	52.9	99.8	0.2
170	42.9	57.1	100.0	0.0
180	38.6	61.4	100.0	0.0
190	34.3	65.7	100.0	0.0
200	27.1	72.9	100.0	0.0

Adapted from Results of Boston diabetes screening evaluation study, Diabetes Program Guide (1960). U.S. Department of Health, Education, and Welfare, Public Health Service, Bureau of State Services, Division of Special Health Services, Chronic Disease Program. Public Health Service Publication no. 506. Washington, DC: U.S. Government Printing Office, p 20.

cost of testing; (2) the physical, emotional, and mental cost to the patient; (3) the cost of follow-up testing; and (4) the consequences of either missing disease or falsely identifying disease when it is absent. Individuals interested in a more in-depth discussion of these issues may wish to consult Galen and Gambino (1975), Fletcher and associates (1988), or Kraemer (1992).

FACTORS INFLUENCING PREDICTIVE VALUES

Predictive values may be extremely useful in situations where the population to which the test is applied is demographically and clinically similar to the reference population (on which the test was developed). Considerable care must be exercised in interpreting predictive values, however, because they are affected by a test's sensitivity and specificity, and also by disease prevalence.

How is the predictive value of a test influenced by its sensitivity and specificity? When the sensitivity of a test increases, it is less likely that an individual with a negative test result will have disease. Thus, the greater the sensitivity of a test, *the greater its negative predictive value*. Similarly, as the specificity of a test increases, *its positive predictive value increases*. The more specific the test, the greater the probability that an individual with a positive test will be diseased, and the less likely that a positive result will be associated with being disease free (Fletcher et al, 1988, p 56).

The predictive value of a test is also influenced by *disease prevalence* in the tested population. Recall that prevalence is the proportion of individuals in a population who have a specific clinical characteristic, such as a disease, at a specific point in time (refer to Chapter 4). When a highly specific test is applied to a population in which disease prevalence is low, positive results will be largely false positives. When a highly sensitive test is applied to a population in which disease prevalence is high, negative results will be largely false negatives. If the formula for the positive predictive value (PPV) is rewritten using the rules of probability, and if the formula is simplified algebraically, the relationship between sensitivity, specificity, and disease prevalence is apparent (Fletcher et al, 1988, p 56; Watson & Tang, 1980, p 497):

$$PPV = \frac{\text{Sensitivity} \times \text{Prevalence}}{(\text{Sensitivity} \times \text{Prevalence}) + (1 - \text{Specificity}) \times (1 - \text{Prevalence})} \qquad 7.7$$

A similar formula for the negative predictive value can be derived. Based on the above formula, *it is obvious that the predictive value of a test is affected, not only by sensitivity and specificity but also by disease prevalence*. Thus, the predictive value is not independent of the setting in which it is used (Fletcher et al, 1988, p 56). Once determined in a broad range of individuals with or without disease, sensitivity and specificity are considered constant (Griner et al, 1980, pp 560–561). Consequently, they are applicable to the study of any given patient as long as the test is uniformly applied, for example, with the same laboratory procedures and cutoff points.

The relationship between disease prevalence and the positive predictive value, $pr(D+|T+)$, is illustrated in Table 7–6. The value of a radioimmunoassay for prostatic acid phosphatase to diagnose prostatic cancer is examined in different populations; disease prevalence ranges from 35 cases per 100,000 to 50,000 cases per 100,000 (Watson & Tang, p 497). The sensitivity and specificity of the assay were established by Foti and co-workers (1977, p 1360), who used a cutoff point of 8 ng per 0.1 mL of serum. Sensitivity is 70% and specificity is 94%. When the prevalence of prostatic cancer is low, as in Caucasian men in the general population (35 cases per 100,000), the positive predictive value of the test approaches zero (0.4%). Thus, only one out of every 244 men (100/0.41 = 243.90) with a positive test has prostate cancer. In men in the general population, age 75 years or older, the prevalence of disease is 500 cases per 100,000; in this group, the test has limited value as a screening tool (PPV = 5.6%). For every 18 patients with a positive test result, only one has cancer (100/5.6 = 17.86). However, when the prevalence of disease is high the positive predictive value is high. When the assay is applied to men who present with a clinically suspicious prostatic nodule (prevalence = 50,000

Table 7–6. Relationship between disease prevalence and positive value of a radioimmunoassay for prostatic acid phosphatase to screen for prostatic cancer (sensitivity = 70%, specificity = 94%).

Clinical Setting	Disease Prevalence (Cases Per 100,000)	Positive Predictive Value (%)
Caucasian men in the general population	35	0.4
General male population, age 75 years or older	500	5.6
Men with a clinically suspicious prostatic nodule	50,000	93.0

Abstracted from 1) Foti A, Cooper J, Herschman H, Malvaez R. Detection of prostatic cancer by solid-phase radioimmunoassay of serum prostatic acid phosphatase. NEJM 1977;297(25):1360. 2) Watson R, Tang D. The predictive value of prostatic acid phosphatase as a screening test for prostatic cancer. NEJM 1980;303(9):497–499.

cases per 100,000), 93% of those who test positive have prostate cancer. Therefore, the test provides clinically useful information in this population (Watson & Tang, 1980, p 499).

In conclusion, the application and interpretation of a test must take into account the clinical and demographic characteristics of the population to which it is applied, including disease prevalence. The major means of interpreting a test is by "accurately intepreting the clinical context through careful observation during the history and physician examination. In an age when laboratory technology offers promise for solving complex diagnostic problems, we must still depend on medicine's oldest process—astute clinical observation" (Fletcher et al, 1988, p 60). A test with a high positive predictive value in one clinical context may be of little predictive utility in another situation, because of differences in disease prevalence in the two populations.

SUMMARY

Clinical laboratory tests are ordered to screen for disease and to manage patients after disease is detected. This chapter focuses on the former purpose. Considerations that figure into selecting a test include (1) its performance characteristics, (2) the reason why the test is ordered (eg, to confirm disease) and (3) the clinical characteristics of the suspected disease (eg, significant morbidity or mortality if not detected and treated). The performance characteristics of a test are:

Sensitivity. The conditional probability that a test is positive if the patient is diseased.

Specificity. The conditional probability that a test is negative if the patient is disease free.

False negative. The conditional probability that a test is negative if the patient is diseased; the complement of sensitivity.

False positive. The conditional probability that a test is positive if the patient is disease free; the complement of specificity.

Positive predictive value. The conditional probability that a patient is diseased if a test is positive.

Negative predictive value. The conditional probability that a patient is disease free if a test is negative.

Diagnostic tests are either qualitative or quantitative. Qualitative tests categorize patients as diseased or disease free, based on whether the clinical sign or symptom is present or absent. Quantitative tests yield results on a numerical continuum. An arbitrarily selected cutoff point differentiates positive (abnormal) from negative (normal) results. The selection of the cutoff point affects the sensitivity and specificity of the test. Lowering the cutoff point (to make it less stringent) increases sensitivity and decreases specificity. In contrast, increasing the cutoff point (to make it more stringent) decreases sensitivity and increases specificity.

Highly sensitive tests are useful when there is an important penalty for missing disease. A sensitive test should be used to detect a serious but treatable condition, such as a sexually transmitted disease or tuberculosis. Highly sensitive tests are useful to screen for disease, especially rare diseases like phenylketonuria. Further, highly sensitive tests are helpful during the early phases of a diagnostic workup, when the goal is to reduce the number of diagnostic possibilities. A highly sensitive test has few false negatives; when a negative result is obtained, the clinician can confidently rule out a disease. Thus, a highly sensitive test is most helpful when the test is negative.

A test with high specificity is selected when a serious condition exists, but cannot be treated effectively or cured (eg, multiple sclerosis). A test with high specificity is useful when knowledge that the disease is absent has psychologic or public health value. In selecting a test with high specificity, the clinician hopes to confirm disease. Because a highly specific test is rarely positive in the absence of disease, the clinician can conclude with confidence that disease is present; the probability of a false-positive result is small. Therefore, a specific test is most helpful when the result is positive.

The predictive value of a test is conditioned on knowledge of the disease status of the patient. For example, the positive predictive value is the conditional probability that a positive test result will occur if the patient is diseased. Predictive values may be extremely useful to the clinician in situations where the population to which the test is applied is demographically and clinically similar to the reference population. We must exercise considerable care in interpreting predictive values, however, because they are affected not only by a test's sensitivity and specificity, but also by disease prevalence. A test with a high positive predictive value in one clinical context may be of little predictive utility in another situation, because of the difference in disease prevalence in the two populations.

Self-study Questions

Part I: Thought Problems

1. Define the following terms in your own words:

   Gold standard   False positive
   Sensitivity   Positive predictive value
   Specificity   Negative predictive value
   False negative   Reference population

2. Identify the two major purposes for which clinical laboratory tests are ordered.
3. Explain how increasing and decreasing the cutoff point to distinguish positive from negative results can affect sensitivity and specificity.
4. Describe the difference between sensitivity and positive predictive value.
5. Describe the difference between specificity and negative predictive value.
6. In which clinical settings is a test with high sensitivity most useful?
7. In which clinical settings is a test with high specificity most useful?

Part II: Calculations

In a community screening program, 3000 healthy adult men had a routine blood test, part of which included determining the percentage of lymphocytes per 100 cells counted. The mean was 34%, with a standard deviation of approximately 4%. Assume that lymphocyte counts follow a Gaussian distribution.

1. Determine the range of normal, based on the central 95% of test results.
2. Determine the range of normal, such that the results yield 3% false-positive outcomes.

Part III: SLE Screening

Explain the meaning of this statement: Antinuclear antibody tests are highly sensitive, but not specific, for the presence of systemic lupus erythematosus (SLE).

Part IV: Test Selection

Clinical Problem 1: Brain Tumors

Radionuclide scanning (RN) and computed tomography (CT) are compared to evaluate their utility for diagnosing brain tumors. A brain tumor is suspected if either test is positive. Both procedures are performed in 100 patients with brain tumors and 100 without brain tumors. Among patients with brain tumors, 87 individuals have positive CT results and 63 patients have positive RN results.

1. Which test, RN or CT, has the higher sensitivity? Explain your answer.
2. Which test, RN or CT, has the higher proportion of false positive results? Explain your answer.

Clinical Problem 2: Procrastinitis

Two tests, PrO and PrU, are available to diagnose procrastinitis, a noncommunicable disease that is usually fatal if not diagnosed and treated. Although some patients with this disease may require long-term treatment, approximately 80% can be cured at modest cost with appropriate intervention. PrO and PrU have the following properties:

Table 7–7. Properties of two tests to diagnose procrastinitis.

Test	Properties
PrO	Positive in 25% of patients who are disease free; negative in 2% of patients who are diseased
PrU	Positive in 2% of patients who are disease free; negative in 25% of patients who are diseased

1. Which test, PrO or PrU, has the higher specificity?
2. If only one test can be selected to diagnosis procrastinitis, which one should be chosen and why?

Part V: Screening for HPV—Computation and Extended Analysis

Many clinicians advocate routine screening for human papillomavirus (HPV) in sexually active women. No symptoms occur in many women infected with HPV (Goldstein & Odom, 1993, p 64). Cervical infection with HPV is associated with a high percentage of all cervical dysplasias and cancers (Margolis & Greenwood, 1993, p 569). Approximately 70% of male partners of women with cervical dysplasias or cancer have HPV-associated warts on the penile shaft or just within the urethra (p 569). Clinicians recommend prompt treatment for HPV-affected women and men.

Many methods have been used to detect HPV. Although Southern blot hybridization is currently considered the most accurate way to detect this virus, this test requires large amounts of DNA, is extremely laborious, and is relatively expensive. Investigators in a west coast laboratory are interested in two new techniques to detect DNA amplification in HPV: VIRA and polymerase chain reaction (PCR). Both tests can be done in the laboratory, are easy to perform, are relatively inexpensive, and are reproducible. However, their use in humans has not been validated.

An investigation was conducted in 1993 at the student health service of a large, west coast university. During a 4-month period in which classes were in session, women who called the health service to make an appointment for routine gynecologic examination were asked to participate in a study to examine the utility of VIRA and PCR in a human population. Ninety-five percent of those invited to participate were enrolled. Of the 467 women who participated, most were Caucasian (71%), young (mean age 21.7 years, standard deviation 3.9 years), single (95%), had never been pregnant (81%), and were or had been involved in heterosexual relationships (96%).

Cervical and genital smears from each participant were evaluated for HPV with Southern blot, PCR, and VIRA determinations. Data from genital smears are summarized in Tables 7–8

Table 7–8. Data from *PCR* determinations in 467 college women.

Test Result	True Infection Status		Total
	D+	D−	
T+	190	23	213
T−	10	244	254
TOTAL	200	267	467

Table 7–9. Data from *VIRA* determinations in 467 college women.

Test Result	True Infection Status		Total
	D+	D−	
T+	45	6	51
T−	155	261	416
TOTAL	200	267	467

and 7–9. Based on Southern blot hybridization (the current gold standard to define HPV status), 200 of the 467 women were infected with HPV. Given the data in Tables 7–8 and 7–9, which test PCR or VIRA, should be used in women with characteristics similar to those included in the study? Consider prevalence and test performance characteristics in developing your response.

Solutions

Part II: Calculations

1. Determine the range of normal based on the central 95% of test results. This problem is like Clinical Example 7 in Chapter 6. Identifying the range of normal based on the central 95% of observations is equivalent to setting the proportion of false-positive outcomes equal to 5%.
   a. Because the normal curve is symmetric, 2.5% of the area falls above the upper and below the lower cutoff point.
   b. Consult Table A–1; look for a two-tailed area of 0.05 or a one-tailed area of 0.025. Identify the z-value: $z = \pm 1.96$.
   c. Use the formula for a standard normal deviate (Formula 6.3), substitute the known z-value, and solve for the 95% central limits:

   $$z = \frac{X - \mu}{\sigma}$$

   $$\pm 1.96 = \frac{X - \mu}{\sigma}$$

   $$X = \mu \pm 1.96\sigma$$

   d. Calculate the upper limit, which is the equivalent of the cutoff point in the right tail of the distribution of lymphocyte counts.

$$X_{Upper} = \mu - 1.96 \, \sigma$$

$$= 34 + (1.96)(4)$$

$$= 41.84\% = 42\%$$

e. Calculate the value of the cutoff point at the lower end of the distribution:

$$X_{Lower} = \mu - 1.96 \, \sigma$$

$$= 34 - (1.96)(4)$$

$$= 26.16 = 26\%$$

Thus, the range of normal in healthy adult men is approximately 26% to 42%.
2. Determine the range of normal such that the results yield 3% false-positive outcomes. Follow the procedure outlined in problem 1 (Part II, above). The z-value is ±2.17. The value of the upper cutoff point is [34 + (2.17)(4) = 42.68, or approximatly 43%]. The value of the lower cutoff point is [34 − (2.17)(4) = 25.32, or approximately 25%]. The range of normal is 25% to 43%. When these cutoff points are utilized, approximately 3% or lymphocyte counts will be identified as abnormal, even though they were obtained from healthy men.

Part III: Screening for SLE

Antinuclear antibody tests are positive in virtually all patients with SLE, but they are also positive in many patients with nonlupus conditions. For example, antinuclear antibodies occur in patients with rheumatoid arthritis, some forms of hepatitis, and interstitial lung disease (Hellman, 1993, p 661).

Part IV: Test Selection

Clinical Problem 1: Brain Tumors

1. Sensitivity is the conditional probability of a positive test, given the presence of disease. To determine sensitivity, we must have data from patients with disease—in this example, patients with brain tumors. Among the 100 patients with brain tumors, 87 individuals have positive CT results and 63 have positive RN results. Thus, the sensitivity of computed tomography is higher than that of radionuclide scanning.
2. The probability of a false-positive outcome is the complement of specificity; both are conditioned on the presence of health (being disease free). Therefore, in order to calculate the probability of a false-positive outcome, data from patients who are disease free must be available. In this problem, data are given only for patients with brain tumors. Consequently, the probability of a false-positive outcome cannot be computed with the available information.

Clinical Problem 2: Procrastinitis
Data in Table 7–10 describe the performance of PrO and PrU. For PrO, a false-negative outcome is obtained only 2% of the time; that is, 2% of patients with disease have a negative

Table 7–10. False negative and positive outcomes for tests to diagnose procrastinitis.

Test	False Negatives (%) $pr(T-|D+)$	False Positives (%) $pr(T+|D-)$
PrO	2%	25%
PrU	25%	2%

test result. In contrast, the percentage of false-negative outcomes is substantially higher for PrU (25%). The reverse is noted for false-positive outcomes, with PrU having a relatively small percentage of false positives (2%) compared to PrO (25%).

Sensitivity is the complement of false negative outcomes; therefore, the sensitivity of PrO is 98%, compared to 75% for PrU. The specificity is 75% for PrO (1 − false positives) and 98% for PrU. Because the disease is usually fatal if not diagnosed and treated, the penalty for missing disease is substantial. Further, treatment is available to alter the natural course of the disease. Therefore, a test with high sensitivity should be selected. Thus, PrO should be used to screen for the disease.

Part V: HPV Screening—Computation and Extended Analysis

Based on the Southern blot technique the prevalence of HPV infection in this group of women is [(200/467) × 100% = 42.83%] or approximately 43 cases per 100 women. Data from Tables 7–8 and 7–9 were used to estimate the prevalence of disease, based on PCR and VIRA determinations, and to calculate the performance characteristics of the tests. The results appear in Box 7–2. The sensitivity and specificity of PCR determinations are quite high (95% and 91.39%, respectively). The specificity of VIRA determinations is high (97.75%), but sensitivity is relatively low (22.50%). Based on the percentage of false-negative outcomes, only 5% of women who have HPV infection will be identified falsely as disease free if PCR determinations are used, compared to 77.50% if VIRA results are used. The predictive values of PCR determinations are relatively high (PPV = 89.2% and NPV = 96.06%). Although the positive predictive value of VIRA is also relatively high (88.24%), its negative predictive value is considerably lower (62.74%) than that of PCR. Note that the positive predictive value of both tests is approximately equal.

For women possessing demographic and clinical characteristics similar to those from whom data were collected, it appears that PCR-DNA amplification is useful as an HPV-screening tool. The clinical utility of VIRA in this population of women is clearly questionable. The prevalence of disease as estimated by PCR determinations is most similar to that determined by Southern blot hybridization (cases per 100 women: PCR, 46; VIRA, 11; Southern blot, 43).

Human papillomavirus infection in women is associated with a high percentage of all cervical dysplasias; the virus can be communicated to the male partner of the sexually active women and cause potentially serious problems; prompt treatment is important for both men and women. Thus, a test with high sensitivity is sought. Both tests are easy to perform, relatively inexpensive, and reproducible. The sensitivity of PCR determinations, however, is clearly superior to that of VIRA determinations. Therefore, PCR-DNA amplification rather than VIRA should be selected.

Box 7–2. Test performance characteristics for PCR and VIRA to diagnose HPV in college women.

Test Characteristic	PCR	VIRA
Estimated prevalence of HPV infection per 100 women	(213/467) × 100 = 45.6 or 46 cases	(51/467) × 100 = 10.93 or 11 cases
Sensitivity (true positive) %	(190/200) × 100% = 95%	(45/200) × 100% = 22.50%
Specificity (true negative) %	(244/267) × 100% = 91.39%	(261/267) × 100% = 97.75%
False negative (%)	(10/200) × 100% = 5%	(155/200) × 100% = 77.50%
False positive (%)	(23/267) × 100% = 8.61%	(6/267) × 100% = 2.25%
Positive predictive value (%)	(190/213) × 100% = 89.20%	(45/51) × 100% = 88.24%
Negative predictive value (%)	(244/254) × 100% = 96.06%	(261/416) × 100% = 62.74%

REFERENCES

Behrman R, Kliegman R: *Nelson Essentials of Pediatrics.* Saunders, 1990.

Fletcher R, Fletcher S, Wagner E: *Clinical Epidemiology: The Essentials,* 2nd ed. Williams & Wilkins, 1988.

Foti A, Cooper J, Herschman H, Malvaez R: Detection of prostatic cancer by solid-phase radioimmunoassay of serum prostatic acid phosphatase. *N Engl J Med* 1977;**297**:1360.

Galen R, Gambino S: *Beyond Normality: The Predictive Value and Efficiency of Medical Diagnoses*. Wiley, 1975.

Goldstein S, Odom R: Skin & appendages. In: *Current Medical Diagnosis and Treatment*. L. Tierney Jr, et al (editors). Appleton & Lange, 1993.

Greenberg R: *Medical Epidemiology*. Appleton & Lange, 1993.

Griner P, Mayewski R, Mushlin A, Greenland P: Selection and interpretation of diagnostic tests and procedures: Principles and applications. *Ann Intern Med* 1981;**94**:553.

Helman D: Arthritis & musculoskeletal disorders. In: *Current Medical Diagnosis and Treatment*. L. Tierney Jr, et al (editors). Appleton & Lange, 1993.

Hennekens C, Buring J: *Epidemiology in Medicine*. Little, Brown, 1987.

Hypertension Detection and Follow-up Program: A Progress Report. *Circ Res* 1977;**40**(suppl I, 5):106.

Kohn J, Weaver P: Serum-alpha$_1$-fetoprotein in hepatocellular carcinoma. *Lancet* 1974:334.

Kraemer H: *Evaluating Medical Tests*. Sage, 1992.

Littenberg B, Garber A, Sox H: Screening for hypertension. *Ann Intern Med* 1990;**112**:192.

Margolis A, Greenwood S: Gynecology & obstetrics. In: *Current Medical Diagnosis and Treatment*. L. Tierney Jr, et al (editors). Appleton & Lange, 1993.

1988 Report of the Joint National Committee on Detection, Evaluation, and Treatment of High Blood Pressure. *Arch Intern Med* 1988;**148**:1023.

Watson R, Tang D: The predictive value of prostatic acid phosphatase as a screening test for prostatic cancer. *N Engl J Med* 1980;**303**:497.

Determining the Probability of Variables with Only Two Outcomes—The Binomial Probability Distribution

8

Clinical Example 1: Automated Clinical Chemistry Determinations

A healthy patient visits her family physician for a yearly check-up. Her physician orders 20 routine chemical determinations from one blood sample (eg, glucose, potassium, calcium, iron). Given the normal range of values for each determination, a total of 5% of values in healthy persons will fall outside the cutoff points. What is the probability that one result will be abnormal for the healthy patient?

Clinical Example 2: Sickle-cell Anemia

An engaged man and woman discover that each is a carrier of the sickle-cell trait. The probability that any child born to them will have sickle-cell anemia (SCA) is 0.25. If the couple were to have three children, how likely is it that all three would have SCA?

Many quantitative variables in medicine are treated as continuous random variables—for example, weight, blood pressure, cholesterol, triglycerides, creatinine, sodium, and potassium. As discussed in Chapter 6, we use the normal curve (Gaussian distribution) to describe the probability of ranges of quantitative observations. Many variables, however, are *qualita-*

tive. Often these variables have only two mutually exclusive outcomes, such as survival (alive/dead), sex (female/male), test result (normal/abnormal), or disease state (present/absent). Variables with two mutually exclusive outcomes are called *dichotomous variables.* In order to determine the probability of one of these two outcomes, we utilize the binomial probability distribution. This distribution is applied commonly in medicine, for example, to determine the probability of obtaining an abnormal test result or to describe the inheritability of a trait.

OBJECTIVES

When you complete this chapter, you should be able to:

- Identify binomial variables and define their characteristics.
- Describe the properties of the binomial probability distribution.
- Use the binomial probability distribution to determine probability.
- Interpret the results of a binomial probability calculation.

DEFINING THE BINOMIAL PROBABILITY DISTRIBUTION

A **probability distribution** is a table or graph showing all possible outcomes of a variable with their respective probabilities (Daniel WW, 1991, p 70). Recall from Chapter 5 that probability is synonymous with *relative frequency.*

A **binomial probability distribution** is generated from a series of *Bernoulli trials,* named in honor of James Bernoulli (1654–1705), whose contributions to probability theory included the binomial distribution (Daniel WW, 1991, p 73). In a Bernoulli trial, an act results in only one of two mutually exclusive outcomes. Examples include selecting a patient from a cancer registry and recording the patient's sex (male or female); observing whether the offspring of a couple who carries the sickle-cell trait has sickle-cell anemia (yes or no); or following a patient who undergoes chemotherapy and radiation therapy for Hodgkin's lymphoma to determine whether he is alive at the end of 5 years (survived or died). A series of Bernoulli trials forms a Bernoulli process from which a binomial distribution is created; this occurs under the following conditions:

1. Only two outcomes are possible on each trial; only one outcome is observed on any given trial. One of the *two mutually exclusive outcomes* is represented by p and the other by q. Because q is the complement of p, q equals $1-p$. The outcome identified by p is sometimes referred to as a "success," while q is designated as a "failure"; these designations do not imply judgments about the worth or merit of findings.

2. There are n independent trials; therefore, an outcome on one trial has no effect on the outcome of any other trial. This is the *independence assumption.* Recall from Chapter 5 that two outcomes are independent if the probability of one does not affect the probability of the other and vice versa. For example, suppose that we sample men with prostate cancer to determine whether nodular involvement is present or absent. The outcome for the first patient does not alter the probability of nodular involvement in the next patient; similarly, the presence or absence of nodular involvement in the second patient does not increase or decrease the chance of nodular involvement in any other patient, and so on. Consequently, the presence or absence of nodular involvement is independent from patient to patient.

3. The probability of a given outcome is constant over all trials. This is the *homogeneity assumption.* For example, if a fair coin is tossed, the probability of obtaining a head is 0.50 on each flip.

4. The number of trials (n) is fixed and specified in advance. For example, prior to selecting patients from the cancer registry and recording whether a patient has survived 5 years following diagnosis (yes/no), we must specify how many patients we will sample.

In summary, the binomial distribution is generated from n *independent trials;* the outcome of each trial consists of only one of *two mutually exclusive outcomes;* the probability of a given outcome is the same on every trial (*homogeneity*); and the number of trials is specified in advance (*predetermined and fixed n*). A variable generated under these conditions is a **binomial variable.**

Next, we discuss how to generate a binomial probability distribution. A coin-tossing experiment is used to demonstrate the relationship between basic rules of probability and the binomial distribution.

Generating a Binomial Probability Distribution

In the next example, a binomial probability distribution is created by tossing a *fair* coin four times (n) and counting the number of heads on each toss. A fair coin is one for which the chance of obtaining a head on each toss of the coin is 0.50. A trial is one toss of the coin. Two *mutually exclusive outcomes* exist; only one (head or tail) will be observed on a given trial. The chance of obtaining a head is the same on each toss (*homogeneity*). Each trial is independent because the outcome on any one trial does not affect the outcome on any other trial (*independence*).

Suppose the coin is tossed four times and three heads are counted. What is the probability of obtaining three heads on four tosses? We can determine the answer in various ways. For example, we could list *all possible sequences of three heads on four tosses* and use rules of probability to calculate the probability. We could also enumerate *all possible sequences of heads and tails,* compute the relative frequencies, and select the relative frequency associated with sequences of three heads on four flips. Alternatively, we could use a formula that describes the distribution that results from a binomial (Bernoulli) process to compute the probability of three heads on four tosses of the coin. Each approach is presented below.

LISTING ALL POSSIBLE SEQUENCES OF HEADS AND TAILS ON FOUR TOSSES

Sequence of Three Heads on Four Tosses of the Coin

If we are interested solely in obtaining the probability of three heads on four tosses of the coin, we could simply list the sequences for this outcome. We begin by determining the number of ways in which three heads can occur on four tosses of the coin. For example, one possible sequence is T H H H; another possible sequence is H T H H. Actually, the total number of ways to obtain X distinct combinations of n objects, irrespective of order, is $\frac{n!}{X!(n-X)!}$ (Hays, 1981, p 114). In our example, n is the number of flips of the coin (n = 4) and X is the number of heads on four tosses of the coin ($X = 3$). Therefore, the number of distinct ways in which three heads can occur from four tosses of the coin is $\frac{4!}{3!(4-3)!} = \frac{4(3!)}{3!(1!)} = 4$. We list these four distinct sequences in Table 8–1. The exclamation point (!) indicates a factorial. For example 4! =(4)(3)(2)(1) = 24; 3! = (3)(2)(1) = 6. By definition, 1! = 1 and 0! = 1.

Listed in the first column are all distinct sequences of three heads in four flips of the coin. Allow p to represent a head and q a tail. Because the trials are independent, we employ the multiplication rule for independent events to calculate the probability of obtaining the first sequence (H H H T): $(p)(p)(p)(q)=p^3q$ (Formula 5.8, Chapter 5). The probability that this specific sequence will result from four flips of the coin is 0.0625. Note that the probability of each distinct sequence of three heads is the same.

Table 8–1. All possible sequences of three heads on four tosses of a fair coin and the probability of each sequence.

Sequence	Probability	Computation
H H H T	$(p)(p)(p)(q) = p^3q$	$0.50^3 (0.50) = 0.0625$
H H T H	$(p)(p)(q)(p) = p^2qp$	$0.50^2 (0.50) (0.50) = 0.0625$
H T H H	$(p)(q)(p)(p) = pqp^2$	$(0.50) (0.50) 0.50^2 = 0.0625$
T H H H	$(q)(p)(p)(p) = qp^3$	$(0.50) 0.50^3 = 0.0625$

If we are interested in the probability of three heads on four tosses of the coin and *not* the probability of a specific sequence, we simply add the probabilities in Table 8–1. The Addition Rule for mutually exclusive events applies because the occurrence of a specific sequence of four tosses of the coin precludes the occurrence of any other sequence on these same tosses (Formula 5.4, Chapter 5):

$$pr(3 \text{ H on 4 tosses}) = pr(H\,H\,H\,T) \text{ or } pr(H\,H\,T\,H) \text{ or } pr(H\,T\,H\,H) \text{ or } pr(T\,H\,H\,H)$$

$$= pr(H\,H\,H\,T) + pr(H\,H\,T\,H) + pr(H\,T\,H\,H) + pr(T\,H\,H\,H)$$

$$= p^3q + p^2qp + pqp^2 + qp^3$$

$$= 4(p^3q)$$

$$= 4(0.0625) = 0.25.$$

Thus, the probability of obtaining three heads on four tosses of the coin is 0.25.

We could employ this approach to answer other questions, such as: What is the probability of obtaining two heads on four tosses of the coin? What is the probability of obtaining one head on four tosses of the coin? To answer these questions, we could enumerate *all possible sequences* of heads and tails and use their respective frequencies to estimate the probabilities of interest. Enumerating all possible sequences is illustrated next.

All Possible Sequences of Heads and Tails

We use the following rule to determine the number of all possible sequences: Given K mutually exclusive outcomes, only one of which can occur on each of n trials, the number of different distinct sequences that may result is K^n (Hays, 1981, p 110). In our example, $K = 2$, the number of mutually exclusive outcomes on one toss of the coin, and $n = 4$, the number of trials. Thus, there are $2^4 = 16$ distinct sequences of heads and tails on four tosses of the coin. Table 8–2 lists all these sequences. The table also contains answers to a question like the following: What is the probability of obtaining two heads on four tosses of the coin? We could use the information more readily if we created a relative frequency distribution from this listing. Table 8–3 contains this distribution. The number of heads on four tosses appears in column one; the frequency appears in column two; and the relative frequency appears in column three. Note that the sum of the relative frequencies is 1.00. Table 8–3 is a probability

Table 8–2. All possible outcomes for tossing a fair coin four times.

Sequence No.	Sequence	Sequence No.	Sequence
1 (4 heads)	H H H H	9 (2 heads)	T T H H
2 (3 heads)	H H H T	10 (2 heads)	T H H T
3 (3 heads)	H H T H	11 (2 heads)	H T T H
4 (3 heads)	H T H H	12 (1 head)	H T T T
5 (3 heads)	T H H H	13 (1 head)	T H T T
6 (2 heads)	H H T T	14 (1 head)	T T H T
7 (2 heads)	H T H T	15 (1 head)	T T T H
8 (2 heads)	T H T H	16 (0 heads)	T T T T

Table 8–3. Relative frequency distribution of the number of heads on four tosses of a fair coin.

No. Heads	Frequency	Relative Frequency
4	1	1 / 16 = 0.0625
3	4	4 / 16 = 0.25
2	6	6 / 16 = 0.3750
1	4	4 / 16 = 0.25
0	1	1 / 16 = 0.0625
		Σ = 1.00

distribution—in particular, a binomial probability distribution. It is easy to determine from Table 8–3 that three heads occur in four of 16 possible sequences. Thus, the probability of obtaining three heads on four coin tosses is 0.25. The probability of obtaining three *or* four heads on four flips of the coin is

$$pr(3\ H\ or\ 4\ H\ on\ 4\ tosses) = pr(3\ H) + pr(4\ H)$$

$$= \left(\frac{4}{16} \right) + \left(\frac{1}{16} \right)$$

$$= \frac{5}{16} = 0.3125.$$

Thus, we expect to obtain three *or* four heads on four tosses of the coin slightly less than one third of the time.

It is relatively easy to enumerate all possible outcomes and determine their respective probabilities when the number of trials is small; the task becomes laborious as n increases significantly. Rather than using the enumeration method, we could employ a formula to describe the distribution of outcomes of trials from a binomial (Bernoulli) process.

Developing the Formula for the Binomial Distribution

The formula for the binomial probability distribution can be developed from the enumeration method illustrated above. We begin by generalizing the formula for the probability of a specific number of heads on four tosses of the coin to X heads on n tosses. For example, the formula for the probability of three heads on four coin tosses is $4(p^3q)$. The number four is the number of distinct sequences in which three heads ($X = 3$) in four tosses (n) can be obtained; the generalized formula is $\frac{n!}{X!(n-X)!}$. The exponent of p (3) is the number of heads; therefore, p^3 is p^x. The exponent on q is actually 1, the number of tails in four tosses of the coin; in its general form q is q^{n-X}. Thus, the probability of X heads on n tosses of the coin is

$$pr(X\ heads\ on\ n\ coin\ flips) = \frac{n!}{X!(n-X)!} p^X q^{n-X} \qquad 8.1$$

Next, to describe the *distribution of all possible sequences* of X heads on n tosses of the coin, we add the probabilities, beginning with $X = 0$ (zero heads) and continuing to n (all heads):

$$\sum_{X=0}^{n} \frac{n!}{X!(n-X)!} p^X q^{n-X} \qquad 8.2$$

Formula 8.2 equals (Bahn, 1972, p 18)

$$\frac{n!}{0!(n-0)!}p^0q^{n-0}+\frac{n!}{1!(n-1)!}p^1q^{n-1}+\ \ldots\ +\frac{n!}{n!(n-n)!}p^nq^{n-n} \qquad \textbf{8.3.}$$

Formula 8.2 and its expanded counterpart, Formula 8.3, describe the binomial probability distribution. We can also develop the binomial probability distribution from the binomial expansion: $(p + q)^n$. Hays (1981, p 122) presents the results of the expansion.

In summary, we can develop the formula for the binomial probability distribution theoretically or by enumerating sequences of X outcomes on n trials. Each approach yields the same outcome. Next, we discuss the calculation of binomial probabilities.

Using the Binomial Formula to Calculate Probabilities

In Box 8–1, we demonstrate the use of the binomial formula to compute probabilities of X heads on four coin flips. The formula for computing the probability of obtaining X heads on n trials is (Formula 8.1):

$$pr(\text{X heads on n trials}) = \frac{n!}{X!(n-X)!}p^Xq^{n-X}.$$

Compare the probabilities in Box 8–1 with the relative frequencies in Table 8–3. Note that they are identical. Keep in mind that a relative frequency is a probability. Unless we are conducting a study that involves a very small sample, it is easier to use the binomial formula to calculate probabilities than to enumerate all possible sequences of outcomes.

Box 8–1. Computating binomial probabilities for the number of heads on four tosses of a fair coin.

No. Heads	Binomial Computation		
4	$pr(4H)$	$=$	$\dfrac{4!}{4!(4-4)!}\ 0.50^40.50^{4-4}$
		$=$	$(1)(0.50^4)(0.50^0)$
		$=$	$0.5^4 = 0.0625$
3	$pr(3H)$	$=$	$\dfrac{4!}{3!(4-3)!}\ 0.50^30.50^{4-3}$
		$=$	$(4)(0.50^3)(0.50^1)$
		$=$	0.25
2	$pr(2H)$	$=$	$\dfrac{4!}{2!(4-2)!}\ 0.50^20.50^{4-2}$
		$=$	$(6)(0.50^2)(0.50^2)$
		$=$	0.3750
1	$pr(1H)$	$=$	$\dfrac{4!}{1!(4-1)}\ 0.50^10.50^{4-1}$
		$=$	$(4)(0.50^9)(0.50^3)$
		$=$	0.25
0	$pr(0H)$	$=$	$\dfrac{4!}{0!(4-0)!}\ 0.50^00.50^{4-0}$
		$=$	$(1)(0.50^0)(0.50^4)$
		$=$	$0.5^4 = 0.0625$

APPLYING THE BINOMIAL FORMULA TO MEDICINE

The Clinical Examples presented at the beginning of the chapter illustrate the use of the binomial formula to solve clinical problems. In Clinical Example 1, does the binomial distribution apply? Let us check to ensure that all assumptions have been met. For each test, one of two mutually exclusive outcomes is possible (normal or abnormal). The probability of an abnormal result is constant from determination to determination (0.05, homogeneity assumption). The number of determinations from a single sample is fixed in advance. Because the values of some tests are related to others, however, we question the independence assumption. For example, patients with a low albumin level are likely to have a low protein level because total protein is the sum of albumin and globulin (Ingelfinger et al, 1987, p 42). Nevertheless, we assume that the tests are independent. We will discuss the reason for this assumption in a moment. Because we believe all assumptions are reasonably satisfied, we apply the binomial formula.

Before we calculate various probabilities, we define n, X, p, and q:

n number of chemical determinations (tests) performed on one blood sample
X number of *abnormal* tests
p probability that a test result will fall outside the range of normal
q probability that a test will fall within the range of normal.

The probability that *exactly one test result* will be abnormal is $pr(X = 1)$:

$$\frac{20!}{1!(20-1)!}0.05^1 0.95^{20-1} = (20)(0.05^1)0.95^{19}$$

$$= 0.3774.$$

Thus, the probability is approximately 0.38 that our healthy patient will have exactly one abnormal test result.

What is the probability that our healthy patient will have *exactly* two abnormal results? The probability is:

$$\frac{20!}{2!(20-2)!}0.05^2 0.95^{20-2} = \frac{20(19)(18!)}{2(18!)}0.05^2 0.95^{18}$$

$$= 190(0.05^2)(0.95^{18})$$

$$= 0.1887.$$

The probability is slightly less than 0.20 that this healthy woman will have exactly two abnormal test results from among 20 routinely ordered chemical determinations.

What is the probability that our healthy patient will have *at least* two abnormal results? This probability equals:

$$pr(X \geq 2) = pr(X = 2) + pr(X = 3) + pr(X = 3) + pr(X = 4) + \ldots + pr(X = 20).$$

We can shorten our computational effort if we recall that the sum of the probabilities of all mutually exclusive events equals one (Formula 5.3, Chapter 5). Note that only two other possible outcomes are not included in the above enumeration; they are $X = 0$ and $X = 1$. Therefore, $pr(X \geq 2) = 1 - [pr(X = 0) + pr(X = 1)]$. Calculate $pr(X = 0)$:

$$\frac{20!}{0!(20-0)!}0.05^0 0.95^{20-0} = (1)(1)0.95^{20}$$

$$= 0.3585.$$

Compute $pr(X = 1)$. (0.3774, calculated previously.) Add $pr(X = 0)$ to $pr(X = 1)$ and subtract from 1.0:

$$pr(X \geq 2) = 1 - [0.3585 + 0.3774] = 0.2641.$$

The probability is approximately 0.26 that a healthy patient will have *at least two* abnormal results, if 20 determinations are made from one blood sample.

Suppose the clinician orders only 10 blood chemistry tests. If the proportion of false positives is the same as in the example above, for a healthy patient, what is the probability that 10 chemical determinations from a single blood sample will yield two abnormal results?

$$pr(X = 2) = \frac{10!}{2!(10-2)!} 0.05^2 0.95^{10-2} = 0.0746$$

Suppose the clinician is even more selective and orders only four chemical determinations from a single blood sample. For a healthy patient, what is the probability that 4 chemical determinations from a single blood sample will yield two abnormal results?

$$pr(X = 2) = \frac{4!}{2!(4-2)!} 0.05^2 0.95^{4-2} = 0.0135$$

The probability is approximately 0.01 that our healthy patient will have exactly two abnormal results, if four chemical determinations are ordered.

The preceding examples show the application of the binomial distribution to a common medical practice—ordering multiple chemical determinations from a single blood sample. The examples also demonstrate that the probability of obtaining an abnormal test result increases with the number of determinations. Therefore, an abnormal test result must be interpreted in light of several factors, including the number of routine determinations ordered. The physician must also consider information from the history and physical examination; data from the patient chart; the cost of follow-up; the cost of missing a diagnosis of disease because an abnormal finding was not followed up; the quality of the test in terms of its operating characteristics; and other factors that affect test results, such as whether the patient fasted prior to the test.

A Comment About the Assumption of Independence

As noted earlier, we may not be able to assume independence of results from one chemical determination to another. By comparing the *theoretical* probability distribution to the distribution of *observed* probabilities, we can assess the adequacy of the binomial distribution to describe the distribution of the number of abnormal results from a single blood sample. We generate the theoretical probability distribution by using the formula for the binomial to compute the probabilities for all possible outcomes. The *observed* probability is created by obtaining a single blood sample from a large number of healthy individuals and running 20 determinations on each blood sample. The number of abnormal results is counted for each example and cast into a relative frequency distribution, like the one displayed in Table 8–3. These relative frequencies are then compared to the theoretical probabilities. On the basis of such a comparison, mathematicians have shown that the observed and theoretical distributions are highly similar (Ingelfinger et al, 1987, p 43). Therefore, even when the assumption of independence is not satisfied totally, the binomial distribution may be used to determine approximate probabilities.

Assessing Inheritability

Using Clinical Example 2 at the start of the chapter, define X as the number of SCA-affected offspring; $n = 3$; $p = 0.25$, the probability that a child will have SCA; and $q = 0.75$, the probability that a child will *not* have SCA. The probability that three of three children will be born with SCA is:

$$pr(X = 3) = \frac{3!}{3!(3-3)!}0.25^30.75^{3-3} = 0.25^3 = 0.0156.$$

If both parents carry the sickle-cell trait, the probability that all three of their children will have sickle cell anemia is less than 0.02. Box 8–2 shows the distribution of all possible outcomes for three offspring of parents who both carry the sickle-cell trait. Based on the calculations displayed in the box, we observe that the probability that none of the three children will have SCA is approximately 0.42. Similarly, the probability is approximately 0.42 that one of the three children will have SCA. The chance that two of the three children will have SCA is slightly greater than 0.14.

Box 8–2. Distribution of children with sickle-cell anemia born to parents who both carry the sickle-cell trait for $n = 3$ and $p = 0.25$.

No. Affected Children	Probability of SCA
0	$\frac{3!}{0!(3-0)!}0.25^00.75^{3-0} = (1)(1)(0.75^3) = 0.4219$
1	$\frac{3!}{1!(3-1)!}0.25^10.75^{3-1} = 3(0.25)(0.75^2) = 0.4219$
2	$\frac{3!}{2!(3-2)!}0.25^2 0.75^{3-2} = 3(0.25^2)(0.75) = 0.1406$
3	$\frac{3!}{3!(3-3)!}0.25^30.75^{3-3} = 0.25^3 = 0.0156$
Sum of the probabilities	$0.4219 + 0.4219 + 0.1406 + 0.0156 = 1.0000$

Computing the Probability of Improvement for a New Treatment

Clinical Example 3: Parkinson's Disease

Patients with Parkinson's disease (PD) are often treated with levodopa and carbidopa, a dopa decarboxylase inhibitor that prevents the metabolism of levodopa until it reaches the brain. When the disease is full blown, drug therapy reduces the severity of symptoms in only 30% of patients. Ten patients with advanced PD undergo an experimental surgery in which a pencil-thin tube is inserted through the patient's skull and small bits of the patient's adrenal gland are pressed onto the brain. Following surgery, 8 patients show improvement comparable to that obtained with L-dopa and carbidopa, but without the side effects associated with drug therapy. If surgery is as likely to lead to improvement as L-dopa and carbidopa, what is the probability of improvement in 8 of 10 Parkinson's patients who undergo the experimental surgery?

Define the following:

$n = 10$ (number of patients who have surgery)
$X = 8$ (number of patients who improve following surgery)
$p = 0.30$ (probability of improvement with L-dopa and carbidopa)
$q = 0.70$ (probability of no improvement with L-dopa and carbidopa).

The probability of improvement in 8 of 10 patients who receive the experimental surgery is

$$\frac{10!}{8!(10-8)!}0.30^80.70^{10-8} = 18(0.30^8)(0.70^2) = 0.0006.$$

Thus, if the experimental surgery proves as effective as L-dopa and carbidopa, we would expect to see improvement in 8 of 10 patients who undergo the experimental surgery approximately 6 times in 10,000.

SUMMARY

The binomial probability distribution is used commonly in medicine, for example, in genetics to assess the inheritability of a trait based on family history. A binomial distribution results from a series of n independent trials; although two mutually exclusive outcomes are possible on each trial, only one is observed. The probability of observing one of the two mutually exclusive outcomes is the same on every trial. The number of trials is fixed and specified in advance.

To use the binomial formula, check first to ensure that all assumptions are satisified. If all assumptions have been met, define n, number of trials; X, the number of observed outcomes; p, the probability of obtaining one outcome; and q, the probability of obtaining the other outcome. Finally, employ the binomial formula to compute the probability of a specified outcome, for example, the probability that two of three siblings will have sickle-cell anemia if both their parents carry the sickle-cell trait.

REFERENCES

Bahn A: *Basic Medical Statistics.* Grune & Stratton, 1972.

Daniel WL: *Genetics and Human Variation.* Stipes, 1991.

Daniel WW: *Biostatistics: A Foundation for Analysis in the Health Sciences,* 5th ed. Wiley, 1991.

Hays W: *Statistics,* 3rd ed. Holt, Rinehart & Winston, 1981.

Ingelfinger J, Mosteller F, Thibodeau L, Ware J: *Biostatistics in Clinical Medicine,* 2nd ed. Macmillan, 1987.

Self-study Questions

Part I: Thought Problems

1. Define a binomial variable.
2. Describe the process used to generate a binomial distribution.

Part II: Binomial Variable?

Read each of the following descriptions and indicate whether the variable described is binomial.

1. The *diastolic blood pressure (mm Hg)* of 60 women, ages 60 to 64 years, is measured as part of a hypertension screening program.
2. The *diastolic blood pressure* of 60 women, ages 60 to 64 years, is measured as part of a hypertension screening program and classified as normal or above normal.
3. The *number of sore throats* is counted over a 12-month period among 75 patients, ages 5 to 18 years, who are seen by a pediatric allergist at a local clinic. Each patient has more than one sore throat.
4. *Progress* following surgery is assessed in 15 patients who underwent a resection for an intestinal obstruction. Progress is categorized as better than expected, about on par with expected, or worse than expected.

5. Seventy-five elementary school children, ages 6 to 12 years, participate in an obesity screening program sponsored by the Wellness Center of a local clinic. The *weight* of each child is measured and categorized as within normal limits or in excess of normal.
6. Seventy-five elementary school children, ages 6 to 12 years, participate in an obesity screening program sponsored by the Wellness Center of a local clinic. The *weight* of each child is reported to the nearest kilogram.
7. *Satisfaction* (satisfied/dissatisfied) with medical care received at a free clinic in an urban area was assessed in a brief interview; 170 patients were queried from July 14 to 18, 1994.
8. The *medical statistics and epidemiology knowledge* of 10,000 practicing physicians across the United States is evaluated by the American Medical Association and rated as adequate or inadequate.
9. *Two-year survival* (yes/no) is determined for 140 patients with an inoperable dissecting abdominal aneurysm.
10. Investigators at the National Institutes of Health evaluated the *effectiveness* (delayed onset of symptoms: yes/no) of early AZT therapy in 450 HIV-positive symptom-free patients with CD4 cell counts at or near 500.

Part III: Computation and Analysis

In the following examples, assume that assumptions of prespecified sample size, homogeneity, and independence are satisfied (unless it is evident that one or more assumptions have been violated).

1. Both Mr. and Mrs. Daniels are carriers of Tay–Sachs disease. The independent probability that any child born to them will have the disease is 0.25. If the couple has two children, what is the probability that both will be born with the disease?
2. The probability of surviving 5 years following surgical removal of a glioma (a type of brain tumor) is 0.40. If 15 successive patients undergo surgical removal of a glioma, what is the probability that exactly 10 patients will be alive at the end of 5 years?
3. Ten percent of individuals, 55 to 60 years of age, who develop a common form of influenza die from it. If 10 individuals in this age group contract this form of influenza, what is the probability that 40% will die?
4. Thirty percent of a particular population are immune to gastroenteritis caused by a retrovirus. If a random sample of 10 patients is selected from this population, what is the probability that it will contain (a) exactly four immune persons? (b) at least two immune persons?
5. Two achondroplasia dwarfs marry and plan to have children. Individuals with achondroplasia have unusually short limbs and normal trunk sizes, giving rise to disproportionate dwarfism (Daniel WL, 1991, p 181). In this case, the chance of a pregnancy terminating in miscarriage or stillbirth of a severely deformed infant is 0.25. If three pregnancies occur, what is the distribution of the number of pregnancies in three that will result in miscarriage or stillbirth of a severely deformed infant?
6. An automated clinical chemistry analyzer is used at a local hospital to provide 20 routinely ordered chemical determinations from a single blood sample. A total of 5% of values in a large group of healthy individuals falls outside the range of normal for each determination.
   (a) What is the probability that a healthy person will have normal results on all 20 tests?
   (b) What is the probability that a healthy person will have at least one abnormal test result?

Part IV: Is the Binomial Appropriate?

A clinician compares the effectiveness of ergotamine tartrate and acetaminophen to relieve migraine headaches. Twelve migraine sufferers participate in a 2-week trial. Each patient takes an appropriate oral dose of ergotamine tartrate immediately after migraine onset, and then records whether relief is experienced (yes/no). Forty-eight headaches are experienced; relief is noted in 18 migraine episodes. If ergotamine tartrate is as effective as acetaminophen in relieving a migraine, 20% of migraine sufferers are expected to experience relief after taking ergotamine tartrate. If ergotamine tartrate has the same chance of yielding relief as acetaminophen, what is the probability of 18 episodes of relief in 44 attacks?

The clinician defines X, n, p, and q:

$X = 18$ (number of episodes of relief)
$n = 44$ (total number of attacks)
$p = 0.20$ (probability of relief)
$q = 0.80$ (probability of no relief)

The binomial model is used next to calculate the probability of relief in 18 of 44 attacks. Comment on the appropriateness of this approach to compute the probability of relief.

Solutions

Part II: Binomial Variable?

1. Diastolic blood pressure (mm Hg) is measured as a quantitative variable.
2. Identified as either normal or above normal, *diastolic blood pressure* is treated as a binomial variable.
3. Although under many circumstances the occurrence of a *sore throat* (yes/no) can be treated as a binomial variable, the condition of *independence* is violated in this example; the presence or absence of a sore throat in a given patient is not independent from episode to episode.
4. *Progress* is treated as a qualitative variable with three mutually exclusive outcomes. Therefore, progress is not a binomial variable.
5. *Weight* is defined as having two mutually exclusive outcomes, either within normal limits or in excess of normal. Weight is a binomial variable.
6. *Weight* is measured and reported to the nearest kilogram. Therefore, weight is a quantitative variable.
7. *Satisfaction* is a binomial variable; it has two mutually exclusive outcomes (satisfied or dissatisfied). Only one can be used to describe the opinion of a patient about medical care.
8. *Medical statistics and epidemiology knowledge* is binomial; two mutually exclusive categories are used to characterize a physician's knowledge (adequate/inadequate).
9. *Two-year survival* is binomial.
10. In this example, *effectiveness* is operationalized as a variable for which only two mutually exclusive outcomes exist. Early AZT therapy will either delay or will not delay the onset of symptoms in these patients.

Part III: Computation and Analysis

Define X, n, p, and q prior to setting up the problem and calculating probabilities. Recall that X is the number of times the outcome of interest is counted and p is the probability of occurrence of this outcome.

1. Tay–Sachs disease.

$X = 2$ (number of children born with the disease)
$n = 2$ (number of children born to the couple)
$p = 0.25$ (probability of Tay–Sachs disease)
$q = 0.75$ (probability of being free of Tay–Sachs disease)

$$pr(X = 2) = \frac{2!}{2!(2-2)!} 0.25^2 0.75^{2-2} = (1)(0.25^2)(1) = 0.0625$$

The chance that both children of such a couple will have Tay–Sachs disease is less than 10%.

2. Five-year survival following surgery.

X = 10 patients (number who survive 5 years)
n = 15 patients (number who underwent surgery)
p = 0.40 (probability of surviving 5 years)
q = 0.60 (probability of not surviving 5 years)

$$pr(\text{10 Surviving in 15 Patients}) = \frac{15!}{10!(15-10)!}0.40^{10}0.60^{15-10}$$

$$= \frac{15(14)(13)(12)(11)10!}{10![5(4)(3)(2)(1)]}0.40^{10}0.60^{15-10}$$

$$= 3(7)(13)(11)0.40^{10}0.60^{5}$$

$$= 0.0245$$

The probability that 10 of 15 patients will survive 5 years is slightly greater than 0.02. Thus, we expect 10 to 15 glioma patients who undergo surgery to survive 5 years approximately two times in 100.

3. Influenza deaths.

X = 4 (number of deaths; 40% of 10 individuals)
n = 10 (number who contract influenza)
p = 0.10 (probability of death)
q = 0.90 (probability of survival)

$$pr(\text{4 Deaths in 10 patients}) = \frac{10!}{4!(10-4)!}0.10^{4}0.90^{10-4}$$

$$= \frac{10(9)(8)(7)6!}{[4(3)(2)(1)]6!}0.10^{4}0.90^{6}$$

$$= (210)0.10^{4}0.90^{6}$$

$$= 0.01116 = 0.01$$

The probability that 4 of 10 influenza patients in this group will die from the illness is approximately 0.01. Thus, we expect 4 deaths in 10 affected patients approximately 1 time in 100.

4. Gastroenteritis caused by retrovirus.

X = number immune
n = 10 patients
p = 0.30 (probability of immunity)
q = 0.70 (probability of no immunity)

a. X = *Exactly Four Immune Persons*

$$pr(\text{4 Immune in 10 Persons}) = \frac{10!}{4!(10-4)!}0.30^{4}0.70^{10-4}$$

$$= \frac{10(9)(8)(7)6!}{[4(3)(2)(1)]6!}0.30^{4}0.70^{6}$$

$$= (210)0.30^{4}0.70^{6}$$

$$= 0.2001 = 0.20$$

The probability is approximately 0.20 that 4 of 10 patients in this population will be immune to gastroenteritis caused by a retrovirus.

b. *At Least Two Immune Persons*

$$pr(X \geq 2) = pr(X = 2) + pr(X = 3) + \ldots + pr(X = 10)$$
$$= 1 - [pr(X = 0) + pr(X = 1)]$$

$$pr(X = 0) = \frac{10!}{0!(10-0)!} \, 0.30^0 0.70^{10-0} = (1)(1)0.70^{10} = 0.0282$$

$$pr(X = 1) = \frac{10!}{1!(10-1)!} \, 0.30^1 0.70^{10-1} = (10)(0.30)(0.70^9) = 0.1211$$

$$pr(X \geq 2) = 1 - (0.0282 + 0.1211) = 0.8507$$

The probability is approximately 0.85 that *at least* 2 in 10 patients in this population will be immune to gastroenteritis caused by a retrovirus.

5. Achondroplasia dwarfs.

$X =$ Number of pregnancies ending in miscarriage or stillbirth
$n = 3$ (total number of pregnancies)
$p = 0.25$ (probability of miscarriage or stillbirth of severely deformed infant)
$q = 0.75$ (probability of no miscarriage or stillbirth of severely deformed infant)

Probability Distribution Calculations

$$pr(X = 0) = \frac{3!}{0!(3-0)!} \, 0.25^0 0.75^{3-0} = (1)(1)0.75^3 = 0.4219$$

$$pr(X = 1) = \frac{3!}{1!(3-1)!} \, 0.25^1 0.75^{3-1} = (3)(0.25)0.75^2 = 0.4219$$

$$pr(X = 2) = \frac{3!}{2!(3-2)!} \, 0.25^2 0.75^{3-2} = (3)(0.25^2)0.75 = 0.1406$$

$$pr(X = 3) = \frac{3!}{3!(3-3)!} \, 0.25^3 0.75^{3-3} = (1)(0.25^3)(1) = 0.0156$$

Distribution of number of pregnancies in three resulting in miscarriage or stillbirth of a *severely deformed infant.*

Number	Probability
0	0.4219
1	0.4219
2	0.1406
3	0.0156
	$\Sigma = 1.0000$

For example, the probability that none of the pregnancies will result in a miscarriage or stillbirth of a severely deformed infant is approximately 0.42. The probability that one pregnancy in three will end in a miscarriage or stillbirth is approximately 0.42. The probability that all three pregnancies will end in a miscarriage or stillbirth is slightly less than 0.02.

6. Chemical determinations.

X = Number of *abnormal* results
n = 20 (number of determinations from one blood sample)
p = 0.05 (probability of a false positive)
q = 0.95 (probability of a normal result)

a. *Normal Results on All 20 Tests*

$$pr(X = 0) = \frac{20!}{0!(20-0)!}0.05^0 0.95^{20-0} = (1)(1)0.95^{20} = 0.3585$$

The probability is slightly less than 0.36 that all test results from the 20 determinations will be normal.

Students frequently ask what would occur if X were defined as the number of *normal* results; thus, X = 20 because all results are normal. The resulting probability is the same as the one just computed:

$$pr(X = 20) = \frac{20!}{20!(20-20)!}0.95^{20} 0.05^{20-20} = (1)(0.95^{20})(1) = 0.3585$$

The key is to remember that p is the probability of the outcome of interest and X corresponds to the number of occurrences of that outcome.

b. *At Least One Abnormal Test Result*

$$pr(X \geq 1) = pr(X = 1) + pr(X = 2) + \ldots + pr(X = 20)$$
$$= 1 - [pr(X = 0) + pr(X = 1)]$$

$$pr(X = 0) = \frac{20!}{0!(20-0)!} \ 0.05^0 0.95^{20-0} = (1)(1)0.95^{20} = 0.3585$$

$$pr(X = 1) = \frac{20!}{1!(20-1)!}0.05^1 0.95^{20-1} = (20)(0.05)0.95^{19} = 0.3774$$

$$pr(X \geq 1) = 1 - (0.3585 + 0.3774) = 0.2641$$

The probability that a healthy patient will have *at least one abnormal result* in 20 chemical determinations is approximately 0.26.

Part IV: Appropriateness of Binomial

This clinician has made a common error: the assumption of *independence* of outcomes does not apply in this case. If a patient responds favorably to ergotamine tartrate during the first migraine attack, he or she will likely experience relief during subsequent episodes. Thus, responses within the same patient *are not independent* from episode to episode. The design of this investigation precludes use of the binomial model.

9

Developing the Foundation for Testing Hypotheses

Clinical Example 1: Renal Cell Cancer

Approximately 27,000 new cases of renal cell cancer are diagnosed annually in the United States (Haas et al, 1993, p 177). One third of patients present with metastatic disease. Suppose that the mean survival time of patients with metastases who receive hormonal treatment and chemotherapy is 8 months (standard deviation of 4.4 months). Sixty patients with metastatic renal cell cancer were treated with interleukin-2 (IL-2) and followed until all died; the mean survival was 14.6 months. Did the use of IL-2 increase mean survival?

Clinical Example 2: Breast Cancer

The effectiveness of lumpectomy plus radiation and lumpectomy alone in preventing recurrence of breast tumors in women with ductal carcinoma in situ was examined. Eight hundred women with ductal carcinoma in situ were assigned randomly to receive either a lumpectomy alone or a lumpectomy plus radiation. After 5 years, 56 of the 400 women who received a lumpectomy alone had a recurrence of cancer in the surgically treated breast; 16 of 400 women who had lumpectomies plus radiation had recurrence in the treated breast. Does the frequency of tumor recurrence differ in women with ductal carcinoma who underwent lumpectomy and radiation compared to those who had lumpectomy alone?

What process should be used to determine if IL-2 therapy increased survival time in metastatic renal cell cancer patients, or if lumpectomy plus radiation differs from lumpectomy alone in preventing tumor recurrence in women with ductal carcinoma in situ? To address these questions, we turn our attention to **statistical inference**, a branch of statistics in which conclusions are drawn from a sample and extended to a population. The principles of statistical inference are considered in this chapter. These principles are illustrated in the next several chapters.

OBJECTIVES

When you complete this chapter, you should be able to:

- Explain the process used to test a hypothesis.
- Identify the scientific and statistical hypotheses from a description of a study.
- Describe the basis for rejecting or retaining the null hypothesis.
- Explain why retaining or rejecting the null hypothesis is *not* equivalent to asserting it is true or false.
- Discuss the difference between statistical significance and clinical importance.

REVIEW OF SELECTED CONCEPTS

To understand hypothesis testing, we must first understand certain basic concepts, such as population, sample, statistic, parameter, and probability. These concepts are reviewed below.

STATISTICAL INFERENCE

Statistical inference is a formal process that uses information from a sample to draw conclusions about a population. The terms **statistical inference, hypothesis testing,** and **significance testing** are often used interchangeably.

POPULATION

A population is the *complete set* of observations, patients, entities, or measurements about which we would like to draw conclusions (Minium et al, 1993, p 15). The **sampled population** is the population from which a sample is drawn. The **target population** is the population to which generalizations are made (Daniel, 1991, p 131). Findings from the sampled population can be extended to the target population only when the two populations closely resemble each other. For example, suppose a clinical trial is conducted to determine if a particular calcium channel blocker is effective in treating angina and high blood pressure in men. If 75 men with angina and high blood pressure are sampled randomly, generalizations should be extended to men with angina and high blood pressure. The sampled and target populations would differ if the results are extended to *men and women* with angina and high blood pressure.

SAMPLE

A sample is a subset of the population. The 75 men with angina and high blood pressure comprise the sample in the example above. One important assumption of hypothesis testing is that the sample is selected randomly from the population. A random sample represents all those who could have been included in a study. Random versus nonrandom sampling is discussed later in the chapter.

RANDOM SAMPLE

A random sample is selected from a population by any process governed by chance, such as drawing from a table of random numbers, rolling a die, flipping a coin, or spinning a roulette wheel. In a **simple random sample,** every possible sample of size n has the same probability of being selected from a population of size N (Daniel, 1991 p 103). In an **equiprobable sample**, every element in the population has an equal probability of selection. Two types of sampling plans exist: **sampling with** and **without replacement.** When **sampling with replacement** occurs, every element in the population is available for selection at each draw, regardless of whether the element has already been chosen. When **sampling without replacement** occurs, an element is not returned to the population once it has been chosen; therefore, it can be included only once in the sample. Keep in mind that sampling in medicine almost always occurs without replacement.

PARAMETER

A parameter is a numerical index that characterizes a population. Greek letters generally are used to designate parameters. For example, μ (mu) is the population mean; π (pi) is the population proportion, σ (sigma) is the population standard deviation.

STATISTIC

A statistic is a numerical index that characterizes the sample. Roman characters designate statistics. For example, $\overline{X}$ is the mean of a sample of X observations; p is the sample proportion, s is the sample standard deviation. Statistics estimate parameters. The sample mean, for example, is an estimate of the population mean; the sample proportion is an estimate of the population proportion. An **estimator** is a rule, such as a formula, that indicates how an estimate is computed. For example, the following formula is an **estimator** of the population mean, μ:

$$\overline{X} = \frac{\sum_{i=1}^{n} X_i}{n}$$

The value that results from the calculation is an estimate of the population mean (Daniel, 1991, p 130).

PROBABILITY

Probability is the relative frequency of an outcome from a very large number of independent trials.

PROBABILITY DISTRIBUTION

A probability distribution is a table or graph showing all possible outcomes of a variable, with their respective probabilities (Daniel, 1991, p 70).

VALIDITY

The validity of a study is discussed in terms of **internal and external** validity. An investigation is **valid internally** if differences between treatment groups or conditions can be attributed to the independent variable(s). Sampling procedures, operational definition of outcomes, experimental methods, and statistical analyses must be appropriate for a study to be valid internally. Internal validity is essential if findings are to be generalized beyond the sample from which they were obtained. **External validity** refers to the extent to which findings from a specific study can be extended or generalized from the sample to the target population. External validity depends upon the extent to which the sampled and target populations resemble each other with respect to important clinical and demographic characteristics.

HYPOTHESIS TESTING

Observation of phenomena leads to questions about what was observed. Questions are often formulated as hypotheses and additional observation is conducted to examine these hypotheses. Conclusions typically are generalized beyond the specific sample from which they were developed. The formalized procedures used to evaluate hypotheses and to generalize findings are referred to as **statistical inference**, **hypothesis testing**, or **significance testing.**

Six Step Process of Hypothesis Testing

Here are the 6 steps to test hypotheses:

1. State the scientific hypothesis.

2. Formulate the statistical hypotheses.

3. Specify the decision rule to evaluate the null hypothesis.
   a. Specify the test statistic.
   b. Identify the relevant sampling distribution and distribution of the test statistic.

    c. Identify the level of significance.
    d. Determine the critical region.

4. Analyze the data.

5. Evaluate the statistics.

6. Interpret the statistics.

We will now discuss each step in some detail.

Step 1: State the Scientific Hypothesis

The **scientific hypothesis**, also known as the research hypothesis, is a *testable* statement of findings anticipated, or hoped for, by the investigator. Developed from published studies or extensive clinical observation, the scientific hypothesis may be stated in general terms or in highly technical language, depending on the field of study. The following are examples of scientific hypotheses:

Early detection of prostate cancer will increase the proportion of men with prostate cancer who survive 5 years.

Use of a widely prescribed calcium channel blocker will lower the diastolic blood pressure of men with high blood pressure.

Administration of protease inhibitors to individuals with precancerous growths of the mouth will arrest progress of cells from precancerous to malignant.

Step 2: Formulate the Statistical Hypotheses

A *statistical hypothesis* is a statement about one or more population *parameters*. Hypothesis testing juxtaposes two contradictory statistical hypotheses: the **null** and **alternative** hypothesis.

The **null hypothesis**, designated H_0, is a statistical statement that a parameter equals a specified value or that the difference between two parameters is zero. The statistical statement indicates that no response, change, or difference is occurring. The null hypothesis is set up to be discredited or nullified, if possible, by data from a sample of observations. The null hypothesis is rejected or retained based on criteria specified before a study begins.

The **alternative hypothesis**, written H_A, is a statistical statement that addresses the same parameters given in the null hypothesis. The alternative hypothesis parallels the scientific hypothesis and contradicts the null hypothesis; and states that the value of a parameter is *different from, less than,* or *greater than* the value specified in the null hypothesis. When sample data are incompatible with the null hypothesis, we reject H_0. Then we conclude that the sample outcome supports the alternative hypothesis.

EXAMPLES OF SCIENTIFIC AND STATISTICAL HYPOTHESES

Example 1: Treating Parkinson's Disease

Scientific Hypothesis: The proportion of Parkinson's disease patients with full-blown disease who undergo an experimental surgical procedure and experience symptom improvement will be *greater than* the proportion in the population of Parkinson's disease patients with full-blown disease who receive L-dopa and carbidopa.

Statistical Hypotheses   Allow π (pi) to represent the proportion in the population of Parkinson's disease patients with full-blown disease who improve after receiving L-dopa and carbidopa. Assume that $\pi = 0.30$. Ten patients, selected randomly from the population of Parkinson's disease patients with full-blown disease, undergo experimental surgery in which pieces of the patient's own adrenal gland are pressed onto the brain. Eight of the 10 improve following surgery. The statistical hypotheses are:

$$H_0: \pi = 0.30$$

$$H_A: \pi > 0.30$$

The null hypothesis states, in essence, that the experimental surgery has the same chance of yielding improvement as drug therapy, that is, that 30% of patients will improve. The alternative hypothesis postulates that the proportion of patients who improve after surgery is greater than 0.30. The objective of hypothesis testing is to determine if the sample result is compatible with the null hypothesis.

Example 2: Metastatic Renal Cell Carcinoma

Scientific Hypothesis: Patients with metastatic renal cell cancer who are treated with interleukin-2 (IL-2) will live longer following diagnosis than patients with metastatic renal cell cancer who receive hormonal treatment and chemotherapy.

Statistical Hypotheses: Consider that it is well established that individuals who receive hormonal treatment and chemotherapy survive a mean of 8 months following diagnosis; therefore, the mean survival of 8 months is treated as the parameter of interest; that is, $\mu = 8$ months. Twenty-five individuals were randomly selected from the population of patients with metastatic renal cell cancer. After receiving IL-2, study participants were followed until all died; their mean survival was 14.8 months. The null and alternative hypotheses are:

$$H_0: \mu = 8 \text{ months}$$

$$H_A: \mu > 8 \text{ months}$$

Example 3: Lumpectomy Versus Lumpectomy Plus Radiation

Scientific Hypothesis: Among women with ductal carcinoma in situ who undergo a lumpectomy alone or lumpectomy plus radiation, a difference will exist between the proportion experiencing tumor recurrence in the treated breast within five years after treatment.

Statistical Hypotheses: Eight hundred women with ductal carcinoma in situ were sampled and assigned randomly to have lumpectomy alone or lumpectomy plus radiation. Within 5 years, 56 of the 400 women who had lumpectomy alone had recurrence of cancer in the treated breast; 16 of 400 women who had lumpectomies plus radiation had recurrence in the treated breast. Allow π to represent the proportion of women who experience tumor recurrence, L to indicate lumpectomy alone, and L/R to designate lumpectomy plus radiation. The statistical hypotheses are:

$$H_0: \pi_{L/R} - \pi_L = 0$$

$$H_A: \pi_{L/R} - \pi_L \neq 0$$

The null hypothesis postulates that no treatment differences exist between lumpectomy alone and lumpectomy plus radiation in the population of women with ductal carcinoma in situ. The alternative hypothesis postulates that a difference in tumor recurrence exists, but the direction of that difference (greater or less than) is unspecified. Sample data are used to determine if the null hypothesis is credible; if it is discredited, we rule in favor of the alternative hypothesis and conclude that a treatment difference exists.

Examples 1 and 2 differ from example 3 in two important ways:

1. In the first two examples, we compare a treatment outcome from one sample, representing one patient population, to the known value of a population parameter. The null hypothesis states that the sample outcome is compatible with the population parameter specified in the null hypothesis. In contrast, in example 3 we compare outcomes from two samples representing two treatment populations. The null hypothesis indicates *no difference between the two parameters,* in this case, no difference in efficacy between the two treatments.

2. The alternative hypotheses in examples 1 and 2 are *directional.* The alternative hypothesis in example 1 indicates that the proportion of patients demonstrating improvement following surgery will be greater than 0.30. Similarly, the alternative hypothesis in example 2 postulates that patients who receive IL-2 will survive longer, on average, than patients who receive hormonal treatment and chemotherapy. In contrast, the alternative hypothesis in example 3 is *nondirectional.* A difference in effectiveness is postulated, but the direction of that difference is not specified. In this case, there is no indication whether the difference between the two groups will be greater than zero (favoring lumpectomy plus radiation) or less than zero (favoring lumpectomy alone). We discuss the basis for developing directional and non-directional alternative hypotheses in "One- Versus Two-Tailed tests" later in the chapter.

Step 3: Specify the Decision Rule Used to Evaluate the Null Hypothesis

To specify the decision rule, identify the (1) test statistic, (2) relevant sampling distribution and the distribution of the test statistic, (3) level of significance, and (4) critical region of the sampling distribution or the distribution of the test statistic.

IDENTIFY THE TEST STATISTIC

The **test statistic** is computed from sample data and used to determine whether the null hypothesis should be rejected or retained. The test statistic may assume many values, depending on the sample selected. According to Daniel (1991, p 193), the general form of a test statistic is:

$$\text{Test Statistic} = \frac{\textbf{Sample Statistic} - \textbf{Hypothesized Parameter}}{\textbf{Standard Error of the Sample Statistic}}.$$

Standard error refers to the standard deviation of the distribution of the sample statistic. Several different test statistics, such as the z statistic and the Student's t, and their standard error are discussed in the next few chapters.

DETERMINE THE RELEVANT SAMPLING DISTRIBUTION AND DISTRIBUTION OF THE TEST STATISTIC

A **sampling distribution** is a relative frequency distribution of all possible values that could be assumed by some statistic. The sampling distribution is computed from all possible samples of the same size, drawn randomly from the same population (Daniel, 1991, p 106). In example 2 above, the sampling distribution is the relative frequency distribution of sample means that could result if all possible samples of size 25 were drawn randomly from the population of patients with metastatic renal cell cancer. The sampling distribution for example 1 is the relative frequency distribution of all possible sample proportions that could be computed from the population of Parkinson's disease patients with full-blown disease who are treated with

L-dopa and carbidopa. In contrast, if we are evaluating a null hypothesis about the difference between two means, as in example 3, the sampling distribution is the relative frequency distribution of all possible differences between two sample means. Keep in mind that sampling distributions are used to retain or reject the null hypothesis.

Sampling distributions can be created by enumeration or with formulae; both approaches are illustrated in Chapter 8. For example, we created a sampling distribution by arraying the relative frequency of the number of heads from all possible sequences of heads and tails on four tosses of a fair coin (Table 8–3). Because it is not feasible to sample human populations repeatedly to construct a sampling distribution by enumeration, we use formula-generated sampling distributions with well-documented properties. Sampling distributions are discussed further in the next chapter.

Like the sampling distribution, the *distribution of the test statistic* can be employed to evaluate the null hypothesis. The distribution consists of all possible values of the test statistic, plus their respective probabilities (relative frequencies). We compare the value of the test statistic computed from the sample to the critical value, in order to retain or reject the null hypothesis. This critical value is based in part on whether the alternative hypothesis is directional or nondirectional and the level of significance. The critical value is analogous to a cutoff point in diagnostic testing.

DETERMINE THE LEVEL OF SIGNIFICANCE

The **level of significance**, referred to as alpha and designated α, is used to determine values of the test statistic that cause us to reject or retain the null hypothesis. Alpha is the conditional probability of rejecting a true null hypothesis:

$$\alpha = pr(\text{Rejecting } H_0 | H_0 \text{ True}).$$

This conditional probability is known as a Type I error. Because rejecting a true null hypothesis is an error, α is set to a relatively small value, typically 0.05 or 0.01, or less frequently, 0.10. We discuss a Type I error in "Correct Decisions and Errors" later in this chapter.

IDENTIFY THE CRITICAL REGION

The **critical region**, also referred to as the **region of rejection**, is an area in the tail or tails of the distribution of the test statistic. This area is specified by α; thus, α is an area under the curve of the distribution of the test statistic. The region of rejection contains values of the test statistic that are relatively improbable, given the null hypothesis. Because values in this region deviate sufficiently from what is expected under the null hypothesis, they lead us to reject the null hypothesis. The values are probable, however, within the context of the alternative hypothesis. A sample result falling in the region of rejection is considered *significant,* that is, *statistically significant.*

The **region of retention** also resides under the curve of the distribution of the test statistic; this region contains values of the test statistic that are compatible with the null hypothesis. A sample result falling in this region causes us to retain the null hypothesis; in this case, we conclude that no effect, change, or difference exists. The *critical value* of the test statistic is the cutoff point that separates the region of rejection from the region of retention. The regions of rejection and retention, illustrated in Figures 9–1 to 9–3, are discussed further in "One- Versus Two-tailed Tests" later in the chapter.

Step 4: Analyze the Data

Data analysis begins when we check all data to verify their accuracy. We compute and examine descriptive statistics appropriate to the respective variables, for example, sample means and standard deviations for quantitative variables. Often we construct and examine graphs to identify interesting patterns. We also check assumptions underlying statistical tests to be used to analyze the data. Alternative statistical procedures are selected if key assumptions are violated. Finally, we analyze the data so that we may determine whether the data support the null or the alternative hypotheses.

Step 5: Evaluate the Statistics

The statistical results (step 4) are evaluated in light of the decision rules (step 3). The investigator rejects or retains the null hypothesis. If the null hypothesis is rejected, the investigator declares statistical significance. If the null hypothesis is retained, the researcher concludes that no significant difference exists between treatments, drugs, or procedures. These choices are illustrated in Table 9–1.

Step 6: Interpret the Statistics

The final step in testing hypotheses is to translate findings into appropriate clinical language.

Table 9–1. Interpretation of significance in test results.

Computed Value of Test Statistic	Statistical Decision	Status of the Null Hypothesis	Compatibility of Sample Value With Null Hypothesis	Interpretation of Sample Value
Falls in the region of rejection.	Results are significant statistically.	Reject the null hypothesis.	Sample value is not compatible with null hypothesis value.	Samples of data like those observed would occur rarely, if the null hypothesis were true.
Falls in the region of retention.	Results are not statistically significant.	Retain the null hypothesis.	Sample value is compatible with the null hypothesis value.	Samples of data like those observed would occur fairly often, if the null hypothesis were true.

OTHER CONSIDERATIONS IN HYPOTHESIS TESTING

We now consider some common questions about hypothesis testing. When can population parameters be specified, given that it is impossible in most situations to survey the entire population? What are the common decisions and errors in hypothesis testing? When we retain the null hypothesis, are we also accepting it as a true statement? Is rejecting the null hypothesis equivalent to saying it is false? When should we formulate a nondirectional alternative hypothesis, instead of a directional one? The answers to these questions are explored below.

Specifying Population Parameters

Statistical hypotheses are phrased in terms of population parameters. Because it is seldom possible to study an entire population to determine the value of the parameter(s) of interest, population parameters are determined from a large number of patients—hundreds, thousands, or hundreds of thousands, depending on the phenomenon of interest. Values computed from large numbers of individuals are employed as population parameters. Phrases like "based on extensive observation," "based on extensive data," or "analysis of charts of thousands of patients" often precede such values.

Correct Decisions and Errors

In hypothesis testing, two errors are possible. A true hypothesis can be rejected or a false hypothesis can be retained. These are referred to as a Type I and Type II error, respectively. A **Type I error** occurs when a true null hypothesis is rejected; the probability of such an error is noted by α:

$$\alpha = pr(\text{Reject } H_0 | H_0 \text{ True}).$$

The statement $\alpha = 0.05$ means that 5 times in 100, we will reject a true null hypothesis, that is, we will conclude erroneously that a significant difference exists. For example, a Type I error would be committed in clinical example 1 at the start of the chapter if we were to conclude that IL-2 administered to patients with metastatic renal cell cancer prolongs survival, when in actuality the mean survival of individuals who received IL-2 (14.8 months) results from chance fluctuation and *not* IL-2. When repeated samples are taken from the same population, chance or sampling fluctuation occurs because outcomes vary from sample to sample.

The **Type II error** occurs when a false null hypothesis is retained. A Type II error is represented by β:

$$\beta = pr(\text{Retain } H_0 | H_0 \text{ False}).$$

For example, we would commit a Type II error if we concluded that protease inhibitors administered to individuals with precancerous growths of the mouth do *not* arrest the progress of cells from precancerous to malignant, when in fact they do. In this case, it would be incorrect to retain the null hypothesis of no effect. Although investigators control the probability of a Type I error by the selection of α, they generally do not control the probability of a Type II error, even though it exceeds α in most cases (Daniel, 1991, p 194).

ANALOGIES TO DIAGNOSTIC TESTING

Potential decisions an investigator may make about the null hypothesis appear in Table 9–2. A Type I error (bottom left) occurs when a true null hypothesis is rejected. This error resembles a *false positive outcome,* which occurs when a clinical test result incorrectly indicates the presence of disease. A Type II error (top right cell) results when a false null hypothesis is retained. A Type II error is similar to a *false negative outcome,* in which a test result incorrectly signals the absence of disease. The complement of a Type II error, the bottom right cell, is **power.**

$$\text{Power} = 1 - \beta$$

Power if the ability of a statistical test to detect true differences when they occur. Power is analogous to sensitivity. A sensitive test accurately signals the presence of disease.

Table 9–2. Conditions of the null hypothesis and possible decisions an investigator may make.

	True Condition of H_0	
Possible Decision	H_0 True (No Difference Exists)	H_0 False (Differences Exist)
Retain H_0	Correct decision	Type II error (β)
Reject H_0	Type I error (α)	Correct decision (Power = $1 - \beta$)

Retaining Versus Rejecting the Null Hypothesis

If we retain the null hypothesis, what conclusions can we draw? Is the null hypothesis true? *Not necessarily!* Two possibilities exist when the null hypothesis has been retained. The null hypothesis is (1) true and should be retained or (2) false and should be rejected. In the first case, a correct decision occurs; in the latter, a Type II error is made because a false null hypothesis is retained. A Type II error may occur because they study design and experimental methods are not sufficiently powerful to detect a true difference.

A study that does not detect true differences may lack power because the experimental design is not optimal, the sample size is too small, measurement procedures result in large random or systematic error, or the sample does not represent the target population. If the evidence does not lead us to reject the null hypothesis, we have two options: we may retain the null hypothesis because it remains credible, or we may suspend judgment and repeat the study with a more powerful design.

If we reject the null hypothesis, can we conclude that it is false? *No!* Whenever an investigator rejects a null hypothesis, he or she runs the risk of committing a Type I error. In most studies, investigators select a value of α that is relatively small, frequently 0.05 or 0.01. Therefore, if we reject the null hypothesis, "we can take comfort from the fact that we made α small and, therefore, the probability of committing a type I error was small" (Daniel, 1991, p 194). Because of this fact, many individuals believe incorrectly that the null hypothesis is false. In short, the true condition of H_0 is never known. Therefore, we can never claim that a null hypothesis is true if retained or false if rejected. Thus, in every study, we run the risk of committing Type I and Type II errors.

One-Versus Two-tailed Tests

Alternative hypotheses are statistical statements that parallel the scientific hypothesis; they may be nondirectional or directional. A nondirectional alternative hypothesis indicates that the value of a parameter or the difference between two parameters is different from or not equal to the value in the null hypothesis. Scientific hypotheses like the following signal a nondirectional alternative hypothesis: "A *difference* will exist between . . . ," "An *association* will exist between . . . ," "A *relationship* will exist between . . . ," "A *change* will be noted in . . . ," or "The [value of the dependent variable] in the group receiving the experimental treatment *will differ* from . . . ." Nondirectional alternative hypotheses require **two-tailed statistical tests**. The region of rejection is divided equally between the upper and lower tails of the distribution of the test statistic. The area in each tail is $\alpha / 2$; the combined area equals α.

Figure 9–1 depicts the sampling distribution for the ductal carcinoma in situ research. This example illustrates the use of a two-tailed test.

Based on principles to be introduced in the next chapter, it is appropriate to draw the sampling distribution so that it resembles a normal curve. We can state the scientific hypothe-

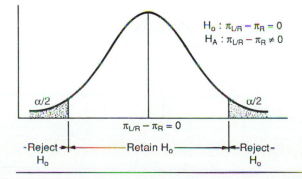

$$H_0 : \pi_{L/R} - \pi_R = 0$$
$$H_A : \pi_{L/R} - \pi_R \neq 0$$

$\alpha/2$ $\alpha/2$

$\pi_{L/R} - \pi_R = 0$

-Reject→|←—Retain H_0—→|←Reject-
  H_0 H_0

Figure 9–1. Sampling distribution for a two-tailed test of tumor recurrence.

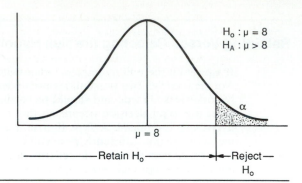

Figure 9–2. Sampling distribution for a one-tailed test of months survived.

sis this way: "Among women with ductal carcinoma in situ who undergo a lumpectomy alone or lumpectomy plus radiation, a difference will exist between the proportion experiencing tumor recurrence in the treated breast within 5 years after treatment." Observe that the mean of the sampling distribution is the value specified in the null hypothesis; in this example, the mean is zero (H_0: $\pi_{L/R} - \pi_L = 0$). The level of significance, α, is apportioned equally in each tail, so that the area in each tail is $\alpha/2$. Any difference between the two sample proportions that falls within the shaded area in either tail of the sampling distribution leads us to reject the null hypothesis and to conclude that a significant difference exists between the two proportions. Alternately, if a difference between the two sample proportions is captured in the unshaded area, we retain the null hypothesis and conclude that no difference exists between the two treatments.

Unlike their nondirectional counterparts, directional alternative hypotheses postulate that the value of the parameter or difference between two parameters will be greater or less than the value postulated in the null hypothesis. Scientific hypotheses that include phrases like "more than," "direct," "indirect," "better than," "worse than," "less than," "decreased," "increased," "longer than," and "fewer than," point to a directional alternative hypothesis. Directional alternative hypotheses lead to **one-tailed statistical tests** in which the entire region of rejection resides in the upper or lower tail of the sampling distribution. Figures 9–2 and 9–3 are examples of sampling distributions for directional alternative hypotheses.

Figure 9–2 corresponds to the study of metastatic renal cell carcinoma cited earlier. In this example, the scientific hypotheses is: "Among patients with metastatic renal cell cancer, those treated with interleukin-2 will live longer following diagnosis than those who receive hormonal treatment and chemotherapy."

Based on extensive data, the investigators chose 8 months to represent the mean survival of all patients who receive hormonal treatment and chemotherapy for ductal carcinoma in situ. Thus, the mean of the sampling distribution is 8 months (H_0: $\mu = 8$ months). Even if it were to fall in the extreme lower tail of the distribution, a sample mean in the unshaded area would lead us to retain the null hypothesis. Any sample mean that falls in the upper tail of the distribution, however, would lead us to reject the null hypothesis; in this latter case, the evidence would support the alternative hypothesis. We would then conclude that the mean survival time of patients receiving IL-2 is significantly greater than 8 months.

Figure 9–3 shows a sampling distribution for a one-tailed test of influenza development.

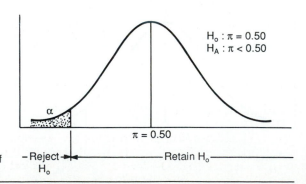

Figure 9–3. Sampling distribution for a one-tailed test of influenza development.

Here we see an alternative hypothesis that postulates a "less than" scenario. Suppose that 50% of individuals, ages 70 to 80 years, contract a particular type of influenza that causes substantial mortality. An experimental vaccine is administered to a random sample of individuals in this age group prior to the beginning of the flu season. It is hypothesized that fewer cases of influenza will occur in vaccinated persons. Note that the region of rejection occurs entirely in the lower tail of the sampling distribution. A sample proportion falling in this region (1) does not support the null hypothesis and (2) suggests a significant decrease in the proportion of vaccinated patients who develop influenza.

We use a one-tailed test when we have sufficient information to formulate a directional scientific hypothesis and a directional alternative hypothesis. Such information usually comes from research, extensive clinical observation, published literature, or pilot studies. A one-tailed test implies that the researcher is not interested in a "deviant" sample value that occurs in the direction *opposite* to that postulated in the alternative hypothesis. Look again at the influenza example depicted in Figure 9–3; suppose that 80% of individuals who receive the experimental vaccine develop influenza. Although this may occur by chance, the result may also be extremely important clinically. According to the formalized rules of hypothesis testing, however, the investigator must retain the null hypothesis, despite this potentially worrisome sample outcome.

Nondirectional alternative hypotheses require a two-tailed statistical test. A two-tailed test is conducted when a researcher wants to determine whether a significant difference exists, regardless of whether the difference exceeds or falls short of the value in the null hypothesis. We formulate a nondirectional alternative hypothesis when literature published on the phenomenon of interest is scarce, and therefore knowledge is not adequate to support a directional statement; published studies contain contradictory results; published investigations are designed poorly and lack validity; or a directional hypothesis may be of interest, but we cannot exclude the possibility of an unexpected and contrary outcome. Because the possibility of an unexpected effect cannot be excluded with 100% certainty, nondirectional alternative hypotheses and two-tailed statistical tests may represent a more ethical choice—unless detection of a paradoxical outcome has no clinical significance.

Unexpected Outcomes With Serious Consequences

Students sometimes argue that unexpected results with serious consequences never occur in the "real world," if animal or small-scale human trials produce promising results. Events that occurred in 1993 suggest otherwise. That year, a major pharmaceutical company released findings about a pilot test of an experimental drug to treat hepatitis B; the test had been conducted in rodents, dogs, and humans. The findings were reported by the Associated Press wire service. Various newspapers in the United States carried the AP report or a version of it. According to an article in the *Champaign-Urbana News-Gazette* (July 7, 1993), results of the pilot study were so promising that "scientists thought they were testing a miracle drug." When researchers at the National Institutes of Health, however, subsequently tested the drug in 15 patients with hepatitis, 3 experienced severe liver damage. Two patients required liver transplants; both died. Seven other patients developed abnormal liver function. Based on these results, the clinical trial was halted. Thus, clinicians and researchers must always be aware that unexpected outcomes may occur. When they do occur, ethical considerations must receive the highest priority.

Random Versus Nonrandom Sampling

Statistical inference rests on the assumption that data have been obtained from a random sample (Daniel, 1991, p 131). Because it often is impossible or impractical to sample randomly from a defined population, medical researchers and investigators in other fields often rely on "convenience" or "grab" samples. A convenience sample contains individuals who are available to participate in a study. A grab sample is synonymous with a convenience sample; the investigator "grabs" readily available participants. Generalizations from studies in which random sampling was not done "may be useful or they may range from misleading to disastrous" because study participants may not represent the target population (Daniel, 1991, p 132). Findings from such studies may have limited external validity. Thus, care must be taken to generalize findings only to populations with clinical and demographic characteristics identical to those of study participants.

In some investigations, the researcher may be able to introduce randomization even though a sample was not selected randomly from the population. Randomization is also referred to as random assignment; study participants are assigned to treatment conditions by chance so that each individual has an equal likelihood of being placed in each condition. Random assignment may be accomplished by using a table of random numbers, flipping a fair coin, rolling a die, or other similar process. Many investigators believe that random assignment permits broad generalization of findings to individuals whose clinical and demographic characteristics are the same as persons who participate in the study.

Statistical Significance

The results of statistical tests must be interpreted and generalized with great care. Keep in mind that grave errors can occur when the appropriateness of a treatment is equated with statistical significance (Hays, 1981, p 265). A significant result indicates only that an unlikely outcome has occurred, given the null hypothesis. Statistical significance does not guarantee that an important or clinically meaningful outcome has occurred. The clinician and researcher must make decisions about the clinical importance of an outcome in light of accumulated experience.

SUMMARY

A statistical test, hypothesis test, or significance test compares two statistical hypotheses, the null and alternative, based on sample evidence. We formulate the null and alternative hypotheses in terms of population parameters. The null hypothesis postulates that no effect, change, or difference exists. The alternative hypothesis may be directional or nondirectional. We formulate directional alternative hypotheses when (1) extant knowledge justifies a "greater" or "less than" statement and (2) detection of a paradoxical outcome has no clinical import. After the scientific and statistical hypotheses are formulated, the sampling distribution and test statistic are specified, the level of significance is stated, and the critical region of the distribution of the test statistic is identified. One or more samples is selected randomly from one or more defined populations. The sample statistic, such as the sample mean or proportion, is computed and used to calculate the test statistic. The computed value of the test statistic is compared to the critical value. If the computed value falls in the region of rejection, we reject the null hypothesis and declare statistical significance. If the computed value falls in the region of retention, we retain the null hypothesis.

Hypothesis testing is based on the assumption that study participants have been chosen randomly. The chance that study participants represent the population increases with random sampling. Assuming an investigation is valid internally, findings obtained from random samples can be extended to the target population with some confidence. Caution is required when interpreting findings from nonrandomized studies because nonrandom samples may not represent the target population.

Statistical significance offers no guarantee that outcomes are clinically meaningful. Therefore, statistical significance should never be equated with the import or worth of an outcome or treatment. Accumulated experience must be combined with results from statistical tests to assess the usefulness of a particular outcome or intervention.

REFERENCES

Champaign-Urbana News-Gazette. Deaths pose mystery in tests of drug. July 7, 1993.

Daniel W: *Biostatistics: A Foundation for Analysis in the Health Sciences,* 5th ed. Wiley, 1991.

Haas G, Hillman G, Redman B, Pontes J: Immunotherapy of renal cell carcinoma. *CA* 1993;**43**:177.

Hays W: *Statistics,* 3rd ed. Holt, Rinehard and Winston, 1981.

Minium E, King B, Bear G: *Statistical Reasoning in Psychology and Education,* 3rd ed. Wiley, 1993.

Self-study Questions

Part I: Definitions

1. Define each of the following terms:

Alternative hypothesis	Scientific hypothesis
Critical region	Statistical hypothesis
Level of significance	Statistical inference
Null hypothesis	(hypothesis testing,
One-tailed test	significance testing)
Power	Test statistic
Region of retention (region	Two-tailed test
of rejection)	Type I error
Sampling distribution	Type II error

2. Describe the six-step process to test hypotheses.

Part II: Study Descriptions

Read each of the following descriptions and write the scientific hypothesis; identify the independent and dependent variables; and indicate whether a one- or two-tailed statistical test is warranted.

1. The proportion of patients who survive 2 years after treatment of colorectal cancer that has metastasized to the liver was evaluated in 2 patient groups. One group received 5-fluorodeoxyuridine (FUDR) intra-arterially (IA); the other group received it intravenously (IV). At the end of 2 years, 20% of patients in the IA group were alive compared to 14% in the IV group.

2. It is well documented that alcoholics have an increased risk of death following accidents involving severe burns. Two clinicians evaluated mortality in alcoholics and nonalcoholics admitted to the burn unit of an urban hospital. Nine of 28 alcoholics died; 8 of 75 nonalcoholics died.

3. Investigators compared the levels of self-reported psychiatric symptomatology in 2 groups of patients with chest pain. One group had coronary artery disease (CAD+); no evidence of coronary artery disease was found in the other group (CAD−). The researchers administered a standardized and reliable psychiatric test to measure depression. The maximum possible score is 100; the higher the score, the more clinically significant the depression. The mean score for CAD+ patients was 86.3 ($s = 11.2$); the mean score in the CAD− group was 68.5 ($s = 9.7$).

4. Investigators studied the use of interferon to treat chronic granulocytic leukemia (CGL). They hypothesized that interferon will reduce the excessive accumulation of leukocytes in the bone marrow, reduce the white blood cell count to the normal range, and decrease the platelet count, if elevated, to the normal range. After 12 months of treatment, 26 to 67 patients exhibited outcomes consistent with hypothesized results.

5. The relationship between parental smoking and number of colds per year was examined in nonsmoking teenagers. Nonsmoking teens in households where both parents smoke had 3 times the number of colds in 1 year compared to nonsmoking teens in households whether neither parent smokes.

6. Researchers hypothesized that men with high blood pressure (HBP) are at greater risk of death than men with low blood pressure (LBP). For 10 years, 1727 men ages 50 to 79 years were followed. In the HBP group, 33% of men died; in the LBP group, 27% of men died.

7. The association between fluid intake and bladder cancer was investigated in men age 55 years or younger. One thousand seventy men were followed for 15 years, beginning in 1975. Men who drank 14 or more cups of fluid per day were 6 times more likely to develop bladder cancer than men who drank 7 cups or less.

8. Clinicians hypothesized that babies born to HIV-positive mothers are less apt to test HIV positive at birth if they are delivered by cesarean section. In one study of children born to HIV-positive mothers, investigators found that 15% of babies delivered by cesarean section were HIV positive, compared to 32% of babies delivered vaginally.

9. Investigators hypothesize that between 1960 and 1990 mortality per 1000 white men in the United States decreased, as average years of education among white males increased. Among 43,000 Caucasian men in 1960, there were 9 deaths per 1000 Caucasion men who did not finish high school, 8 deaths per 1000 Caucasian men who finished high school only, and 5 deaths per 1000 Caucasian men who graduated from college. Among 60,000 Caucasian men in 1990, the deaths per 1000 were 7, 6, and 3, respectively.

10. Extensive research confirms that the well-being of infants and youngsters improved between 1985 and 1990. Therefore, two clinicians hypothesize that the well-being of teenagers will follow the same pattern. The following results come from a 1990 nationwide survey of teenagers. The number of teens finishing high school in 4 years declined to 69% in 1990 from 75% in 1985. Arrests for juvenile violent crime increased from 314 per 100,000 teens in 1986 to 470 per 100,000 in 1990. Teen death from accident, suicide, or homicide increased 15% between 1985 and 1990.

Solutions

Part II: Study Descriptions

1. *Scientific hypothesis:* The proportion of patients who survive 2 years following treatment of colorectal cancer that metastatized to the liver differs between the group of patients receiving 5-fluorodeoxyuridine (FUDR) intra-arterially and those receiving it intravenously.
   Independent variable: 5-fluorodeoxyuridine (FUDR) administered intra-arterially or intravenously.
   Dependent variable: Two-year survival (yes/no).
   One- or two-tailed: Two-tailed because no statement of increased or decreased survival is made.

2. *Scientific hypothesis:* A greater proportion of alcoholics, compared to nonalcoholics, die following accidents in which severe burns are sustained.
   Independent variable: Alcoholic status (alcoholic versus nonalcoholic). (Many individuals believe that the independent variable must be manipulated by the investigator and must have multiple levels, such as different doses of a drug, or many conditions, such as different routes of drug delivery as in question 1, above. The independent variable, however, need not be manipulated experimentally or have multiple levels or conditions; a characteristic or event, such as accidents, may affect an outcome.)
   Dependent variable: Death (yes/no).
   One- or two-tailed: One-tailed because an increased risk of death is hypothesized for alcoholics.

3. *Scientific hypothesis:* The level of psychiatric symptomatology will differ between two groups of patients with chest pain, one group with coronary artery disease and the other without this disease.
   Independent variable: Presence or absence of coronary artery disease in patients with chest pain.
   Dependent variable: Self-reported psychiatric symptomatology, specifically, depression.
   One- or two-tailed: Two-tailed because no direction is specified; the investigators postulated only that a difference exists.

4. *Scientific hypothesis:* In patients with granulocytic leukemia, interferon reduces the excessive accumulation of leukocytes in the bone marrow, white blood cell count to the normal range, and platelet count, if elevated, to the normal range.
   Independent variable: Interferon treatment.
   Dependent variable: There are 3 dependent variables: number of leukocytes in the bone marrow, white blood cell count, and platelet count.
   One- or two-tailed: One-tailed for each dependent variable.

5. *Scientific hypothesis:* A relationship exists between parental smoking (smokers versus nonsmokers) and number of colds per year in nonsmoking teenagers.
   Independent variable: Smoking status of parents (smoker versus nonsmoker).
   Dependent variable: Number of colds in a 12-month period.
   One- or two-tailed: Two-tailed; a relationship is postulated between the independent and dependent variable, but no direction is stated. For example, it is not hypothesized that nonsmoking teens whose parents both smoke will have a greater number of colds per year than nonsmoking teens whose parents are nonsmokers.

6. *Scientific hypothesis:* Men ages 50 to 79 years with high blood pressure are at a greater risk of death than similarly aged men with low blood pressure. The scientific hypothesis could also be stated more specifically: Among men between the ages of 50 and 79 years, a greater proportion who have high blood pressure will die in the next 10 years, compared to the proportion with low blood pressure.
   Independent variable: Blood pressure (high versus low).
   Dependent variable: Death (yes/no) in the 10-year follow-up period.
   One- or two-tailed: One tailed; men with high blood pressure are at greater risk of death than men with low blood pressure.

7. *Scientific hypothesis:* An association exists between fluid intake and bladder cancer in men ages 55 years or younger.
   Independent variable: Fluid intake (14 or more cups per day versus 7 cups or fewer per day).
   Dependent variable: Bladder cancer development (yes/no) during follow-up period.
   One or two-tailed: Two-tailed because no directional findings are hypothesized.

8. *Scientific hypothesis:* Babies born to HIV-positive mothers will be less apt to test HIV positive at birth if they are delivered by cesarean section. The scientific hypothesis may also be written: Among babies born to HIV-positive mothers, the proportion who are HIV positive at birth will be less if the baby is delivered by cesarean section.

9. *Scientific hypothesis:* As average years of education increased, a decrease occured in mortality per 1000 Caucasian males in the United States between 1960 and 1990.
   Independent variable: Years of education (did not finish high school; finished high school only; graduated from college).
   Dependent variables: Mortality per 1000 Caucasian men in 1960 and 1990.
   One- or two-tailed: One-tailed.

10. *Scientific hypothesis:* The well-being of teenagers improved between 1985 and 1990.
    Independent variable: Age group (teenage).
    Dependent variable: Three dependent variables are used as measures of well-being: teen high school completion; teen arrests for juvenile violent crime; and teen death from accident, suicide, or homicide.
    One or two-tailed: One-tailed test for each dependent variable.

10   Testing Hypotheses About One Mean

Clinical Example: Fetal Alcohol Exposure

The relationship between fetal alcohol exposure and infant development was examined in 31 randomly selected, female infants born to women who drank the equivalent of 2 drinks containing 1.5 ounces of alcohol 5 or more times per week, during at least 7 months of their pregnancy. The mean birthweight of these infants was 2.5 kg, with a standard deviation of 0.54 kg, compared to 3.3 kg for female infants in the general population. The fetal-alcohol-exposed infants tripled their birthweight at a mean of 15 months, with a standard deviation of 2.7 months, compared to 12 months for female infants in the general population.

Based on these findings, does the mean birthweight of female, fetal-alcohol-exposed infants differ from that of female newborns in the general population? Does the mean age at which female, fetal-alcohol-exposed infants triple their birthweight differ from the corresponding mean age of female infants in the general population? The statistical tools used to answer questions like these are presented in this chapter.

OBJECTIVES

When you complete this chapter, you should be able to:

- Distinguish between one- and two-tailed statistical tests.
- Differentiate between the use of the z and Student's t statistics and select the appropriate one to test hypotheses about one mean.
- Conduct a test of the hypothesis that H_0: $\mu = \mu_0$.
- Use nonstatistical language to explain the results of hypothesis tests about one mean.

SAMPLING DISTRIBUTION OF MEANS

The **sampling distribution of means** is a relative frequency distribution of all possible values that can be assumed by the sample mean, computed from all possible samples of the same size drawn randomly from the same population. If the population is finite, we generate the sampling distribution by drawing all possible samples of size n from a defined population, computing the mean for each sample, and tabling or graphing the sample means and their respective relative frequencies. As pointed out in Chapter 9, however, it is not feasible to sample human populations repeatedly. Therefore, in statistical inference, we use theoretically generated sampling distributions with well-documented properties.

To describe the sampling distribution of means, we must assess whether the population is distributed normally or nonnormally. Students often ask how they can tell whether a population is distributed normally or nonnormally. Clinical experience is the best guide. For example, the population of ages at onset of Alzheimer's disease is skewed negatively because the disease does not occur until later in life. In this and subsequent chapters, the shape of the population (normal or nonnormal) will be noted, when it is central to selecting the appropriate test statistic.

If the population is distributed normally, the sampling distribution of means will be distributed normally. The **mean of the sampling distribution of means** is $\mu_{\bar{X}}$. We obtain it by summing all sample means and dividing by their number:

$$\mu_{\bar{X}} = \frac{\Sigma \bar{X}}{\textbf{Number of Sample Means}}. \qquad \textbf{10.1}$$

When simplified, Formula 10.1 equals:

$$\mu_{\bar{X}} = \mu_X. \qquad \textbf{10.2}$$

The mean of the sampling distribution of means equals the population mean. The **standard deviation of the sampling distribution of means,** referred to as the **standard error of the mean,** is $\sigma_{\bar{X}}$:

$$\sigma_{\bar{X}} = \sqrt{\frac{\Sigma(\bar{X} - \mu_{\bar{X}})^2}{\textbf{Number of Sample Means}}}. \qquad \textbf{10.3}$$

Formula 10.3, when simplified, equals:

$$\sigma_{\bar{X}} = \frac{\sigma_X}{\sqrt{n}}, \qquad \textbf{10.4}$$

where σ_X is the population standard deviation and n is the sample size. Hays (1981, pp 185–187) demonstrates the algebra used to simplify Formulas 10.1 and 10.3.

In summary, when sampling from a normally distributed population, the sampling distribution of means has the following characteristics (Daniel, 1991, pp 109–110):

- The sampling distribution of means is distributed normally.
- The mean of the sampling distribution of means equals the population mean, $\mu_{\bar{X}} = \mu_X$.
- The standard deviation of the sampling distribution of means, known as the standard error of the mean, equals the population standard deviation divided by the square root of the sample size: $\sigma_{\bar{X}} = \frac{\sigma_X}{\sqrt{n}}$.

What are the characteristics of the sampling distribution, when sampling is from a population that is distributed nonnormally? The **Central Limit Theorem** provides the answer (Hays, 1981, p 217):

> Given a population that is not distributed normally with mean μ and variance σ^2, the distribution of sample means approaches a normal distribution with mean μ and variance σ_n^2 as sample size increases. When the sample size is large, the sampling distribution of means is approximately normal.

The Central Limit Theorem allows us to sample from a population that is not distributed normally, with a guarantee that the sampling distribution will be approximately normal—provided the sample is large. How large is large? Daniel (1991, p 110) indicates: "One rule of thumb states that, in most practical situations, a sample of size 30 is satisfactory."

When sampling from a population that is not distributed normally, the sampling distribution of means has the following characteristics:

- The sampling distribution is approximately normal, if n is equal to or greater than 30. The approximation to normality improves as sample size increases.
- The mean of the sampling distribution of means equals the population mean, $\mu_{\bar{X}} = \mu_X$.
- The standard deviation of the sampling distribution of means, referred to as the standard error of the mean, equals the population standard deviation divided by the square root of the sample size, $\sigma_{\bar{X}} = \frac{\sigma_X}{\sqrt{n}}$.

Thus, the characteristics of the sampling distribution are the same, regardless of whether the population is distributed normally or nonnormally, as long $n \geq 30$. Individuals interested in an illustration of the Central Limit Theorem should consult Colton (1974, pp 106–108). The importance of the Central Limit Theorem will become apparent later in this chapter, when we discuss sampling from a nonnormal population and choosing the appropriate test statistic to examine a hypothesis about the population mean.

We assume in generating the sampling distribution of means that an infinite population is sampled or that sampling is with replacement. In medicine, however, finite populations are sampled, and sampling without replacement is the norm. When finite populations are sampled, the variance of the sampling distribution of means should be multiplied by the finite population correction factor (fpc):

$$\text{fpc} = (N - n)/N - 1) \text{ and}$$

$$\sigma^2_{\bar{X}} = \frac{\sigma^2_X}{n}\left(\frac{N - n}{N - 1}\right).$$

Most statisticians do not use the correction factor unless the sample contains more than 5% of the observations in the population, because its use produces a negligible change in the variance of the sampling distribution of means (Daniel, 1991, p 111). Individuals working with samples containing more than 5% of the observations in the population should consult a statistician to determine if the correction factor should be employed. We do not use the correction factor in this chapter because we assume that the populations are quite large and that samples are small, relative to size of the population.

TESTING HYPOTHESES ABOUT ONE MEAN

Testing hypotheses about one mean is explored under three different conditions: when sampling from a population that is (1) distributed normally with known variance, (2) distributed normally with unknown variance, and (3) distributed nonnormally. Regardless of whether the population is distributed normally or nonnormally, the null hypothesis is:

$$H_0: \mu = \mu_0, \qquad\qquad 10.5$$

where μ_0 is the value of the population mean (eg, 3.3 kg or 12 months) as in the hypothetical clinical example at the beginning of the chapter. The alternative hypothesis may be either nondirectional or directional:

$$H_A: \mu \neq \mu_0 \text{ Nondirectional, not equal to} \qquad\qquad 10.6$$

$$H_A: \mu > \mu_0 \text{ Directional, greater than}$$

$$H_A: \mu < \mu_0 \text{ Directional, less than}$$

In the following sections, we present examples of testing hypotheses under each of the three conditions noted above.

Normally Distributed Population With Known Variance

Clinical Example: Lead Exposure in Children

Twenty-five randomly sampled children who have lived from birth to age 12 years within 2 miles of a lead smelter are studied to determine if chronic exposure to a lead smelting operation adversely affects performance on a standardized intelligence test. Children in the study group are compared to 12-year-old children in the general population. The mean IQ of children in the study group is 90, with a standard deviation of 14; the mean IQ of 12-year-old children in the general population is 100, with a standard deviation of 16.

We will walk through the 6-step process for testing hypotheses. In this hypothetical example, our goal is to determine if the performance of children in the study group is comparable to that of the children in the general population, or if the performance of the study group has been affected adversely.

1. State the Scientific Hypothesis

The performance on a standardized intelligence test of 12-year-old children who have lived from birth to 12 years within 2 miles of a lead smelting operation will be less than that of 12-year-old children in the general population. A directional hypothesis is chosen, because substantial published evidence suggests that lead exposure adversely affects children.

2. Formulate the Statistical Hypotheses

$$H_0: \mu = 100$$
$$H_A: \mu < 100$$

3. Specify the Decision Rule Used to Evaluate the Null Hypothesis

The first step is to identify the test statistic to be used to test the null hypothesis. Because the population distribution is normal and the population variance is known, the z statistic applies. Recall from Chapter 9 that the general form of a test statistic is:

$$\text{Test Statistic} = \frac{\text{Sample Statistic} - \text{Hypothesized Parameter}}{\text{Standard Error of the Sample Statistic}}$$

The sample statistic is $\overline{X}$; the hypothesized parameter is μ. The standard error of the sample statistic is the standard error of the mean, $\sigma_{\overline{X}}$. The z statistic is, therefore:

$$z = \frac{\overline{X} - \mu_0}{\sigma_{\overline{X}}}, \text{ where } \sigma_{\overline{X}} = \frac{\sigma_X}{\sqrt{n}}. \qquad 10.7$$

Note that although the sample standard deviation is known, it does not figure into Formula 10.7.

Next, identify the relevant sampling distribution and the distribution of the test statistic. The relevant sampling distribution is the sampling distribution of means. The test statistic, z, is distributed as a standard normal deviate. Thus, the distribution of the test statistic is the standard normal curve. The table of the standard normal curve is used to identify the critical value of z that separates the region of retention from rejection.

Identify the level of significance and determine the critical region. Allow α, the level of significance, to equal 0.05. The critical value of z is obtained from Table A–1 in the appendix of statistical tables. Look for the area of 0.05 in the column labeled "one-tailed area" and identify the corresponding value of z. The area of 0.05 is halfway between the one-tailed areas of 0.0505 ($z = 1.64$) and 0.0495 ($z = 1.65$). Therefore, the critical value of z is -1.645. This value is negative because the alternative hypothesis is a "less than" statement. Figure 10–1 contains the distribution of the test statistic for this example.

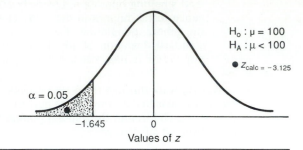

Figure 10–1. Standard normal distribution to examine children's exposure to a lead smelting operation, $\alpha = 0.05$.

4. Analyze the Data

Summary data and calculations appear in Box 10–1. The standard error of the mean is calculated and used in the denominator of the z test. The calculated value of z is -3.1250.

5. Evaluate the Statistics

The calculated value of z is shown in Figure 10–1. Compare it (z_{calc}) to the critical value (z_{crit}) and make a decision about the hypotheses. The null hypothesis is rejected, because the calculated value of z falls in the region of rejection. Thus, the data support the alternative hypothesis.

A decision about the null hypothesis can also be made by comparing the probability of the sample result to α. The obtained probability, known as a **p-value**, is the probability of obtaining a result as extreme or more extreme than the sample value, assuming that the null hypothesis is true (Rosner, 1986, p 187). Decisions are made about the null hypothesis as follows:

$$p - \text{value} \le \alpha \Rightarrow \text{Reject } H_0$$

$$p - \text{value} > \alpha \Rightarrow \text{Retain } H_0$$

To determine the p-value for our example, use Table A–1. Find the absolute value of z_{calc} and identify the appropriate area. Remember that areas for negative and positive values of z are the same because the normal curve is symmetric. If H_A is directional, use the one-tailed

Box 10–1. Analysis of data from 12-year-old children living in close proximity to a lead smelter.

Hypotheses	$H_0 : \mu = 100$
	$H_A : \mu < 100$
Population distribution	Normal
Population mean	100
Population standard deviation	16
Sample mean	90
Sample standard deviation[a]	14
Sample size	25
Standard error of the mean	$\sigma_{\bar{x}} = \dfrac{16}{\sqrt{25}} = 3.20$
Critical value of z for a one-tailed test with $\alpha = 0.05$	-1.645
Test statistic	$z = \dfrac{90 - 100}{3.2} = -3.1250$
p-value	$p \approx 0.0009$
Decision	Reject the null hypothesis

[a]Sample standard deviation is not used because the population standard deviation is known.

area; if H_A is nondirectional, select the two-tailed area. Keep in mind that the area in the tail is the probability of obtaining a result as extreme or more extreme than the sample value, given the null hypothesis. In our example, the calculated value of z is -3.125. Round down to -3.12; find 3.12 in Table A–1 and read the corresponding one-tailed area, which is 0.0009. This area (0.0009) is the p-value. Thus, the chance of obtaining a sample mean of 90 or less is approximately 9 times in 10,000, if the true population mean is 100. Because the p-value is less than α (0.05), we reject the null hypothesis.

6. Interpret the Statistics

The mean score on a standardized intelligence test of 12-year-old children who have lived from birth to age 12 years within 2 miles of a lead smelter is significantly less than that of 12-year-olds in the general population (p-value ≈ 0.0009).

Note the p-value in parentheses in our conclusion. An increasing number of journals require that investigators include p-values in their manuscripts. When p-values are given, we are able to compare this probability to our own decision rule and make an independent decision about statistical significance. For example, consider that an individual wishes to evaluate the lead smelter results with $\alpha = 0.01$. By comparing the p-value (0.0009) to α (0.01), she determines that the results are still significant statistically, even using a decision rule that is more conservative than $\alpha = 0.05$.

Normally Distributed Population With Unknown Variance

We repeat the example from the beginning of the chapter and use it to illustrate a second type of one-mean hypothesis test.

Clinical Example: Fetal Alcohol Exposure

The relationship between fetal alcohol exposure and infant development was examined in 31 randomly selected, female infants born to women who drank the equivalent of 2 drinks containing 1.5 ounces of alcohol 5 or more times per week, during at least 7 months of their pregnancy. The mean birthweight of these infants was 2.5 kg, with a standard deviation of 0.54 kg, compared to 3.3 kg for female newborns in the general population. The fetal-alcohol-exposed infants tripled their birthweight at a mean of 15 months, with a standard deviation of 2.7 months, compared to 12 months for female infants in the general population.

1. State the Scientific Hypothesis

Because the study was conducted before clinicians understood the effects of fetal alcohol exposure on birthweight and development, the investigators believed that nondirectional scientific and alternative hypotheses were appropriate. Therefore they hypothesized that, compared to female infants in the general population, female infants born to mothers who consumed 2 drinks containing 1.5 ounces of alcohol (or the equivalent) 5 or more times per week, during at least 7 months of their pregnancy, will differ in mean birthweight and the mean age at which birthweight triples.

2. Formulate the Statistical Hypotheses

Birthweight	Age at Which Birthweight Triples
H_0: μ = 3.3 kg	H_0: μ = 12 months
H_A: $\mu \neq$ 3.3 kg	H_A: $\mu \neq$ 12 months

3. Specify the Decision Rule to be Used to Evaluate the Null Hypothesis

Although the relevant population distributions are normal, the z statistic (Formula 10.7) cannot be used in this example because the population variance is unknown. A relative of the z statistic, the t statistic or Student's t, is employed when the population variance is not known and is estimated from sample data. Because σ_x is unknown, the standard error of the mean is also estimated from sample data. In this case, then, it is written $s_{\bar{X}}$, rather than $\sigma_{\bar{X}}$. The Student's t statistic is:

$$t = \frac{\bar{X} - \mu_0}{s_{\bar{X}}} \text{ with df} = n - 1 \text{ and } s_{\bar{X}} = \frac{s_X}{\sqrt{n}} \qquad 10.8$$

The concept of degrees of freedom, designated df, is discussed in the next section. The sampling distribution is the sampling distribution of means. The distribution of the test statistic is the Student's t distribution with $n-1$ degrees of freedom. Table A–2 in the appendix of statistical tables is used to identify the critical value of t. The calculated value of t is compared to the critical value and a decision is made about the null hypothesis. An explanation of how to use the Student's t table follows a brief description of the Student's t distribution.

Degrees of Freedom **Degrees of freedom** refers to the number of values free to vary when computing a statistic (Vogt, 1993, p 64). For example, in computing the sample variance, we indicate that there are $n-1$ degrees of freedom, and place this quantity in the denominator of the formula. The sample variance is $s_X^2 = \frac{\Sigma(X - \bar{X})^2}{(n - 1)}$. We know from Chapter 3 that $\Sigma(X - \bar{X}) = 0$, that is, the sum of deviations of values about their mean is zero. When the value of $n - 1$ of the observations is known, the value of the nth observation is determined, because the n deviations about the mean must add to zero. Suppose that four observations ($n = 4$) are drawn from a population; their mean is 10 and variance is 1.6330. Consider that the first observation in our sample of four values equals 10; the second equals 8; the third equals 10. The value of the fourth observation must equal 12. Thus, in computing the sample variance for this problem, we have three degrees of freedom.

Student's t Distribution The t distribution was used first by W. S. Gosset, who published his results in 1908 under the pen name "Student" (Hays, 1981, p 275). Thus, the distribution is often referred to as the Student's t distribution. The t distribution has the following characteristics (Daniel, 1991, p 139; Hays, 1981, pp 276–277).

1. The t distribution is a probability distribution. It is a family of distributions, each characterized by its degrees of freedom. Figure 10–2 contains t distributions for 4, 12, and an infinite number of degrees of freedom.

2. All t distributions are unimodal, symmetric, and bell-shaped about a mean of zero. The variance of a t distribution is greater than that of the standard normal curve. The variance of the t distribution approaches the variance of the standard normal curve, as sample size increases.

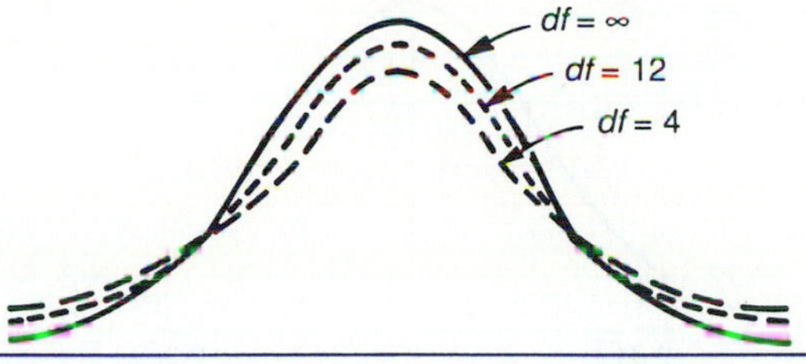

Figure 10–2. The *t* distribution as a function of different degrees of freedom. (Adapted with permission from Minium E: *Statistical Reasoning in Psychology and Education*, 2nd ed. Wiley, 1978.)

3. The *t* distribution is less peaked (flatter) in the center and plumper in the tails than the standard normal curve.

4. Values of *t* range from $+\infty$ to $-\infty$.

5. The *t* distribution approaches the standard normal distribution as degrees of freedom increase. The *t* distribution is identical to the standard normal distribution when there is an infinite number of degrees of freedom.

Using a t Table   Table A–2 in the appendix of statistical tables is the theoretical distribution of *t*. This table gives the critical value of *t* for different degrees of freedom, α, and one- and two-tailed tests. The panel along the top of the table is for two-tailed tests; the one beneath it is for one-tailed tests. No distinction is made between negative and positive values of *t*, because the *t* distribution is symmetric. Let us locate the critical value of *t* (t_{crit}) to be used in our example. Recall that the test is two-tailed, $df = 30$, and $\alpha = 0.05$. To find t_{crit}, scan down column one to $df = 30$. Read across this row to the intersection of $df = 30$ and the two-tailed area of 0.05: $t_{crit} = \pm 2.042$. Now use the *t* table to identify the critical value for the following examples:

df	α	One- or Two-tailed Test	Critical Value of t
20	0.01	One (greater than)	2.528
25	0.05	One (less than)	−1.708
40	0.05	One (greater than)	1.684
20	0.01	Two	±2.845
25	0.05	Two	±2.060
40	0.05	Two	±2.021

   Now that we have defined Student's *t* distribution and used the *t* table, we can return to answering the question about the relationship between fetal alcohol exposure and (1) infant birthweight and (2) age at which birthweight triples.

3. Specify the Decision Rule to be Used to Evaluate the Null Hypothesis (Continued)

   Define the level of significance and determine the critical region. Allow $\alpha = 0.05$. The critical value of *t* is ±2.042 for a two-tailed test with $df = 30$ and $\alpha = 0.05$. The *t* distribution is shown in Figure 10–3. The same distribution and decision criteria apply to both sets of hypotheses.

4. Analyze the Data

   The researchers obtained the following results. Designate birthweight as *X* and age at which birth weight triples as *Y*. Sample size equals 31.

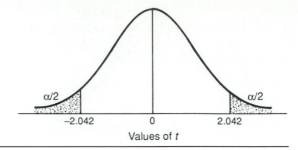

Figure 10–3. Student's t distribution to study questions about the effect of fetal exposure to alcohol; $df = 30$ and $\alpha = 0.05$.

Birthweight	Age at Which Birthweight Triples
$\overline{X} = 2.50$ kg	$\overline{Y} = 15$ months
$s_X = 0.54$	$s_Y = 2.7$

The Student's t statistic is used. Calculations appear in Box 10–2. The calculated value of t for the birthweight data is -8.25; t_{calc} for the age at which the birthweight triples is 6.19.

5. Evaluate the Statistics

Compare the calculated and critical values. Birthweight: $t_{calc} = -8.25$, $t_{crit} = \pm2.042$. Age at which birthweight triples: $t_{calc} = 6.19$, $t_{crit} = \pm2.042$. Based on these statistics, we reject both null hypotheses.

We can also make a decision about the null hypothesis by comparing the p-value to α. The exact p-values for our example cannot be determined from Table A–2, because no t values greater than 3.646 are given for a two-tailed test with $df = 30$. Consequently, we estimate the p-value. Select the two-tailed area corresponding to the largest t value in the table (3.646) for $df = 30$; this two-tailed area is 0.001. We say, then, that the p-value is less than 0.001. The null hypothesis is rejected because the p-value $\leq \alpha$.

6. Interpret the Statistics

The mean birthweight of female infants born to women who drink the equivalent of 2 drinks containing 1.5 ounces of alcohol 5 or more times per week, during at least 7 months of their

Box 10–2. Analysis of data from 31 infants exposed to alcohol during at least 7 months of their mother's pregnancy.

	Birthweight (kg)	Age at Which Birthweight was Tripled (months)
Hypotheses	$H_0 : \mu = 3.3$ kg $H_A : \mu \neq 3.3$ kg	$H_0 : \mu = 12$ months $H_A : \mu \neq 12$ months
Population distribution	Normal	Normal
Population mean	2.5 kg	12 months
Population variance	Unknown	Unknown
Sample mean	3.3 kg	15 months
Sample standard deviation	0.54 kg	2.7 months
Sample size	31 infants	31 infants
Standard error of the mean	$s_{\overline{X}} = \dfrac{0.54}{\sqrt{31}} = 0.0970$	$s_{\overline{Y}} = \dfrac{2.7}{\sqrt{31}} = 0.4849$
Critical value of t for a two-tailed test with $\alpha = 0.05$ and $df = 30$	±2.042	±2.042
Test statistic	$t = \dfrac{2.5 - 3.3}{0.0970} = -8.2484$	$t = \dfrac{15 - 12}{0.4849} = 6.1868$
p-value	$p < 0.001$	$p < 0.001$
Decision	Reject the null hypothesis	Reject the null hypothesis

pregnancy, differs significantly from the mean birthweight of female infants in the general population (p-value < 0.001). Similarly, the mean age at which the fetal-alcohol-exposed infants triple their birthweight differs significantly from female infants in the general population (p-value < 0.001).

Nonnormally Distributed Population

We next demonstrate how to test a one-mean hypothesis when the population is distributed nonnormally, perhaps as with the distribution of age-at-onset of Alzheimer's disease in the adult population. The Student's t distribution and t statistic cannot be used if the population is distributed nonnormally. However, the Central Limit Theorem ensures that the sampling distribution will approximate a normal distribution when the sample size is 30 or greater. Therefore, the z statistic and standard normal distribution are employed. If the population variance is known, the z statistic is:

$$z = \frac{\overline{X} - \mu_0}{\sigma_{\overline{X}}}, \text{ where } \sigma_{\overline{X}} = \frac{\sigma_X}{\sqrt{n}}. \qquad 10.9$$

If the population variance is unknown, the z statistic is modified to reflect that sample data have been used to estimate the population variance and standard error of the mean:

$$z = \frac{\overline{X} - \mu_0}{s_{\overline{X}}}, \text{ where } s_{\overline{X}} = \frac{s_X}{\sqrt{n}} \text{ and } n \geq 30. \qquad 10.10$$

Investigators working with data from small samples ($n < 30$) and a nonnormally distributed population should consult a statistician for appropriate alternative analyses. The use of Formula 10.10 is illustrated in the next example.

Clinical Example: Congestive Heart Failure

Clinicians and researchers note that despite medical advances since 1948, the mean survival time following diagnosis for patients with congestive heart failure remains 2.5 years. An experimental drug undergoing Food and Drug Administration (FDA) review is administered to 50 randomly selected patients with congestive heart failure; all are then followed until death. Their mean survival is 3.3 years, with a standard deviation of 1.8 years. Does the use of this drug affect survival in patients with congestive heart failure?

1. State the Scientific Hypothesis

Although investigators believe the experimental drug will prolong survival, they are concerned that unexpected side effects may decrease survival after patients take the drug for several weeks or months. Therefore, the investigators formulate a nondirectional scientific hypothesis and conduct a two-tailed statistical test. If increased survival time is found in several human clinical trials, a directional scientific hypothesis (survival time increases) and a one-tailed test may be warranted in future research.

2. Formulate the Statistical Hypotheses

$$H_0 : \mu = 2.5 \text{ years}$$
$$H_A : \mu \neq 2.5 \text{ years}$$

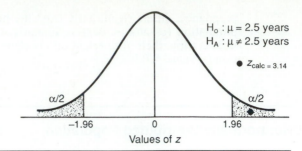

Figure 10–4. Standard normal curve to assess survival of patients with congestive heart failure; $\alpha = 0.05$.

3. Specify the Decision Rule to be Used to Evaluate the Null Hypothesis

The z statistic is used. The sampling distribution is the sampling distribution of means; the distribution of the test statistic is the standard normal curve. Allow $\alpha = 0.05$. To identify the critical value of z, consult Table A–1, find the two-tailed area of 0.05, and locate the corresponding value of z. The critical value of z is ± 1.96. The distribution of the test statistic appears in Figure 10–4.

4. Analyze the Data

Mean survival in the 50 randomly selected patients who receive the experimental drug is 3.3 years, with a standard deviation of 1.8 years. The analysis appears in Box 10–3. The calculated value of z also appears in Figure 10–4. The calculated value of $z = 3.14$.

5. Evaluate the Statistics

We reject the null hypothesis: $z_{calc} = 3.14$ versus $z_{crit} = \pm 1.96$. The p-value is 0.0016. A common mistake occurs in identifying the two-tailed p-value; the p-value is often given as the area in only the tail containing the observed result. Because this test is two-tailed, however, we must allow for the possibility of a computed statistic in the opposite tail. Therefore, we use the p-value that corresponds to the two-tailed area. Hence, the p-value is 0.0016.

6. Interpret the Statistics

The mean survival time of patients who receive the experimental drug differs significantly from 2.5 years (p-value $= 0.0016$). The observed mean survival of 3.3 years is consistent with

Box 10–3. Analysis of survival time in 50 congestive heart failure patients.

Hypotheses	$H_0 : \mu = 2.5$ **years**
	$H_A : \mu \neq 2.5$ **years**
Population distribution	Nonnormal
Population mean	2.5 years
Population variance	Unknown
Sample mean	3.3 years
Sample standard deviation	1.8 years
Sample size	50 patients
Standard error of the mean	$s_{\bar{x}} = \dfrac{1.8}{\sqrt{50}} = 0.2546$
Critical value of z for a two-tailed test with $\alpha = 0.05$	± 1.96
Test statistic	$z = \dfrac{3.3 - 2.5}{0.2546} = 3.1422$
p-value	$p = 0.0016$
Decision	Reject the null hypothesis

anticipated results. These preliminary results are promising; however, continued investigation is recommended before the drug can be administered widely to congestive heart failure patients.

SUMMARY

Testing hypotheses about one mean is summarized in Table 10–1 and Figure 10–5. The z statistic is used when (1) the population is distributed normally and population variance is known; (2) population is distributed nonnormally and population variance is known; and (3) population is distributed nonnormally, population variance is unknown, and $n \geq 30$. In the latter case, the Central Limit Theorem allows us to utilize the z statistic and the standard normal curve because the sampling distribution of means is distributed approximately normally when n is large (ie, $n \geq 30$), even though the population is distributed nonnormally.

The Student's t statistic and t distribution are applied when the population is distributed normally and population variance is unknown. In this case, the sample variance is used to estimate the population variance and the standard error of the mean. The t statistic is evaluated with $n - 1$ degrees of freedom.

The null hypothesis is rejected if the calculated value of the test statistic falls in the region of rejection. Alternately, the null hypothesis is rejected if the p-value associated with the sample result is less than or equal to α (p-value $\leq \alpha$).

Table 10–1. Summary of testing hypotheses about one mean.

Hypothesis	Assumptions	Test Statistic	Tables
$H_0 : \mu = \mu_0$	Population distributed normally Population variance known	$z = \dfrac{\bar{X} - \mu_0}{\sigma_{\bar{x}}}$ with $\sigma_{\bar{x}} = \dfrac{\sigma_X}{\sqrt{n}}$	Normal curve
$H_0 : \mu = \mu_0$	Population distributed normally Population variance unknown	$t = \dfrac{\bar{X} - \mu_0}{s_{\bar{x}}}$ with $df = n - 1$ and $s_{\bar{x}} = \dfrac{s_X}{\sqrt{n}}$	Student's t
$H_0 : \mu = \mu_0$	Population distributed nonnormally Population variance known	$z = \dfrac{\bar{X} - \mu_0}{\sigma_{\bar{x}}}$ with $\sigma_{\bar{x}} = \dfrac{\sigma_X}{\sqrt{n}}$	Normal curve
$H_0 : \mu = \mu_0$	Population distributed nonnormally Population variance unknown $n \geq 30$	$z = \dfrac{\bar{X} - \mu_0}{s_{\bar{x}}}$ with $s_{\bar{x}} = \dfrac{s_X}{\sqrt{n}}$	Normal curve

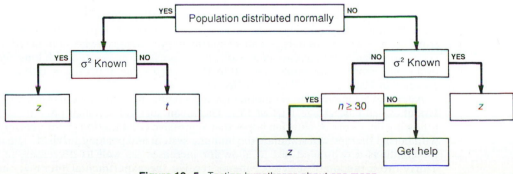

Figure 10–5. Testing hypotheses about one mean.

REFERENCES

Colton T: *Statistics in Medicine.* Little, Brown, 1974.
Daniel W: *Biostatistics: A Foundation for Analysis in the Health Sciences,* 5th ed. Wiley, 1991.
Hays W: *Statistics,* 3rd ed. Holt, Rinehart and Winston, 1981.
Minium E, *Statistical Reasoning in Psychology and Education,* 2nd ed. Wiley, 1978.
Rosner B: *Fundamentals of Biostatistics,* 2nd ed. Duxbury Press, 1986.
Vogt W: *Dictionary of Statistics and Methodology.* Sage, 1993.

Self-study Questions

Part I: Definitions

Define each of the following terms:

Central Limit Theorem	Sampling distribution of means
Degrees of freedom	Standard error of the mean
Mean of the sampling distribution of means	(standard deviation of the sampling dis-
p-value	tribution of means)

Part II: Are the Researchers' Conclusions Warranted?

Read each of the following descriptions and evaluate the conclusion in light of the information provided. Assume that calculations and supporting information (eg, *p*-values) are correct.

1. *Prostate Specific Antigen as a Serologic Marker for Metastases*
   Clinicians examined the value of prostate specific antigen (PSA) as a serologic marker for prostate cancer that has metastasized. The researchers hypothesized that PSA will be elevated in men whose cancer has metastasized, compared to the population of men with prostate cancer without metastases. The mean PSA is 12 ng/mL in the population of men whose prostate cancer is confined to the prostate gland. The mean PSA is 15 ng/mL ($s = 1.5$ ng/mL) in 35 randomly selected men whose cancer has metastasized. The investigators concluded that mean PSA levels rise significantly in men whose prostate cancer has metastasized, compared to men whose cancer is confined to the gland (population nonnormal; $z_{calc} = 11.83$, $z_{crit} = 1.645$, $\alpha = 0.05$). These findings suggest that PSA may be a serological marker of metastases in men who have prostate cancer.

2. *Oral Contraceptive Use and Hypertension*
   Concern exists that long-term use of oral contraceptives may contribute to hypertension. Fifty women, ages 40 to 45 years, were sampled randomly; they had used oral contraceptives for at least 5 consecutive years and had no history of hypertension before oral contraceptive use. Diastolic blood pressure in the general population of women in this age category is distributed approximately normally, with a mean of 85 mm Hg (standard deviation of 13 mm Hg). The mean diastolic blood pressure of the 50 women in the study group was 87 mm Hg. The obstetrician/gynecologist who conducted the study reported a significant increase in diastolic blood pressure associated with long-term use of oral contraceptives in women, ages 40 to 45 years (*p*-value < 0.14, $\alpha = 0.05$).

3. *Survival in Patients With Hodgkin's Disease*
   Aggressive combination chemotherapy is recommended for patients with disseminated Hodgkin's disease (stage IIIB or IV). The mean survival for such patients is 2.2 years following diagnosis. A clinician hopes that aggressive combination chemotherapy coupled with herbal therapy will stimulate the immune system and prolong survival. The investigator conducts a two-tailed test to allow for increases, as well as decreases, in survival. Thirty-three randomly selected patients receive the experimental therapy; their mean survival following diagnosis is 2.4 years, with a standard deviation of 0.9 years. The

investigator concludes that no significant change in survival accrues from the experimental therapy (nonnormal population; $z_{calc} = 1.2763$, $z_{crit} = 1.645$, $\alpha = 0.05$).

4. *The Effects of Exposure to Environmental Tobacco Smoke in Nonsmoking Women*

   Autopsy data were obtained from 22 randomly selected women who died between the ages 40 and 60 years and who had been married to smokers. Their data were compared to information from thousands of women who died at a similar age, were nonsmokers, and were married to nonsmokers. Nonsmoking women married to smokers were exposed for 15 years or more to environmental tobacco smoke. All women died of causes other than respiratory failure or cancer. The researchers hypothesized that pathologic indicators thought to be risk factors for the development of lung cancer will be present to a greater degree in nonsmoking women married to smokers. The mean pathologic indicator for deceased nonsmoking women married to nonsmokers is 41.26; the mean is 61.43, with a standard deviation of 19.04, for the 22 deceased nonsmokers married to smokers. The higher the score, the more likely the pathological entities indicate precancerous lesions in the main and lobar bronchi and parenchyma. According to the investigators, their results provide additional support to the body of growing evidence linking passive smoking to lung cancer risk (population normal; $t_{calc} = 4.97$, $t_{crit} = 2.518$, $df = 21$, p-value < 0.0005, $\alpha = 0.01$).

5. *Iron Status in Breastfed Infants*

   The iron status of 25 randomly sampled infants, breastfed exclusively from birth to age 6 months, was compared to extensive data from formula-fed infants to determine if the iron status of breastfed infants is higher than that of their formula-fed counterparts. Total body iron for the population of formula-fed infants was 271 mg, compared to 254 mg ($s = 37$ mg) for the 25 breastfed infants. The investigators concluded that the iron status of the breastfed infants was superior to that of formula-fed infants (normal population, $t_{calc} = -2.2973$, $t_{crit} = 1.711$, $df = 24$, $\alpha = 0.05$).

Part III: Which Statistical Test Should Be Used?

Read each of the following descriptions. For each, identify the statistical hypothesis and the statistical test that should be used to evaluate the hypothesis.

1. *Micrometastatic Tumor Cells*

   Disease-free survival is assessed in 40 randomly selected patients with radically resected colorectal carcinoma, whose bone marrow aspirates are positive for CK18. The presence of this protein in the bone marrow is thought to suggest malignant disease. It is postulated that disease-free survival in such patients is less than that of the population of patients with radically resected colorectal carcinoma, whose bone marrow aspirates are negative for CK18. The population disease-free survival is 24 months; it is 18 months ($s = 7$ months) in the sample. Assume population disease-free survival is nonnormal.

2. *Fertility Among Female Dental Assistants Exposed to Nitrous Oxide*

   Fifteen randomly selected, married female dental assistants, age 20 to 25 years, who are exposed in their workplace to nitrous oxide are followed to determine time to conception. All work full time and have been exposed to nitrous oxide in the workplace for at least 1 year. The investigators suggest that time to conception will be greater for these women than for similarly aged counterparts in the population of healthy women. For similarly aged healthy married women in the population, the time to conception is distributed approximately normally, with a mean of 6 menstrual cycles and standard deviation of 2 cycles. The mean among these dental assistants is 7.1 cycles.

3. *Recurrent Episodes of Otitis Media*

   In one of the first investigations of the effects of recurrent episodes of otitis media with effusion (9 or more bouts per year), it was hypothesized that language development of affected youngsters would differ from that of the healthy population. It is well established that healthy children routinely use sentences at a mean age of 36 months. In 10 randomly sampled children referred for recurrent episodes of otitis media with effusion, the mean age at which sentences were used routinely was 47 months, with a standard deviation of 12 months. Assume the population age distribution is normal.

4. *Deaths from Stroke Due to Subarachnoid and Intracerebral Hemorrhage*

Clinicians investigating risk factors of death from stroke due to subarachnoid and intracerebral hemorrhage hypothesize that deceased, affected men had a documented history of hypertension. The mean diastolic blood pressure, determined from chart review, of 19 randomly selected Caucasian men who died from stroke due to subarachnoid and intracerebral hemorrhage was 110 mm Hg; in 22 randomly selected deceased African-American men, the mean was 115 mm Hg. Mean diastolic blood pressure in the general population is distributed approximately normally, with a mean of 85 mm Hg and standard deviation of 13 mm Hg.

5. *Foreign Bodies and Blood Lead Levels in Children*

Emergency room physicians at an inner-city hospital hypothesized that children who present with foreign bodies have a variant of pica and are at increased risk of elevated blood lead levels. Thirty-seven randomly selected children who presented with foreign bodies in their gastrointestinal tract were screened for blood lead levels. The mean was 15.7 μg/dL for these 37 children, compared to a mean of 14 μg/dL, with a standard deviation of 2 μg/dL, for the population of healthy children. Assume population blood lead levels are distributed normally.

Part IV: Analysis

Read each of the following descriptions, write the statistical hypotheses, identify the decision-rule criteria, conduct the statistical test, and make a decision about the statistical hypotheses. Allow $\alpha = 0.05$.

1. *Systolic Blood Pressure in Male Nursing Home Residents*

It is well documented that nursing home residents are at increased risk for many different health outcomes (eg, memory impairment, stroke, depression) compared to their nonresident nursing home counterparts. Two geriatricians studied male nursing home residents, ages 65 to 79 years, and hypothesized that they will have a greater systolic blood pressure than males in this age category in the general population. Consider that the population distribution of systolic pressures of men in this age group is approximately normal, with a mean of 122.4 mm Hg and standard deviation of 11.9 mm Hg. A random sample was obtained of 253 male nursing home residents, ages 65 to 79 years. Their mean systolic blood pressure was 145.2 mm Hg.

2. *Systolic Blood Pressure in Female Nursing Home Residents*

As part of their study of male nursing home residents, the clinicians also sought to describe the health status of female residents in this same age group. It was hypothesized that their systolic blood pressure will differ from that of the population of comparably aged females. The systolic blood pressure of females, ages 65 to 79 years, in the general population is distributed approximately normally with a mean of 115.7 mm Hg. The mean systolic blood pressure of 31 randomly selected female nursing home residents, ages 65 to 79 years, was 142.1 mm Hg ($s = 15.8$ mm Hg).

3. *Serum Cholesterol and Diet*

The relationship between diet and serum cholesterol was investigated in 23 females, ages 30 to 35, sampled randomly from the general population of women in this age classification. Women in the study group followed a 3-month diet having optimal lipid and caloric content. Serum cholesterol was measured and compared to that of the general population of women in this age range. The mean serum cholesterol in the general population of women is distributed normally, with a mean of 196 mg/dL. The mean serum cholesterol in the study sample was 176.9 mg/dL ($s = 28.7$ mg/dL).

4. *Gastrointestinal Malignancy*

Two gastroenterologists believe that leucine metabolism may decrease in patients with advanced gastric and colorectal cancer. The researchers hope to establish that leucine metabolism is a serologic marker of advanced gastric and colorectal cancer. In the population of healthy adults, leucine metabolism is distributed normally with a mean of 2.3 mL/kg/day and standard deviation of 0.32 mL/kg/day. In a random sample of 10 adults with advanced gastric and colorectal cancer, the mean is 1.71 mL/kg/day.

5. *Maternal Hypertension*
   The relationship between maternal hypertension and systolic blood pressure in daughters was examined in 35 randomly selected girls, ages 8 to 12 years, whose mothers have clinically diagnosed hypertension. It was thought that the blood pressure for girls in the study group will be higher than that of comparably aged girls in the population. Population systolic blood pressure values in this age group are distributed nonnormally with a mean of 102.5 mm Hg. The mean systolic blood pressure in the sample is 112.0 with a standard deviation of 11.4 mm Hg.

Solutions

Part II: Are the Researchers' Conclusions Warranted?

1. *Prostate Specific Antigen as a Serologic Marker for Metastases*
   The conclusion is supported by the statistical analyses. The population of PSA values in men with prostate cancer is distributed nonnormally. Therefore, the Student's *t* statistic is not used. The *z* statistic is appropriate because (1) the population is distributed nonnormally and (2) $n \geq 30$. The calculated value of *z* (11.83) falls in the region of rejection ($z_{crit} = 1.645$ for a one-tailed test with $\alpha = 0.05$). The null hypothesis is rejected; sample data support the alternative hypothesis of elevated PSA levels in men whose cancer has metastasized.

2. *Oral Contraceptive Use and Hypertension*
   The conclusion is not supported by the statistical analyses because the *p*-value is greater than α ($p < 0.14$, $\alpha = 0.05$). The null hypothesis is retained, not rejected, when the *p*-value is greater than α.

3. *Survival in Patients With Hodgkin's Disease*
   The conclusion is supported by the statistical analyses. The *z* statistic is applied because (1) the population is distributed nonnormally and (2) $n \geq 30$. The calculated value of *z* (1.2763) falls in the region of retention ($z_{crit} = 1.645$ for a one-tailed test with $\alpha = 0.05$). Coupling aggressive combination chemotherapy with herbal therapy does not increase survival significantly.

4. *The Effects of Exposure to Environmental Tobacco Smoke in Nonsmoking Women*
   The conclusion is supported by the statistical analyses. The Student's *t* statistic and distribution are appropriate because the population of pathologic indicator scores is distributed normally. The calculated value of *t* falls in the region of rejection; the *p*-value is considerably smaller than α ($t_{calc} = 4.97$, $t_{crit} = 2.518$, $df = 21$, $p < 0.0005$, $\alpha = 0.01$). Therefore, reject the null hypothesis. The mean indicator score for deceased nonsmoking women married to smokers is significantly greater than that of deceased nonsmoking women married to nonsmokers.

5. *Iron Status in Breastfed Infants*
   The conclusion is not supported by the statistical analysis. The Student's *t* statistic and distribution are used appropriately. However, the alternative hypothesis is a directional "greater than" statement. The sample mean is less than the population value. The null hypothesis must be retained according to the decision rule criteria. (It is inappropriate for the investigators to change the decision rule criteria after the data are analyzed.)

Part III: Which Statistical Test Should Be Used?

1. *Micrometastatic Tumor Cells*
   The population disease-free survival is nonnormal and $n \geq 30$. The population variance (standard deviation) is unknown and is estimated from sample data. The *z* statistic having the following form is used: $z = \frac{(\bar{X} - \mu_0)}{s_{\bar{X}}}$ and $s_{\bar{X}} = \frac{s_X}{\sqrt{n}}$.

2. *Fertility Among Female Dental Assistants Exposed to Nitrous Oxide*
   The Student's *t* statistic and distribution are used, because the population of time to

conception is distributed approximately normally and the population variance is esti-mated from sample data.

3. *Recurrent Episodes of Otitis Media*

   The Student's t statistic and distribution are employed, because the population of ages is distributed normally and the population variance is unknown and is determined from sample data.

4. *Deaths from Stroke Due to Subarachnoid and Intracerebral Hemorrhage*

   Systolic blood pressure is distributed approximately normal in the general population and the population standard deviation is known. The z statistic is used to examine both sets of data. It has the following form: $z = \frac{(\bar{X} - \mu_0)}{\sigma_{\bar{X}}}$. The standard error of the mean equals $\sigma_{\bar{X}} = \frac{\sigma_X}{\sqrt{n}}$.

5. *Foreign Bodies and Blood Lead Levels in Children*

   The population is distributed normally and the population standard deviation is known. The z statistic and standard normal distribution apply: $z = \frac{(\bar{X} - \mu_0)}{\sigma_{\bar{X}}}$ and $\sigma_{\bar{X}} = \frac{\sigma_X}{\sqrt{n}}$.

Part IV: Analysis

1. *Systolic Blood Pressure in Male Nursing Home Residents*

$$H_0 : \mu = 122.4$$

$$H_A : \mu > 122.4$$

Population: Distributed approximately normally.
Population standard deviation: Known, $\sigma = 11.9$ mm Hg.
Sampling distribution: Sampling distribution of means.
Test statistic: $z = \frac{(\bar{X} - \mu_0)}{\sigma_{\bar{X}}}$
Distribution of the test statistic: Standard normal curve.
Decision rule: $\alpha = 0.05$; one-tailed test; $z_{crit} = 1.645$.
Calculation:

$$z = \frac{145.2 - 122.4}{11.9/\sqrt{253}} = 30.48$$

Decision: Reject the null hypothesis.
Interpretation: The systolic blood pressure of males, ages 65 to 79 years, who live in nursing homes is significantly higher than the systolic blood pressure of the general population of males in this age category who do not live in nursing homes ($p < 0.0005$, $\alpha = 0.05$).

2. *Systolic Blood Pressure in Female Nursing Home Residents*

$$H_0 : \mu = 115.7$$

$$H_A : \mu \neq 115.7$$

Population: Distributed approximately normally.
Population standard deviation: Unknown, estimated from sample data, $s = 15.8$ mm Hg.
Sampling distribution: Sampling distribution of means.
Test statistic: $t = \frac{(\bar{X} - \mu_0)}{s_{\bar{X}}}$
Distribution of the test statistic: Student's t distribution.
Decision rule: $\alpha = 0.05$; two-tailed test; $df = 30$; $t_{crit} = \pm 2.042$.
Calculation:

$$z = \frac{142.1 - 115.7}{15.8/\sqrt{31}} = 9.30$$

Decision: Reject the null hypothesis.

Interpretation: The systolic blood pressure of female nursing home residents, ages 65 to 79 years, differs significantly from the systolic blood pressure of the females in this age category in the general population who do not live in nursing homes ($p < 0.001$, $\alpha = 0.05$).

3. *Serum Cholesterol and Diet*

$$H_0 : \mu = 196 \text{ mg/dL}$$

$$H_A : \mu < 196 \text{ mg/dL}$$

Population: Distributed approximately normally.
Population standard deviation: Unknown, estimated from sample data, $s = 28.7$ mm Hg.
Sampling distribution: Sampling distribution of means.
Test statistic: $t = \frac{(\bar{X} - \mu_0)}{s_{\bar{X}}}$
Distribution of the test statistic: Student's t distribution.
Decision rule: $\alpha = 0.05$; one-tailed test; $df = 22$; $t_{crit} = 1.717$.
Calculation:

$$t = \frac{176.9 - 196}{28.7/\sqrt{23}} = -3.19$$

Decision: Reject the null hypothesis.

Interpretation: The mean serum cholesterol of females, ages 30 to 35 years, who consume a diet having optimal lipid and caloric content is significantly lower than the mean serum cholesterol of women in this age category in the general population ($p < 0.005$, $\alpha = 0.05$).

4. *Gastrointestinal Malignancy*

$$H_0 : \mu = 2.3 \text{ mL/kg/day}$$

$$H_A : \mu < 2.3 \text{ mL/kg/day}$$

Population: Distributed normally.
Population standard deviation: Known, $\sigma = 0.32$ mL/kg/day.
Sampling distribution: Sampling distribution of means.
Test statistic: $z = \frac{(\bar{X} - \mu_0)}{\sigma_{\bar{X}}}$
Distribution of the test statistic: Standard normal curve.
Decision rule: $\alpha = 0.05$; one-tailed test; $z_{crit} = -1.645$.
Calculation:

$$z = \frac{1.71 - 2.3}{0.32 \div \sqrt{10}} = -5.83$$

Decision: Reject the null hypothesis.

Interpretation: The mean level of leucine metabolism is significantly lower in patients with advanced gastric and colorectal cancer, compared to the population of healthy adults ($p < 0.000032$, $\alpha = 0.05$). Before the level of leucine metabolism can be established as a serologic marker of advanced gastric and colorectal cancer, the investigators must demonstrate that lowered levels of leucine metabolism are not markers of other diseases. They must also demonstrate that decreased leucine metabolism is not associated with other stages of gastric and colorectal cancer.

5. *Maternal Hypertension*

$$H_0 : \mu = 102.5 \text{ mm Hg}$$

$$H_A : \mu > 102.5 \text{ mm Hg}$$

Population: Distributed nonnormally.
Population standard deviation: Unknown, estimated from sample data, $s = 11.4$ mm Hg, $n \geq 30$.
Sampling distribution: Sampling distribution of means.
Test statistic: $z = \frac{(\bar{X} - \mu_o)}{s_{\bar{X}}}$
Distribution of the test statistic: Standard normal curve.
Decision rule: $\alpha = 0.05$; one-tailed test; $z_{\text{crit}} = 1.645$.
Calculation:

$$z = \frac{112.0 - 102.5}{11.4/\sqrt{35}} = 4.93$$

Decision: Reject the null hypothesis.
Interpretation: Girls ages 8 to 12 years whose mothers have clinically diagnosed hypertension have a mean systolic blood pressure that is significantly higher than that of comparably aged girls in the general population ($p < 0.000032$, $\alpha = 0.05$).

11

Estimating One Mean

Clinical Example: Fetal Alcohol Exposure

Clinicians concluded that the birthweight of 31 randomly selected female infants born to women who consume the equivalent of 2 drinks containing 1.5 ounces of alcohol, 5 or more times per week during at least 7 months of their pregnancy, differs significantly from that of female infants in the general population ($\bar{X} = 2.5$ kg, $s = 0.54$ kg, $\mu = 3.3$ kg, $t = -8.25$, $df = 30$, p-value < 0.001).

The above conclusion derives from a test of the null hypothesis that $\mu = 3.3$ kg. After comparing the calculated and critical value of the test statistic, the investigators rejected the null hypothesis. They ruled in favor of the alternative hypothesis that $\mu \neq 3.3$ kg. Based on these results, we recognize that the mean birthweight of the fetal-alcohol-exposed infants differs significantly from 3.3 kg. We know little else, however, about the value of the mean birthweight of these infants. Because sample statistics estimate population parameters, we might ask whether it is appropriate to use the sample mean of 2.5 kg to estimate the population mean. Although the answer is yes, a caveat exists: We must keep in mind that outcomes vary from sample to sample. Thus, if another group of fetal-alcohol-exposed infants is studied, it is highly unlikely that their mean birthweight will equal 2.5 kg; instead, it might be 2.8 kg or 2.7 kg or 2.4 kg. Therefore, rather than using a specific sample value to estimate the parameter, we might estimate a range of values within which the parameter is likely to occur. In this chapter, we address procedures to estimate this range.

OBJECTIVES

When you complete this chapter, you should be able to:

- Identify the purposes of confidence intervals.
- Describe similarities and differences between confidence intervals and hypothesis tests.
- Choose between the z and t statistics to construct a confidence interval about a mean.
- Interpret a confidence interval.

ESTIMATION

We focused in the previous chapter on one of two areas known as statistical inference, that is, hypothesis or significance testing. The second area, **estimation**, is addressed in this chapter. In many situations, populations are so large that it is impossible to describe their central tendency and dispersion by studying 100% of their members, or by studying a sufficiently large portion of the population to justify treating sample statistics as population parameters. In other situations, clinicians may study a new phenomenon or process with little or no basis to specify a population parameter. For example, gastroenterologists might investigate the response of Crohn's disease patients to an experimental drug designed to minimize chronic intestinal inflammation. Crohn's disease is a chronic inflammatory disease of the alimentary tract; the ileum is the principal site, either alone or in conjunction with the colon and jejunum (Knauer, 1993, p 480). Because insufficient data exist to identify the value of the mean response in a population of Crohn's patients, the researchers describe a range of values in which the population mean response is likely to occur.

Two types of estimates of a population parameter can be developed, a point estimate and an interval estimate. A **point estimate** is a single numerical value of a sample statistic used to estimate the corresponding population parameter. For example, the sample mean, $\overline{X}$, estimates the population mean, μ. In the hypothetical clinical example at the beginning of the chapter, 2.5 kg is an estimate of the population mean birthweight of female, fetal-alcohol-exposed infants. Point estimates are not used widely because the value of some statistic, such as the sample mean, varies from sample to sample. Consequently, we cannot conclude with any degree of certainty that a single point estimate equals the population parameter (Hays, 1981, p 191). Therefore, an **interval estimate** is typically favored over a point estimate. An interval estimate is a range of values within which the parameter is likely to occur.

INTERVAL ESTIMATION

Interval estimates, known as **confidence intervals**, reflect a range of values with a specified high probability of containing the population parameter (Hays, 1981, p 191). Because medical studies frequently include two-tailed confidence intervals, we focus on them in this chapter. Individuals interested in one-tailed intervals are directed to Rosner (1986, pp 214–215).

All confidence intervals have the same general form, regardless of the parameter estimated:

Sample Statistic ± Critical Value × Standard Error.

The sample statistic is the estimator of the unknown population parameter. The critical value corresponds to the two-tailed value of the test statistic (eg, t or z) that leads us to reject the null hypothesis. The formula also includes the standard error of the sample statistic. For example, if $\overline{X}$ is the sample statistic, the standard error of the mean is used.

The confidence interval about the population mean, μ, is constructed from Formula 11.1 (a or b) if the population is distributed normally and has a known population variance:

$$100(1 - \alpha)\% = (\overline{X} - z_{\alpha/2}\,\sigma_{\overline{X}} \leq \mu \leq \overline{X} + z_{\alpha/2}\sigma_{\overline{X}}) \qquad \textbf{11.1a}$$

$$100(1 - \alpha)\% = \overline{X} \pm z_{\alpha/2}\sigma_{\overline{X}} \qquad \textbf{11.1b}$$

where $100(1 - \alpha)\%$ is the confidence coefficient or confidence level. For example, if $\alpha = 0.05$, the interval is referred to as the 95% confidence interval, with 95% being the confidence coefficient or confidence level. If $\alpha = 0.01$, the interval is the 99% confidence interval. Interpretation of a confidence interval follows a definition of its components, which include:

$\overline{X}$	Sample mean; estimates the unknown population mean
μ	Population mean
$z_{\alpha/2}$	Critical value of the test statistic for a two-tailed test
$\sigma_{\overline{X}}$	Standard error of the mean computed from the population standard deviation, $\frac{\sigma_X}{\sqrt{n}}$
$\overline{X} - z_{\alpha/2}\sigma_{\overline{X}}$	Lower limit of the confidence interval
$\overline{X} + z_{\alpha/2}\sigma_{\overline{X}}$	Upper limit of the confidence interval

As noted above, we use Formula 11.1 if the population is distributed normally and has a known population variance. We also use this formula if (1) the population is distributed nonnormally, (2) the population variance is known, and (3) $n \geq 30$. Recall that the Central Limit Theorem discussed in Chapter 9 allows us to sample from a population that is distributed nonnormally with a guarantee that the sampling distribution will be approximately normal, provided the sample is large. We used $n \geq 30$ as our definition of "large" (Daniel, 1991, p 110). If the variance of the nonnormally distributed population is unknown and $n \geq 30$, we modify Formula 11.1 to indicate that the sample variance is used to estimate the population variance. Therefore, $s_{\overline{X}}$ replaces $\sigma_{\overline{X}}$, as follows: $\overline{X} \pm z_{\alpha/2}s_{\overline{X}}$.

Confidence intervals have two interpretations, probabilistic and practical. The *probabilistic interpretation* is as follows.

In repeated random sampling from a normally distributed population with known variance, $100(1 - \alpha)\%$ of all intervals of the form $\overline{X} \pm z_{\alpha/2}\sigma_{\overline{X}}$ will, in the long run, include the population mean, μ (Daniel, 1991, p 134).

Consider that all possible random samples of size n are drawn from a normally distributed population with known variance, σ^2. The sample mean, $\overline{X}$, is computed for each sample. Next, confidence intervals are constructed for every possible value of $\overline{X}$. A large number of intervals of the form $\overline{X} \pm z_{\alpha/2}\sigma_{\overline{X}}$ results. If $\alpha = 0.05$, approximately 95% of these intervals will have centers falling within the $\pm z_{\alpha/2}\sigma_{\overline{X}}$ interval about μ. This probabilistic interpretation is illustrated in Figure 11–1. Although the values of μ, and hence $\mu_{\overline{X}}$, remain unknown, we recognize that μ is the center of the sampling distribution of means. In Figure 11–1, values of sample means appear along the x-axis. The interval constructed about each sample mean is

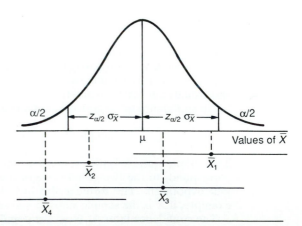

Figure 11–1. Four confidence intervals constructed about the population mean. (Adapted with permission from Daniel W: *Biostatistics: A Foundation for Analysis in the Health Sciences*, 5th ed. Wiley, 1991.)

indicated by a vertical line, with ● marking the sample mean. Note that $\overline{X}_1$, $\overline{X}_2$, and $\overline{X}_3$ fall within the $\pm z_{\alpha/2}\sigma_{\overline{X}}$ interval about the unknown population mean, μ. Thus, the $\pm z_{\alpha/2}\sigma_{\overline{X}}$ intervals about these sample means include μ. Examine the interval about $\overline{X}_4$. Note that its center falls in the lower tail beyond the $-z_{\alpha/2}\sigma_{\overline{X}}$ lower limit of the interval; therefore, the interval does not capture μ.

The practical interpretation of a confidence interval is as follows:

We are 100 $(1 - \alpha)$% confident that a single interval of the form $\overline{X} \pm z_{\alpha/2}\sigma_{\overline{X}}$ contains the population mean, μ (Daniel, 1991, p 134).

For example, consider that 36 patients are given an experimental treatment to delay the progression of Alzheimer's disease, following early identification of symptoms. The population of time-to-symptom progression is assumed to be distributed approximately normally, with a standard deviation of 9 months. The researchers find that symptom progression in the study group is delayed a mean of 27 months. In this case, the 95% confidence interval is (24.06 months $\leq \mu \leq$ 29.94 months). Thus, the investigators are 95% confident that the mean symptom delay for patients in the target population is between approximately 24 and 30 months

If the population is distributed normally and its variance is unknown, we alter Formula 11.1. We use the sample variance to estimate the population variance. In addition, the Student's t distribution rather than the standard normal curve applies. Formula 11.2 (a or b) results:

$$100\ (1 - \alpha)\% = (\overline{X} - t_{\alpha/2}s_{\overline{X}} \leq \mu \leq \overline{X} + t_{\alpha/2}s_{\overline{X}}) \qquad \textbf{11.2a}$$

$$100\ (1 - \alpha)\% = \overline{X} \pm t_{\alpha/2}s_{\overline{X}} \qquad \textbf{11.2b}$$

CONSTRUCTING TWO-SIDED CONFIDENCE INTERVALS

Population Distribution Normal, Population Variance Known

Let us return to the hypothetical research on Alzheimer's disease and construct the 95% confidence interval. Symptom progression is delayed a mean of 27 months in Alzheimer's disease patients who receive an experimental treatment after early symptom identification. The population is distributed normally, with a standard deviation of 9 months. Follow these steps to construct the confidence interval:

1. Identify α (=0.05).

2. Determine if the standard normal curve or Student's t distribution applies. The standard normal curve and, therefore, z is employed because the population is distributed normally and its variance is known.

3. Use Table A–1 in the appendix of statistical tables to obtain the two-tailed critical value of z: $z_{\alpha/2} = \pm 1.96$

4. Calculate the standard error of the mean:

$$\sigma_{\overline{X}} = \frac{\sigma_X}{\sqrt{n}} = \frac{9}{\sqrt{36}} = 1.5$$

5. Construct the lower limit:

$$\overline{X} - z_{\alpha/2}\sigma_{\overline{X}} = 27 - 1.96\ (1.5) = 24.06$$

6. Construct the upper limit:

$$\overline{X} + z_{\alpha/2}\sigma_{\overline{X}} = 27 + 1.96(1.5) = 29.94$$

7. Assemble the information:

$$\overline{X} \pm z_{\alpha/2}\sigma_{\overline{X}}$$

$$95\% = (24.06 \le \mu \le 29.94) \text{ or } 27 \pm 1.96\ (1.5) = 27 \pm 2.94 = (24.06,\ 29.94)$$

The 95% confidence interval extends from approximately 24 to 30 months. We are 95% confident that the mean delay in symptom progression is between approximately 24 and 30 months in the population of Alzheimer's disease patients receiving the experimental treatment.

Population Distribution Nonnormal and $n \ge 30$

The following hypothetical example, developed from actual clinical research, illustrates the construction of a confidence interval when the population distribution is nonnormal and $n \ge 30$.

Clinical Example: Directional Atherectomy

> The directional atherectomy catheter tunnels through artery blockages with a tiny, razor-sharp blade that whirls at 2500 rpm. Use of the device as an alternative to balloon angioplasty interests cardiologists and other clinicians. Fifty-four patients undergoing atherectomy to open clogged coronary arteries are followed to determine how long it takes for stenosis to recur. The mean time to artery renarrowing is 6 months, with a standard deviation of 2.3 months. It is assumed that the population of months to recurrence is distributed nonnormally.

Within what central 95% limits will the population mean time to recurrence fall? The confidence interval is constructed as follows:

1. Identify α (=0.05).

2. Determine if the standard normal curve or Student's t distribution applies. The standard normal curve and z are used, because the population is distributed nonnormally and $n \ge 30$. Note, however, that the sample standard deviation estimates the population standard deviation. Therefore, Formula 11.1 is modified to reflect the inclusion of $s_{\overline{X}}$.

3. Obtain the critical value of z for a two-tailed test:

$$z_{\alpha/2} = \pm 1.96$$

4. Determine the standard error of the mean:

$$s_{\overline{X}} = \frac{s_X}{\sqrt{n}} = \frac{2.3}{\sqrt{54}} = 0.3130$$

5. Construct the lower limit:

$$\overline{X} - z_{\alpha/2}s_{\overline{X}} = 6 - 1.96\ (0.3130) = 5.3865$$

6. Construct the upper limit:

$$\overline{X} + z_{\alpha/2}s_{\overline{X}} = 6 + 1.96\ (0.3130) = 6.6135$$

7. Assemble the information:

$$\overline{X} \pm z_{\alpha/2}s_{\overline{X}}$$

$$95\% = (5.39 \le \mu \le 6.61) \text{ or } 6 \pm 1.96\,(0.3130) = 6 \pm 0.6135 = (5.39, 6.61)$$

The 95% confidence interval extends from approximately 5.4 to 6.6 months. We are 95% confident that the mean time to artery renarrowing is between approximately 5.4 and 6.6 months, in the population of patients having atherectomy to open clogged coronary arteries.

Normally Distributed Population, Population Variance Unknown

In the next hypothetical clinical example, developed from actual studies, we focus on the construction of a confidence interval when the variance of a normally distributed population is unknown.

Clinical Example: Ulcers in Textile Mill Workers

Health officials in the southern United States received reports of an increased incidence of gastric and duodenal ulcers in textile mill workers. Officials randomly sampled the records of 97 permanent, full-time textile workers to determine the mean time between beginning to work in the mill and subsequent development of either a gastric or duodenal ulcer. The mean is 7.8 years, with a standard deviation of 4.3 years. Assume that the population of time to ulcer development is distributed normally.

Construct the 95% confidence interval to estimate the range of values within which the population mean time is likely to occur.

1. Identify α (=0.05).

2. Determine if the standard normal curve or Student's t applies. The Student's t distribution and t apply, because the population is distributed normally and its variance is unknown. Use Formula 11.2 to construct the interval.

3. Obtain the critical value of t for a two-tailed test from Table A–2 in the appendix of statistical tables:

$$t_{\alpha/2} = \pm 1.98, \text{ df} = 96$$

4. Calculate the standard error of the mean:

$$s_{\overline{X}} = \frac{s_X}{\sqrt{n}} = \frac{4.3}{\sqrt{97}} = 0.4366$$

5. Construct the lower limit:

$$\overline{X} - t_{\alpha/2}s_{\overline{X}} = 7.8 - 1.96\,(0.4366) = 6.9443$$

6. Construct the upper limit:

$$\overline{X} + t_{\alpha/2}s_{\overline{X}} = 7.8 + 1.96\,(0.4366) = 8.6557$$

7. Assemble the information:

$$\overline{X} \pm t_{\alpha/2}s_{\overline{X}}$$

$$95\% = (6.94 \le \mu \le 8.66) \text{ or } 7.8 \pm 1.96 \,(0.4366) = 7.8 \pm 0.8557 = (6.94, 8.66)$$

We are 95% confident that the mean time between beginning to work in the textile mill and the development of gastric or duodenal ulcers is between approximately 6.9 and 8.7 years in the population of textile mill workers.

FACTORS AFFECTING THE WIDTH OF THE CONFIDENCE INTERVAL

Clinicians and researchers typically want to develop narrow, rather than wide, confidence intervals. Sample size, standard deviation, and α affect the width of a confidence interval. To illustrate the effect of manipulating these three factors, we consider the mean total cholesterol among a group of randomly sampled vegetarians who include milk products and eggs in their diet. Because we assume that the population distribution of total cholesterol values is approximately normal and its variance is unknown, each interval has the following form:

$$\overline{X} \pm t_{\alpha/2}s_{\overline{X}}$$

Table 11–1 contains three panels. The sample size is manipulated in the top panel; the standard deviation and α remain constant. The standard deviation varies in the second panel, while sample size and α remain unchanged. In the bottom panel, α is changed, while the sample size and standard deviation remain unaffected. Note the effect of manipulating these three factors:

- As sample size increases [Top panel], the width of the confidence interval decreases (assuming the standard deviation and α do not change).
- As the standard deviation decreases [Middle panel], the width of the confidence interval decreases (assuming the sample size and α are constant).
- As α decreases [Bottom panel], the width of the confidence interval increases (assuming the sample size and standard deviation remain unchanged).

Table 11–1. The effect of varying the sample size, standard deviation, and α on the width of a two-sided confidence interval.

Sample Size	Standard Deviation	α	$s_{\overline{X}}$	$t_{\alpha/2}$	$(\overline{X} \pm t_{\alpha/2}s_{\overline{X}})$
$n = 24$	35	0.05	7.1443	±2.069	(160.22, 189.78)
$n = 31$	35	0.05	6.2862	±2.042	(162.16, 187.84)
$n = 24$	35	0.05	7.1443	±2.069	(160.22, 189.78)
$n = 24$	25	0.05	5.1031	±2.069	(164.44, 185.56)
$n = 24$	35	0.05	7.1443	±2.069	(160.22, 189.78)
$n = 24$	35	0.01	7.1443	±2.807	(154.95, 195.05)

HYPOTHESIS TESTING AND CONFIDENCE INTERVALS

Confidence intervals and tests of hypotheses provide similar information about the null hypothesis. We reject the null hypothesis if the confidence interval does not contain the value of the parameter specified in the null hypothesis; we retain the null hypothesis if the confidence interval captures the null hypothesis value. The following hypothetical example illustrates the relationship between a two-sided confidence interval and a two-tailed hypothesis test.

Clinical Example: Otitis Media With Effusion

In a pioneering investigation of recurrent episodes of otitis media with effusion (9 or more bouts per year), researchers hypothesize that language development of affected youngsters differs from that of healthy children. It is well established that healthy children routinely use sentences at a mean age of 36 months. In 10 randomly sampled children who experience recurrent episodes of otitis media with effusion, the mean age at which sentences are used routinely is 47 months, with a standard deviation of 12 months. (Assume the population age distribution is normal.)

Box 11–1. Test of the hypothesis that recurrent otitis media with effusion affects language development

Hypothesis Test	Confidence Interval
$H_0 : \mu = 36$ months	$\alpha = 0.05$
	Distribution of age is approximately normal.
$H_A : \mu \neq 36$ months	Population variance is unknown.
	Use Student's t statistic and distribution.
$\alpha = 0.05$	$n = 10$, $df = 9$, $t_{\alpha/2} = \pm 2.262$
Distribution of age is approximately normal.	
Population variance is unknown.	$\bar{X} = 47$ months, $s = 12$ months
Use Student's t statistic and distribution.	
$n = 10$, $df = 9$, $t_{crit} = \pm 2.262$	
$\bar{X} = 47$ months, $s = 12$ months	$s_{\bar{x}} = \dfrac{12}{\sqrt{10}} = 3.7947$
$s_{\bar{x}} = \dfrac{12}{\sqrt{10}} = 3.7947$	$(\bar{X} \pm t_{\alpha/2}s_{\bar{x}}) = 47 \pm (2.262)(3.7947)$
$t = \dfrac{47 - 36}{3.7947} = 2.8988$	95% interval = (38.4164, 55.5836)
Conclusion: Reject the null hypothesis.	Conclusion: The 95% confidence interval extends from approximately 38.42 to 55.58 months.
Interpretation: The mean age at which youngsters who experience recurrent bouts of otitis media with effusion use sentences routinely differs significantly from 36 months, the mean age at which healthy children employ sentences routinely.	Interpretation: We are 95% confident that the mean age at which children who have recurrent bouts of otitis media with effusion use sentences routinely is between approximately 38.42 and 55.58 months.

The hypothesis test appears in Box 11–1. The scientific hypothesis is: Language development of youngsters who experience recurrent otitis media with effusion differs from that of the population of healthy children. Construction of a confidence interval is also outlined in Box 11–1.

In conducting the hypothesis test, we calculate the Student's t statistic. The calculated value of t (2.8988) leads us to (1) reject the null hypothesis and (2) conclude that the mean age at which language development occurs in children who experience chronic otitis media with effusion differs significantly from the corresponding mean age in the population of healthy children (p-value < 0.02). We also construct the 95% confidence interval, which extends from approximately 38.42 to 55.58 months. Thus, we are 95% confident that the mean age at which children who have recurrent otitis media with effusion use sentences routinely is between approximately 38.42 and 55.58 months. Because the null hypothesis value of 36 months falls outside this interval, we reject H_0; we conclude that this value (36 months) does not describe the population of youngsters who experience chronic otitis media with effusion.

Confidence Interval or Hypothesis Test?

We construct confidence intervals for two general purposes: to estimate a parameter and to test a hypothesis.

ESTIMATING A PARAMETER

Investigators studying a new phenomenon may have little or no basis to specify the value of a particular parameter, such as the population mean. In this case, they estimate a range of values within which the parameter is likely to occur. In other situations where very large populations exist, researchers cannot (1) study 100% of the members to calculate central tendency and dispersion or (2) examine a sufficiently large portion of the population to justify treating sample statistics as population parameters. In such cases, we construct a confidence interval to estimate the range of values within which a parameter is likely to occur. In addition, in other contexts clinicians may be more interested in estimating a parameter rather than testing an hypothesis. For example, the clinicians who conducted the otitis media study sampled 200 children who had experienced 2 or more bouts of otitis media with effusion. The investigators grouped the youngsters according to the number of bouts, and constructed an interval to estimate the mean age at which sentences were first used routinely in each group (2 to 4 bouts, 5 to 7 bouts, and 8 or more bouts). In this example, the goal is estimation, not hypothesis testing.

TESTING HYPOTHESES

For the following reasons, many statisticians and clinicians recommend that confidence intervals supplement or replace hypothesis tests:

A confidence interval and an hypothesis test provide the same information about the null hypothesis. If the value of the parameter specified in the null hypothesis falls outside the confidence interval, we reject the null hypothesis. If the value of the parameter specified in the null hypothesis resides in the confidence interval, we retain the null hypothesis.

Confidence intervals offer more information than a hypothesis test. For example, in the research on children with recurrent otitis media with effusion, we can interpret the 95% confidence interval as a rejection of all null hypotheses associated with values less than 38.42 months and greater than 55.58 months. A sample mean of 37.0 months leads us to reject the null hypothesis that $\mu = 36$ months. Further, when the null hypothesis is rejected, the confidence interval describes a range of values within which the parameter is likely to occur in the population indicated by the alternative hypothesis.

Confidence intervals make clear that outcomes vary from sample to sample. Therefore, confidence intervals emphasize that results from one study may not be replicated exactly if others repeat the investigation. Confidence intervals, however, allow clinicians to determine readily if their results are consistent with findings reported by other investigators.

Confidence intervals highlight the role of sample size. For example, small differences that are not meaningful clinically will be significant statistically, if the sample is sufficiently large. Although the difference may be small, the confidence interval shows plainly the magnitude of the difference.

Confidence intervals reflect the amount of variability associated with an outcome of interest. Thus, a difference that may appear large takes on a clearer meaning when cast into a confidence interval. Recall how the standard deviation affects the width of an interval. For example, a confidence interval is wide when the standard deviation is large. Large standard deviations occur when sample size is small, biologic variability is large, or measurement and other types of systematic or random error are relatively large.

In summary, confidence intervals are central to the interpretations of results. Consequently, because of the valuable information provided by confidence intervals, many journals require that investigators include confidence intervals and hypothesis tests, when appropriate.

SUMMARY

Hypothesis testing and estimation belong to the branch of statistics known as inferential statistics. Procedures of estimation allow investigators to develop a point or an interval estimate about a population parameter. A point estimate is a single numerical value of a sample statistic that is used to estimate the corresponding population parameter. Interval estimates, also known as confidence intervals, reflect a range or interval of values in which the parameter is likely to occur. Because outcomes vary from sample to sample, interval estimates are preferred over point estimates.

Confidence intervals are used for two purposes: to estimate the value of a parameter and to test an hypothesis. Clinicians who study a new phenomenon have no solid foundation to specify the value of a particular parameter; therefore, they cannot test an hypothesis. Instead, they estimate a range of values within which the parameter is likely to occur. In other situations, researchers conduct an hypothesis test to determine if an experimental treatment is more effective than standard therapy. In such cases, the investigators may use a confidence interval because it can provide the same information as the hypothesis test—plus other useful data. We reject the null hypothesis if the value of the null hypothesis parameter falls outside the boundaries of the confidence interval. If we reject the null hypothesis, we use the confidence interval to identify a range of values within which the parameter is likely to occur, in the population identified by the alternative hypothesis.

Beyond determining if a null hypothesis should be retained or rejected, confidence intervals (1) make clear that results vary from study to study, (2) allow investigators to determine more readily if their findings are consistent with those of other clinicians, and (3) facilitate the interpretation of results by clarifying the role of sample size and variation in the dependent variable; thus clinical significance can be assessed more readily in light of the number of observations and their variability. For all these reasons, many journals require that investigators present hypothesis tests and confidence intervals.

Formulae to construct confidence intervals and related assumptions are summarized in Table 11–2.

Table 11–2. Summary of confidence intervals about one mean.

Assumptions	Probability Distribution	Confidence Interval
Population distributed normally Population variance known	Standard normal curve	$(\bar{X} - z_{\alpha/2}\sigma_{\bar{X}} \leq \mu \leq \bar{X} + z_{\alpha/2}\sigma_{\bar{X}})$ $\bar{X} \pm z_{\alpha/2}\sigma_{\bar{X}}$
Population distributed nonnormally Population variance known	Standard normal curve	$(\bar{X} - z_{\alpha/2}\sigma_{\bar{X}} \leq \mu \leq \bar{X} + z_{\alpha/2}\sigma_{\bar{X}})$ $\bar{X} \pm z_{\alpha/2}\sigma_{\bar{X}}$
Population distributed nonnormally Population variance unknown $n \geq 30$	Standard normal curve	$(\bar{X} - z_{\alpha/2}s_{\bar{X}} \leq \mu \leq \bar{X} + z_{\alpha/2}s_{\bar{X}})$ $\bar{X} \pm z_{\alpha/2}s_{\bar{X}}$
Population distributed normally Population variance unknown	Student's t distribution	$(\bar{X} - t_{\alpha/2}s_{\bar{X}} \leq \mu \leq \bar{X} + t_{\alpha/2}s_{\bar{X}})$ $\bar{X} \pm t_{\alpha/2}s_{\bar{X}}$

References

Daniel W: *Biostatistics: A Foundation for Analysis in the Health Sciences,* 5th ed. Wiley, 1991.

Hays W: *Statistics,* 3rd ed. Holt, Rinehart and Winston, 1981.

Knauer CM: Alimentary tract. In: *Current Medical Diagnosis and Treatment.* Tierney L Jr, et al (editors). Appleton & Lange, 1993.

Rosner B: *Fundamentals of Biostatistics,* 2nd ed. Duxbury Press, 1986.

Self-study Questions

Part I: Definitions

Define each of the following terms:

Confidence coeficient
Estimation
Interval estimate
Point estimate

Part II: Extended Answer Questions

1. Identify the purposes and uses of confidence intervals.
2. Identify factors that affect the width of a confidence interval. Describe how each factor affects the width of the interval.
3. Describe how confidence intervals help clinicians to evaluate the clinical meaning of findings.
4. Explain how a confidence interval can be used to evaluate a null hypothesis.
5. Describe situations in which (1) an hypothesis test cannot or should not be conducted and (2) a confidence interval is warranted.

Part III: Problems and Analysis

Complete each problem as directed.

Clinical Example for Problems 1 to 3: Lead Exposure and Calcium

Exposure to lead before birth or during childhood can significantly impair a child's intellectual development. Many clinicians believe that lead absorbed by the body is deposited in the skeleton. Consequently, as lead-exposed pregnant women draw calcium from their bodies to nourish the fetus, they also draw lead. For this reason, clinicians believe that lead enters the fetus from the mother's skeleton. Investigators have found that blood levels in fetal rats are reduced if lead-exposed pregnant rats are fed a diet high in calcium.

Forty-nine pregnant women who live close to a lead smelting operation consume diets high in calcium during their entire pregnancy. The mean blood lead level of their infants at birth is 5 μg/dL, with a standard deviation of 1.2 μg/dL. Assume that blood lead levels are distributed nonnormally in the population of infants born to lead-exposed pregnant women who consumed an enriched calcium diet during pregnancy.

1. Construct and interpret the 95% confidence interval about the mean blood lead level.
2. Based on previous research, the mean serum lead level of infants born to women living near a lead smelting operation is 20 μg/dL. Assume serum lead levels are distributed nonnormally.
   a. Test the null hypothesis that the mean serum lead level of the sample of newborns differs significantly from the population mean of 20 μg/dL. Allow $\alpha = 0.05$.
   b. Compare the results of the hypothesis test to the 95% confidence interval constructed in problem 1, above.
3. The 49 infants born to the lead-exposed pregnant women continued to live near the lead smelting plant. The infants are placed on a calcium-enriched diet at birth and followed until they are 7 years old, to determine if the calcium-rich diet might alter the impact of continued lead exposure on intellectual development. The mean intelligence test score of these children at age 7 years is 100. The mean intelligence test score in a population of similarly exposed, comparably aged children is 90, with a standard deviation of 14. Does a significant difference exist between the mean score of children who eat a calcium-enriched diet until age 7 years and the mean score of similarly exposed, comparably aged children whose diet is not calcium enriched? Assume the population of test scores is nonnormal. Construct the 95% confidence interval to evaluate the null hypothesis.

Clinical Example for Problems 4 and 5: Experimental Drug to Alter Cholesterol Levels

Researchers investigated the effectiveness of an experimental drug undergoing FDA testing in 36 patients with elevated low-density lipoprotein levels (LDL > 160 mg/dL) and diminished high-density lipoprotein levels (HDL < 40 mg/dL). The investigators want to estimate post-therapy mean change in LDL and HDL levels. After 8 weeks of drug therapy, the mean LDL level is 120 mg/dL, with a standard deviation of 18 md/dL. The mean HDL level is 41 mg/dL, with a standard deviation of 6 mg/dL. Assume LDL and HDL levels are distributed non-normally in the population of such patients.

4. Construct and interpret the 95% confidence interval about the mean LDL level.
5. Construct and interpret the 95% confidence interval about the mean HDL level.

Clinical Example for Problem 6: Smoking Relapse and Alcohol Intake

Substance abuse counselors attempt to describe characteristics of 61 individuals who quit smoking after attending a 7-week program in a "stop smoking clinic," then resumed smoking within 6 months after completing the program. Several characteristics are studied, including weekly alcohol intake. The mean alcohol intake is 42.0 ounces or its equivalent; the standard deviation is 7.8 ounces. Assume alcohol intake is distributed normally in the population of smokers who quit and then resumed smoking within 6 months.

6. Construct and interpret the 99% confidence interval about the mean.

Solutions

Part III: Problems and Analysis

Problems 1–3: *Lead Exposure and Calcium*

1. *Confidence Interval*
$\alpha = 0.05$
Distribution of serum lead levels is nonnormal.
Population variance is unknown, $n \geq 30$.
Use z and standard normal distribution.
$n = 49$, $z_{\alpha/2} = \pm 1.96$
$\bar{X} = 5\mu g/dL$, $s = 1.2\ \mu g/dL$

$$s_{\bar{X}} = \frac{1.2}{\sqrt{49}} = 0.1714\ \mu g/dL$$

$$(\bar{X} - z_{\alpha/2}\sigma_{\bar{X}} \leq \mu \leq \bar{X} + z_{\alpha/2}\sigma_{\bar{X}})\ \text{or}\ \bar{X} \pm z_{\alpha/2}\sigma_{\bar{X}}$$

$$5 \pm 1.96\ (0.1714) = 5 \pm 0.3359 = (4.6641, 5.3359)$$

Interpretation: We are 95% confident that the mean serum lead level at birth of the population of infants born to lead-exposed women who consume high-calcium diets during their entire pregnancy is between approximately 4.66 and 5.33 μg/dL.

2. *Hypothesis Test*

$$H_0: \mu = 20\ \mu g/dL$$

$$H_A: \mu \neq 20\ \mu g/dL$$

$\alpha = 0.05$
Distribution is nonnormal.
Population variance is unknown, $n \geq 30$.
Use z statistic and standard normal curve.
$n = 49$, $z_{crit} = \pm 1.96$

$$\bar{X} = 5\ \mu g/dL,\ s = 1.2\ \mu g/dL$$

$$s_{\bar{X}} = \frac{1.2}{\sqrt{49}} = 0.1714$$

$$z = \frac{5 - 20}{0.1714} = -87.5146$$

Conclusion: Reject the null hypothesis.

Interpretation: The mean serum lead level at birth of infants born to women living near a lead smelting operation differs significantly, depending upon whether an infant's mother consumed a high-calcium diet during pregnancy.

Confidence Interval

If we use the confidence interval to test the null hypothesis that $H_0 : \mu = 20$ µg/dL, we reject the null hypothesis because the 95% confidence interval (4.6641, 5.3359) does not contain the population mean. Because the null hypothesis is not tenable, we conclude that a significant difference exists in mean serum lead levels at birth in infants in these 2 populations.

3. *Confidence Interval to Test the Null Hypothesis*

$$H_0 : \mu = 90$$

$$H_A : \mu \neq 90$$

$\alpha = 0.05$
Distribution is nonnormal.
Population standard deviation is known, $\sigma = 14$ and $n \geq 30$.
Use z statistic and standard normal curve.
$n = 49$, $z_{\text{crit}} = \pm 1.96$
$\bar{X} = 100$, $\sigma_{\bar{X}} = 14$

$$\sigma_{\bar{X}} = \frac{14}{\sqrt{49}} = 2.0$$

$$(\bar{X} - z_{\alpha/2}\sigma_{\bar{X}} \leq \mu \leq \bar{X} + z_{\alpha/2}\sigma_{\bar{X}}) \text{ or } \bar{X} \pm z_{\alpha/2}\sigma_{\bar{X}}$$

$$100 \pm (1.96)(2.0) = 100 \pm 3.92 = (96.08, 103.92)$$

Interpretation: The 95% confidence interval extends from approximately 96 to 104; it does not capture the value of 90, the mean of the population of children who lived from birth to age 7 years near a lead smelter. Therefore, a significant difference exists in mean intelligence test scores between exposed children who eat a calcium-enriched diet and those who do not. The calcium-enriched diet appears promising in altering the impact of chronic lead exposure.

Problems 4 and 5: *Experimental Drug to Alter Cholesterol Levels*

4. *Confidence Interval About LDL Level*
   $\alpha = 0.05$
   Distribution of blood lead levels is nonnormal.
   Population variance is unknown, $n \geq 30$.
   Use z and standard normal distribution.
   $n = 36$, $z_{\alpha/2} = \pm 1.96$
   $\bar{X} = 120$ mg/dL, $s = 18$ mg/dL

$$s_{\bar{X}} = \frac{18}{\sqrt{36}} = 3.0 \text{ mg/dL}$$

$$(\overline{X} - z_{\alpha/2}s_{\overline{X}} \le \mu \le \overline{X} + z_{\alpha/2}s_{\overline{X}}) \text{ or } \overline{X} \pm z_{\alpha/2}s_{\overline{X}}$$

$$120 \pm 1.96 \,(3.0) = 120 \pm 5.88 = (114.12, 125.88)$$

Interpretation: We are 95% confident that the mean LDL level of a population of individuals with elevated LDL and diminished HDL levels who took an experimental drug for 8 weeks is between approximately 114 and 126 mg/dL.

5. *Confidence Interval about HDL Level*
   $\alpha = 0.05$
   Distribution of blood lead levels is distributed nonnormally.
   Population variance is unknown, $n \ge 30$.
   Use z and standard normal distribution.
   $n = 36$, $z_{\alpha/2} = \pm 1.96$
   $\overline{X} = 41$ mg/dL, $s = 6$ mg/dL

$$s_{\overline{X}} = \frac{6}{\sqrt{36}} = 1.0 \text{ mg/dL}$$

$$(\overline{X} - z_{\alpha/2}s_{\overline{X}} \le \mu \le \overline{X} + z_{\alpha/2}s_{\overline{X}}) \text{ or } \overline{X} \pm z_{\alpha/2}s_{\overline{X}}$$

$$41 \pm 1.96 \,(1.0) = 41 \pm 1.96 = (39.04, 42.96)$$

Interpretation: We are 95% confident that the mean HDL level of a population of individuals with elevated LDL and diminished HDL levels who took an experimental drug for 8 weeks is between approximately 39 and 43 mg/dL.

Problem 6: *Smoking Relapse and Alcohol Intake*

6. *99% Confidence Interval*
   $\alpha = 0.0$
   Distribution of alcohol intake is normal.
   Population variance is unknown.
   Use Student's t distribution and t statistic.
   $n = 61$, $df = 60$, $t_{\alpha/2} = \pm 2.66$
   $\overline{X} = 42$ ounces, $s = 7.8$ ounces

$$s_{\overline{X}} = \frac{7.8}{\sqrt{61}} = 0.9987$$

$$(\overline{X} - t_{\alpha/2}s_{\overline{X}} \le \mu \le \overline{X} + t_{\alpha/2}s_{\overline{X}}) \text{ or } \overline{X} \pm t_{\alpha/2}s_{\overline{X}}$$

$$42 \pm 2.66 \,(0.9987) = 42 \pm 2.6565 = (39.3435, 44.6565)$$

Interpretation: We are 99% confident that the mean alcohol intake of smokers who participate in a "stop smoking clinic" and begin smoking again within 6 months after completing the program is between approximately 39 and 45 ounces per week of alcohol, or its equivalent.

12 Testing and Estimating the Difference Between Two Means

Clinical Example 1: Breast Cancer and Dietary Fiber

Suppose the association between breast cancer and dietary fiber is investigated in two groups of randomly selected women. Mean daily fiber consumption in women with breast cancer ($n_{BC} = 25$) is 15 g, with a standard deviation of 5 g. Mean daily fiber consumption in women without breast cancer ($n_{NC} = 41$) is 17 g, with a standard deviation of 6 g. Is the difference in mean daily fiber consumption statistically significant?

Clinical Example 2: Over-the-Counter Home Cholesterol Test

Suppose the Food and Drug Administration evaluates an over-the-counter home cholesterol test in 10 randomly selected individuals. Patients fast for 12 hours and measure their total cholesterol level using the home test. Total cholesterol level is also assessed in a certified clinical laboratory. Mean total cholesterol determined from the home test is 201.50 mg/dL. The mean level obtained by laboratory analysis is 200.6 mg/dL. Is the home test a viable tool to monitor total cholesterol?

In the last two chapters, we explored procedures to test hypotheses about one mean. In this chapter, we extend one-mean procedures to questions about the difference between two means. To select the appropriate test statistic, we address several questions. For example, how are the two samples formed? Are the populations distributed normally? Are population variances known? Are population variances equal? Answers to these questions help us select the appropriate statistical test and construct the appropriate confidence interval.

OBJECTIVES

When you complete this chapter, you should be able to:

• Differentiate between independent and dependent groups designs.
• Select the appropriate test statistic or confidence interval to test an hypothesis about the difference between two means.
• Conduct a test of a null hypothesis about the difference between two means and construct a confidence interval.
• Interpret the findings from a statistical test and confidence interval.

INDEPENDENT VERSUS DEPENDENT GROUPS DESIGNS

The first step in identifying the appropriate test statistic is to determine whether an independent or dependent groups design is used. An **independent groups design** involves random selection and random assignment of study participants to groups. A **dependent groups design** may be one of three types: within-subject, naturally occurring pairs, or investigator-created pairs. Dependent groups designs are used to control extraneous factors thought to influence the outcome of interest. When pairs of subjects are created, members of a pair are as similar as possible with regard to extraneous factors. By controlling these factors, investigators infer that differences between groups are associated with the independent variable, not initial differences among study participants. Within the context of two mean studies, dependent groups paradigms are frequently referred to as matched/paired designs.

In *within-subject* designs, each study participant is measured under two different conditions. Within-subject paradigms involve "self-pairing," because each participant serves as his or her own control. Clinical Example 2 illustrates a within-subject design; the total cholesterol level of each participant is measured twice, from an over-the-counter home test and by a clinical laboratory. A common type of a within-subject paradigm is the *pre-post design,* in which study participants are assessed before (pretreatment) and after treatment (posttreatment). For example, suppose the effectiveness of a beta-adrenergic blocking agent developed to control hypertension is evaluated in randomly selected, hypertensive patients. Blood pressure is measured before the patient takes the medication (pretreatment) and again after the patient has taken it for a specified period of time (posttreatment). The difference between pre- and posttreatment blood pressures is then evaluated to assess drug efficacy.

Naturally occurring pairs is another type of dependent groups design. For example, twins are naturally occurring pairs. Investigators design "twin studies" to try to untangle genetic and nongenetic contributions to an outcome of interest, such as disease development or gender identification. Another example of naturally occurring pairs is found in many laboratory experiments, where two animals from the same litter are selected; one animal is assigned randomly to one treatment and the other is then allocated automatically to the other condition. The pairs may or may not contain animals of the same sex, depending on the purpose of the study.

Investigator-created pairs result when an investigator creates pairs of participants by matching on one or more extraneous characteristics thought to influence the dependent variable. The goal is to create pairs in which the two members are as alike as possible with respect to these characteristics. One member of the pair is assigned randomly to one group; the other is assigned by default to the other group. For example, suppose a study is done on postpartum weight loss and primary method of infant feeding (breast versus formula) during the first 6 months after delivery. Because breastfeeding requires more calories than formula feeding, investigators believe that postpartum weight loss during the first 6 months differs between women who breastfeed and those who use formula (Potter et al, 1991). Because the number of pregnancies, family income, woman's education, and age appear to be associated with postpartum weight loss, study participants are matched on these factors. Thus, the two women who form a pair are as similar as possible with respect to age, number of pregnancies, family income, and education. They differ in primary method of infant feeding. One member of the pair breastfed her infant for the first 6 months; the other member of the pair formula-fed her infant. Any differences in weight loss are then attributed to differences in infant feeding method, assuming other life style variables beyond the control of the investigators are similar (eg, postpartum exercise levels).

In summary, the first step in selecting the appropriate test statistic is to determine if groups are independent or dependent. In an independent groups design, study participants are selected randomly and assigned randomly to groups. The hallmark of dependent groups designs, often called *matched/paired designs,* is matching or pairing study participants to control extraneous variation. Dependent groups designs include within-subject comparisons and comparisons between naturally occurring or investigator-created pairs.

INFERENCES FROM INDEPENDENT GROUPS DESIGNS

The mean from the first population is designated μ_1; the mean from the second population is identified as μ_2. The null and alternative hypothesis take one of the following forms:

$$H_0 : \mu_1 - \mu_2 = 0 \qquad H_0 : \mu_1 - \mu_2 = 0 \qquad H_0 : \mu_1 - \mu_2 = 0$$

$$H_A : \mu_1 - \mu_2 \neq 0 \qquad H_A : \mu_1 - \mu_2 > 0 \qquad H_A : \mu_1 - \mu_2 < 0$$

The first set of hypotheses produces a nondirectional or two-tailed test. The second and third set yield a directional or one-tailed test, with one resulting in a *greater than* and the other a *less than* alternative hypothesis.

Before we present statistical tests and confidence intervals, we describe the random sampling distribution of the difference between two independent means.

Random Sampling Distribution of the Difference Between Two Means

The random sampling distribution of the difference between two means is a relative frequency distribution of the difference between all possible pairs of means calculated from independent random samples that are drawn from two populations. Although we would not attempt to enumerate the difference between all possible pairs of sample means, we can conceptualize the process as follows:

1. Identify two finite populations.

2. Draw all possible random samples of size n_1 from population one and all possible random samples of the same size (n_2) from population two.

3. Compute the mean for each sample from population one and for each sample from population two.

4. Take all possible pairs of sample means, one mean from population one and one mean from population two, and determine the difference, $\bar{X}_1 - \bar{X}_2$.

5. List or graph these differences and their relative frequency.

The result is the random sampling distribution of the difference between two independent means. According to Daniel (1991, p 115), the characteristics of this sampling distribution are as follows.

> Given two normally distributed populations with means μ_1 and μ_2, and variances σ_1^2 and σ_2^2, the sampling distribution of the difference between the means of independent random samples $\bar{X}_1 - \bar{X}_x$, of size n_1 and n_2, drawn from these two populations is (1) normally distributed with (2) a mean of $\mu_1 - \mu_2$ and (3) variance of $\left[\left(\frac{\sigma_1^2}{n_1} \right) + \left(\frac{\sigma_2^2}{n_2} \right) \right]$.

The mean of this sampling distribution, written as $\mu_1 - \mu_2$ or $\mu_{\bar{X}_1} - \mu_{\bar{X}_2}$, equals zero. The standard deviation of this sampling distribution is the square root of its variance, referred to as the *standard error of the difference between two independent means*. This standard error, symbolized as $\sigma_{\bar{X}_1 - \bar{X}_2}$, equals $\sqrt{\left(\frac{\sigma_1^2}{n_1} \right) + \left(\frac{\sigma_2^2}{n_2} \right)}$.

Testing the Difference Between Two Independent Means

We noted in Chapter 10 that many test statistics have the same general form:

$$\text{Test Statistic} = \frac{\text{Sample Statistic} - \text{Hypothesized Parameter}}{\text{Standard Error of the Sample Statistic}}.$$

If we extend the general form of the test statistic, as well as that of the z statistic in Chapter 10 (Formula 10.7), we develop a comparable statistic to test the difference between two independent means:

$$z = \frac{(\bar{X}_1 - \bar{X}_2) - (\mu_1 - \mu_2)}{\sqrt{\left(\dfrac{\sigma_1^2}{n_1}\right) + \left(\dfrac{\sigma_2^2}{n_2}\right)}} . \qquad \textbf{12.1a}$$

Because $\mu_1 - \mu_2 = 0$, this expression can be omitted from the numerator of Formula 12.1a to produce Formula 12.1b:

$$z = \frac{(\bar{X}_1 - \bar{X}_2)}{\sqrt{\left(\dfrac{\sigma_1^2}{n_1}\right) + \left(\dfrac{\sigma_2^2}{n_2}\right)}} . \qquad \textbf{12.1b}$$

When we sample from populations whose form is unknown or from populations distributed nonnormally, the Central Limit Theorem applies if each sample is "sufficiently large." If the samples are large, the random sampling distribution will be approximately normal, with a mean and variance of $\mu_1 - \mu_2$ and $\left[\left(\dfrac{\sigma_1^2}{n_1}\right) + \left(\dfrac{\sigma_2^2}{n_2}\right)\right]$, respectively. The rule-of-thumb for "sufficiently large" is $n_1 \geq 30$ and $n_2 \geq 30$ (Winer, 1971, p 41).

As described in Chapter 11, we can also extend the general form of the confidence interval to the difference between two independent means. The general form of a confidence interval is: (sample statistic $\pm$ critical value $\times$ standard error). The statistic of interest is the difference between sample means. The two-sided confidence interval about the difference between two independent means is:

$$(\bar{X}_1 - \bar{X}_2) \pm z_{\alpha/2} \sqrt{\frac{\sigma_1^2}{n_1} + \frac{\sigma_2^2}{n_2}} \qquad \textbf{12.2}$$

where $z_{\alpha/2}$ is the two-tailed critical value of z for a given α. This critical value is determined from Table A–1 in the appendix of statistical tables. Formula 12.2 applies if sampling has been from nonnormally distributed populations, $n_1 \geq 30$, and $n_2 \geq 30$. The conditions under which formulas 12.1 and 12.2 apply are summarized in panels A and E in Table 12–1.

These formulas do not enjoy widespread use because population variances are typically unknown. The formulas are important, however, because they provide a basis for generalizing to other applications in which the difference between two independent means is sought. These applications are illustrated in the following sections.

Normally Distributed Populations With Unknown Population Variances

When populations are distributed normally or approximately normally and their variance is unknown, we do not use the z statistic (Formula 12.1a or b). Instead, we employ the Student's t statistic. This statistic was introduced first in Chapter 10. We now discuss its application to two means.

The Student's t test for the difference between two independent means rests on two assumptions: (1) populations are distributed normally or approximately normally and (2) each population has the same variance, that is, $\sigma_1^2 = \sigma_2^2 = \sigma^2$. When the population variances are equal, they are called **homogeneous**. Thus, the second requirement is known as **homogeneity or equality of variance**. When population variances are unknown, sample values are used to estimate the population variances—s_1^2 estimates σ_1^2 and s_2^2 estimates σ_2^2. Homogeneity of variance can be tested formally; the null hypothesis is $H_0: \sigma_1^2 - \sigma_2^2 = 0$. The test, called an F-test, is

$$F = \left(\frac{s_{larger}^2}{s_{smaller}^2}\right) .$$

Table 12–1. Summary of Inference About Two Means.[a]

Hypothesis Tested: $H_0 : \mu_1 - \mu_2 = 0$

Panel	Assumptions/Conditions	Test Statistic	Two-sided Confidence Interval
A	Two independent groups Normally distributed populations Known population variances	$z = \dfrac{\bar{X}_1 - \bar{X}_2}{\sqrt{\dfrac{\sigma_1^2}{n_1} + \dfrac{\sigma_2^2}{n_2}}}$	$(\bar{X}_1 - \bar{X}_2) \pm z_{\alpha/2}\sqrt{\dfrac{\sigma_1^2}{n_1} + \dfrac{\sigma_2^2}{n_2}}$

B	Two independent groups
	Normally distributed populations
	Population variances unknown,
	  but assumed equal based on
	  sample data—rule-of-thumb:
	$(s^2_{larger}/s^2_{smaller} < 4)$
		$t = \dfrac{\bar{X}_1 - \bar{X}_2}{s_p\sqrt{\dfrac{1}{n_1} + \dfrac{1}{n_2}}}$
		
		$s_p^2 = \dfrac{(n_1 - 1)s_1^2 + (n_2 - 1)s_2^2}{n_1 + n_2 - 2}$
		
		$s_p = \sqrt{s_p^2}$
		
		$df = n_1 + n_2 - 2$
			$(\bar{X}_1 - \bar{X}_2) \pm t_{\alpha/2}\left(s_p\sqrt{\dfrac{1}{n_1} + \dfrac{1}{n_2}}\right)$
			
			$df = n_1 + n_2 - 2$

C	Two independent groups
	Normally distributed populations
	Population variances unknown,
	  but assumed unequal based on
	  sample data—rule-of-thumb:
	$(s^2_{larger}/s^2_{smaller} \geq 4)$
	Sample sizes equal or approxi-
	mately equal—rule-of-thumb:
	$(n_{larger}/n_{smaller} < 2)$
		$t = \dfrac{\bar{X}_1 - \bar{X}_2}{s_p\left(\sqrt{\dfrac{1}{n_1} + \dfrac{1}{n_2}}\right)}$
		
		$s_p^2 = \dfrac{(n_1 - 1)s_1^2 + (n_2 - 1)s_2^2}{n_1 + n_2 - 2}$
		
		$s_p = \sqrt{s_p^2}$
		
		$df = n_1 + n_2 - 2$
			$(\bar{X}_1 - \bar{X}_2) \pm t_{\alpha/2}\left(s_p\sqrt{\dfrac{1}{n_1} + \dfrac{1}{n_2}}\right)$
			
			$df = n_1 + n_2 - 2$

D	Two independent groups
	Normally distributed populations
	Population variances unknown,
	  but assumed unequal based on
	  sample data—rule-of-thumb:
	$(s^2_{larger}/s^2_{smaller} \geq 4)$
	Sample sizes unequal—
	rule-of-thumb:
	$(n_{larger}/n_{smaller} \geq 2)$
		$t = \dfrac{\bar{X}_1 - \bar{X}_2}{\sqrt{\dfrac{s_1^2}{n_1} + \dfrac{s_2^2}{n_2}}}$
		
		$df_{Adjusted} = \dfrac{\left[\left(\dfrac{s_1^2}{n_1}\right) + \left(\dfrac{s_2^2}{n_2}\right)\right]^2}{\left[\dfrac{(s_1^2/n_1)^2}{(n_1 - 1)}\right] + \left[\dfrac{(s_2^2/n_2)^2}{(n_2 - 1)}\right]}$
			$(\bar{X}_1 - \bar{X}_2) \pm t_{\alpha/2}\sqrt{\dfrac{s_1^2}{n_1} + \dfrac{s_2^2}{n_2}}$
			
			$df = \dfrac{\left[\left(\dfrac{s_1^2}{n_1}\right) + \left(\dfrac{s_2^2}{n_2}\right)\right]^2}{\left[\dfrac{(s_1^2/n_1)^2}{(n_1 - 1)}\right] + \left[\dfrac{(s_2^2/n_2)^2}{(n_2 - 1)}\right]}$

E	Two independent groups Nonnormally distributed populations Known population variances	$z = \dfrac{\bar{X}_1 - \bar{X}_2}{\sqrt{\dfrac{\sigma_1^2}{n_1} + \dfrac{\sigma_2^2}{n_2}}}$	$(\bar{X}_1 - \bar{X}_2) \pm z_{\alpha/2}\sqrt{\dfrac{\sigma_1^2}{n_1} + \dfrac{\sigma_2^2}{n_2}}$
F	Two independent groups Nonnormally distributed populations Population variances unknown $n_1 \geq 30$ *and* $n_2 \geq 30$	$z = \dfrac{\bar{X}_1 - \bar{X}_2}{\sqrt{\dfrac{s_1^2}{n_1} + \dfrac{s_2^2}{n_2}}}$	$(\bar{X}_1 - \bar{X}_2) \pm z_{\alpha/2}\sqrt{\dfrac{s_1^2}{n_1} + \dfrac{s_2^2}{n_2}}$

Hypothesis Tested: $H_0: \mu_d = 0$

Panel	Assumptions/Conditions	Test Statistic	Two-sided Confidence Interval

G	Matched/paired groups or within-
	  subject design
	
	Population of differences
	  distributed normally
	Population variance of the
	  differences known
		$z = \dfrac{\bar{d} - \mu_d}{\sigma_{\bar{d}}}$
		
		$\sigma_{\bar{d}} = \dfrac{\sigma_d}{\sqrt{n}}$
			$\bar{d} \pm z_{\alpha/2}\sigma_{\bar{d}}$
			
			$\sigma_{\bar{d}} = \dfrac{\sigma_d}{\sqrt{n}}$

H	Matched/paired groups or within-
	  subjects design
	
	Population of differences
	  distributed normally
	Population variance of the
	  differences unknown
		$t = \dfrac{\bar{d} - \mu_d}{s_{\bar{d}}}$
		
		$s_{\bar{d}} = \dfrac{s_d}{\sqrt{n}}$
		
		$df = n - 1$
			$\bar{d} \pm t_{\alpha/2}s_{\bar{d}}$
			
			$s_{\bar{d}} = \dfrac{s_d}{\sqrt{n}}$
			
			$df = n - 1$

[a]Shaded panel indicates that this particular application is encountered often.

Routine testing for homogeneity of variance is no longer recommended because (1) the results of the F-test are not useful if the population distributions are nonnormal and (2) the t test is *robust* with respect to moderate departures from homogeneity *if sample sizes are equal or approximately equal* (Hays, 1981, p 287). A statistic that is robust remains useful when its assumptions are violated (Vogt, 1993, p 198).

Because routine testing for homogeneity of variance is not recommended, rules-of-thumb have been developed for situations where unequal variances combine with unequal sample sizes. In such situations, we (1) modify the denominator of the t statistic and (2) adjust either the critical value of the t or its degrees of freedom.

RULES-OF-THUMB TO DETECT VIOLATIONS OF THE ASSUMPTION OF EQUAL POPULATION VARIANCES

When sample sizes are relatively unequal, the t statistic is affected by substantial departures from the assumption of equal population variances. We use the following rules-of-thumb to determine when adjustments are required. Make adjustments when

$$\left(\frac{s^2_{larger}}{s^2_{smaller}} \geq 4 \right) \text{ AND } \left(\frac{n_{larger}}{n_{smaller}} \geq 2 \right).$$

Now we examine the use of these rules-of-thumb within the context of salient, hypothetical problems derived from actual clinical situations.

Clinical Example: Breast Cancer and Dietary Fiber

> Two independently sampled populations
> Populations distributed normally or approximately normally
> Unknown population variances assumed to be equal

A case-control design was used to investigate the association between breast cancer and dietary fiber. Mean daily fiber consumption in randomly selected women with breast cancer ($n_{BC} = 25$) is 15 g, with a standard deviation of 5 g. Mean daily fiber consumption in randomly sampled women without breast cancer ($n_{NC} = 41$) is 17 g, with a standard deviation of 6 g. Is the difference in mean daily fiber consumption significant statistically?

If $\left(\frac{s^2_{larger}}{s^2_{smaller}} < 4 \right)$, we conclude that the unknown population variances are relatively equal

and no adjustments are required. Therefore, we use the t statistic displayed in panel B of Table 12–1. The shading in the first column of the table indicates that this application of the t statistic is common. The t statistic is:

$$t = \frac{\overline{X}_1 - \overline{X}_2}{s_p \sqrt{\frac{1}{n_1} + \frac{1}{n_2}}} \text{ with } df = n_1 + n_2 - 2. \qquad 12.3$$

Note the denominator in Formula 12.3. Because the unknown population variances are thought to be relatively equal, a pooled estimate of the unknown population variance, σ^2, is developed from sample data. The square root of this pooled estimate is s_p:

$$s^2_p = \frac{(n_1 - 1)s^2_1 + (n_2 - 1)s^2_2}{n_1 + n_2 - 2} \qquad 12.4$$

$$s_p = \sqrt{s^2_p}. \qquad 12.5$$

The two-sided confidence interval about the difference between two independent means is also displayed in panel B (column 4) of Table 12–1:

$$(\bar{X}_1 - \bar{X}_2) \pm t_{\alpha/2} \left(s_p \sqrt{\frac{1}{n_1} + \frac{1}{n_2}} \right) \text{ with } df = n_1 + n_2 - 2.$$ 12.6

A test of the null hypothesis of equal daily fiber consumption is shown in Box 12–1. Note that $\left(\frac{s^2_{larger}}{s^2_{smaller}} \right)$ is well within the guideline; we conclude that the population variances are relatively equal and we do not check the sample size rule-of-thumb. We calculate t next. The calculated value, approximately -1.40, falls in the region of retention ($t_{crit} = \pm 1.9987$, $df = 64$, p-value > 0.10, $\alpha = 0.05$). We retain the null hypothesis of no difference. We conclude that women with breast cancer and disease-free women consume approximately equal mean amounts of daily fiber. A prospective cohort investigation to track breast cancer development in groups of women whose diet includes different amounts of dietary fiber may shed more light on this question than a case-control study.

The two-sided confidence interval for this clinical problem is displayed in Box 12–2. The 95% confidence interval for the difference between the population means is approximately

---

Box 12–1. Testing the null hypothesis of equal fiber consumption in two groups of women.

1. *State the scientific hypothesis*
Mean daily dietary fiber consumption (g) differs in two groups of women; one group has breast cancer and the other does not.

2. *Formulate the Statistical Hypotheses*
$H_0 : \mu_{Cancer} - \mu_{No\ Cancer} = 0$
$H_A : \mu_{Cancer} - \mu_{No\ Cancer} \neq 0$

3. *Determine the Decision Rules*
   a. Student's t statistic for the difference between two independent means
   b. Sampling distribution of the difference between two independent means
   c. $\alpha = 0.05$
   d. $t_{crit} = \pm 1.9987$ (based on interpolation) for $df = 25 + 41 - 2 = 64$

4. *Analysis*

   Group With Cancer $\quad\quad$ Cancer-free Group
   $\bar{X}_{Cancer} = 15\ g \quad\quad\quad \bar{X}_{No\ Cancer} = 17\ g$
   $s_{Cancer} = 5\ g \quad\quad\quad\quad s_{No\ Cancer} = 6\ g$
   $n_{Cancer} = 25 \quad\quad\quad\quad n_{No\ Cancer} = 41$

   Check the variance rule-of-thumb:

   $$\left(\frac{6^2}{5^2} \right) = 1.44 < 4 \text{ (Satisfied)}$$

   Obtain pooled estimate, s_p, for denominator of t statistic:

   $$s_p^2 = \frac{(25 - 1)5^2 + (41 - 1)6^2}{25 + 41 - 2} = 31.8750$$

   $$s_p = \sqrt{31.8750} = 5.6458$$

   Calculate denominator of t statistic:

   $$s_p \sqrt{\frac{1}{n_{Cancer}} + \frac{1}{n_{No\ Cancer}}} = 5.6458 \sqrt{\frac{1}{25} + \frac{1}{41}} = 1.4326$$

   Calculate the t statistic:

   $$t = \frac{15 - 17}{1.4326} = -1.3961$$

5. *Evaluate the Statistics*
Retain the null hypothesis that the difference between the two means equals zero.

6. *Interpret the Statistics*
No significant difference exists in mean daily fiber consumption in women who have breast cancer and in women who do not ($t_{calc} = -1.3961$, $t_{crit} = \pm 1.9987$, $df = 64$, p-value > 0.10).

$(-4.86, 0.86)$. Zero, the null hypothesis difference, is captured in this interval. Therefore, we retain the null hypothesis. Note that we reached the same conclusion when we used a conventional hypothesis test.

Now let us consider a clinical example in which the variance rule-of-thumb is not satisfied. However, because the sample size rule-of-thumb is met, we carry out the t test as just demonstrated. Formulae are presented in panel C of Table 12–1. The panel designation is shaded because this application is relatively common.

Box 12–2. Two-sided confidence 95% interval to test null hypothesis of equal fiber consumption in two groups of women.

Write the Statistical Hypotheses
$H_0 : \mu_{Cancer} - \mu_{No\ cancer} = 0$
$H_A : \mu_{Cancer} - \mu_{No\ Cancer} \neq 0$
Construct the 95% Two-sided Interval

$$(\bar{X}_{Cancer} - \bar{X}_{No\ Cancer}) \pm t_{\alpha/2} \left(s_p \sqrt{\frac{1}{n_{Cancer}} + \frac{1}{n_{No\ Cancer}}} \right)$$

$(15 - 17) \pm 1.9987(1.4326) = (15 - 17) \pm 2.8633 = (-4.8633, 0.8633)$

Interpret the Statistics
Retain the null hypothesis because zero is captured in the interval. No significant difference exists between the mean daily fiber consumption of women with breast cancer and women without breast cancer.

Clinical Example: Environmental Exposure to Lead

Two independently sampled populations
Populations distributed normally or approximately normally
Unknown population variances which appear unequal
Similar sample sizes

The effect of environmental exposure to lead on intellectual development is investigated in two randomly selected samples of 7-year-old children from similar demographic, social, and economic backgrounds. Serum lead levels in group 1 children $(n_1 = 61)$ are $> 30\ \mu g/dL$; serum lead levels in group 2 children $(n_2 = 41)$ are $< 10\ \mu g/dL$. Because of conflicting published results, the investigators hypothesize that a difference in intelligence test scores exists between these two groups. A standardized and widely used intelligence test is administered to all children. The mean intelligence test score for group 1 youngsters is 94, with a standard deviation of 17; the mean for group 2 children is 101, with a standard deviation of 8.

Does a significant difference exist between the mean intelligence test score in these two groups? The results of the Student's t test and 95% confidence interval appear in Boxes 12–3 and 12–4, respectively.

Examine Box 12–3; the equal variance rule-of-thumb is not satisfied. Observe, however, that the sample size rule-of-thumb is met. We conduct the t test as outlined in Box 12–1, because the t statistic is robust with respect to moderate departures from the assumption of homogeneity of variance, if sample sizes are equal or approximately equal. We obtain the pooled standard deviation, s_p, and use it in the denominator of the t statistic. Degrees of freedom are $n_1 + n_2 - 2$. The calculated value of t is determined and compared to the critical value $(t_{calc} = -2.4572$ versus $t_{crit} = \pm1.9867)$. Based on these statistics, we reject the null hypothesis of no difference. We conclude that a significant mean difference exists in intelligence scores. We observe that the mean score of children with serum lead levels $> 30\ \mu g/dL$ is lower than that of youngsters with serum lead levels $< 10\ \mu g/dL$ (94 versus 101, respectively). Although we describe the direction of the differences in order to guide other clinicians in formulating hypotheses, we must be careful not to suggest that the current problem involves an *a priori* directional expectation.

Box 12–3. Testing the null hypothesis of equal mean intelligence scores in two groups of children with different serum lead levels.

1. *State the Scientific Hypothesis*
Mean intelligence test scores differ in two groups of 7-year-old children who have different serum lead levels.
2. *Formulate the Statistical Hypotheses*
$H_0 : \mu_1 - \mu_2 = 0$
$H_A : \mu_1 - \mu_2 \neq 0$
3. *Determine the Decision Rules*
   a. Student's t statistic for the difference between two independent means
   b. Sampling distribution of the difference between two independent means
   c. $\alpha = 0.05$
   d. $t_{crit} = \pm 1.9867$ (based on interpolation) for $df = 61 + 41 - 2 = 100$
4. *Analyze the Data*

   Group 1: Blood Lead Level   Group 2: Blood Lead Level
   > 30 µg/dL < 10 µg/dL
   $\overline{X} = 94$ $\overline{X} = 101$
   $s = 17$ $s = 8$
   $n = 61$ $n = 41$

   Check the variance rule-of-thumb:

   $$\left(\frac{17^2}{8^2} \right) = 4.5156 > 4 \text{ (Not satisfied)}$$

   Check sample size rule-of-thumb:

   $$\frac{61}{41} = 1.4878 < 2 \text{ (Satisfied)}$$

   Obtain pooled estimate, s_p, for denominator of t statistic:

   $$s_p^2 = \frac{(61 - 1)17^2 + (41 - 1)8^2}{61 + 41 - 2} = 199.00$$

   $$s_p = \sqrt{199} = 14.1067$$

   Calculate denominator of t statistic:

   $$s_p \sqrt{\frac{1}{n_1} + \frac{1}{n_2}} = 14.1067 \sqrt{\frac{1}{61} + \frac{1}{41}} = 2.8488$$

   Calculate the t statistic:

   $$t = \frac{94 - 101}{2.8488} = -2.4752$$

5. *Evaluate the Statistics*
Reject the null hypothesis.
6. *Interpret the Statistics*
A significant difference exists in mean intelligence test scores in two groups of 7-year-olds who have different mean serum lead levels. The mean score is 94 children with a mean serum lead level > 30 µg/dL, compared to 101 in children with a mean serum lead level < 10 µg/dL ($t_{calc} = -2.4572$, $t_{crit} = \pm 1.9867$, $df = 100$, p-value < 0.02).

Box 12–4. Two-sided confidence 95% interval to test null hypothesis of equal mean intelligence test scores in two groups of children with different serum lead levels.

Write the Statistical Hypotheses
$H_0 : \mu_1 - \mu_2 = 0$
$H_A : \mu_1 - \mu_2 \neq 0$
Construct the 95% Two-sided Interval

$$(\overline{X}_1 - \overline{X}_2) \pm t_{\alpha/2} \left(s_p \sqrt{\frac{1}{n_1} + \frac{1}{n_2}} \right)$$

$(94 - 101) \pm 1.9867 \, (2.8488) = (94 - 101) \pm 5.6597 = (-12.6597, -1.3403)$

Evaluate the Statistics
Reject the null hypothesis of no difference in mean test scores. A significant difference exists between the mean intelligence test scores of children with serum lead levels of > 30 µg/dL and that of children with serum levels of < 10 µg/dL (94 versus 101, respectively). Further, we are 95% confident that the difference between the two means is between approximately -12.7 and -1.3 points, when the difference is constructed as $(\overline{X}_{Higher \, Lead \, Level} - \overline{X}_{Lower \, Lead \, Level})$.

The 95% confidence interval about the difference between the mean intelligence test scores is calculated in Box 12–4. It is not necessary to check the variance and sample size rules-of-thumb, because we considered them when conducting the significance test. Otherwise, we evaluate them before constructing the confidence interval. The 95% confidence interval for the difference between means extends from -12.6597 to -1.3403. Observe that zero is not captured in this interval. Thus, we reject the null hypothesis.

We next explore a hypothetical example, developed from an actual investigation, in which the variance and sample size rules-of-thumb are not met.

Clinical Example: Patient Satisfaction With Medical Care

> Two independently sampled populations
> Populations distributed normally or approximately normally
> Unknown population variances which appear unequal
> Dissimilar sample sizes

Satisfaction with medical care is compared in two groups of randomly selected patients. In one group, patients receive care from clinicians who participate in small multispecialty group practices (MSGs); patients in the other group receive care from clinicians who participate in health maintenance organizations (HMOs). Several indices of patient satisfaction are obtained, including the patient's overall satisfaction with the care received during the last 12 months. Satisfaction is rated on a 100-point scale, with higher ratings indicating greater satisfaction. In MSG patients, the mean level of satisfaction is 80, with a standard deviation of 6 ($n_{MSG} = 20$). In HMO patients, the mean is 63, with a standard deviation of 15 ($n_{HMO} = 50$).

We use the t statistic to examine these data, but we must modify it because, as we see in Box 12–5, the population variances and sample sizes are relatively unequal. We modify the denominator and use each sample variance separately:

$$t = \frac{\overline{X}_1 - \overline{X}_2}{\sqrt{\dfrac{s_1^2}{n_1} + \dfrac{s_2^2}{n_2}}} . \qquad 12.7$$

Statisticians disagree on the next adjustment: whether to adjust the degrees of freedom downward or modify the critical value of t. Results are highly similar regardless of which modification is made (Winer, 1971, p 44). We use the Satterthwaite approach to adjust the degrees of freedom (Rosner, 1986, p 259). The adjusted degrees of freedom are computed as

$$df_{Adjusted} = \frac{\left[\left(\dfrac{s_1^2}{n_1} \right) + \left(\dfrac{s_2^2}{n_2} \right) \right]^2}{\left[\dfrac{(s_1^2/n_1)^2}{(n_1 - 1)} \right] + \left[\dfrac{(s_2^2/n_2)^2}{(n_2 - 1)} \right]} . \qquad 12.8$$

Adjusting the degrees of freedom downward is a penalty for violating the assumption of equal population variances when sample sizes differ considerably. The net effect of reducing the degrees of freedom is to increase the size of the calculated value of t required to reject the null hypothesis (Dawson-Saunders & Trapp, 1994, p 117). Readers interested in how to adjust the critical value of t may wish to consult Winer (1971, pp 42–44) or Daniel (1991, p 147).

The two-sided confidence interval is

$$(\overline{X}_1 - \overline{X}_2) \pm t_{\alpha/2} \sqrt{\frac{s_1^2}{n_1} + \frac{s_2^2}{n_2}} \text{ with } df_{Adj} . \qquad 12.9$$

Is the mean level of satisfaction different between MSG and HMO patients? Calculations are summarized in Boxes 12–5 (*t* test) and 12–6 (confidence interval). We check the equal variance rule-of-thumb first. If it is violated, we next check the sample size rule-of-thumb. If it is violated, we (1) use the separate sample variance estimates to calculate the denominator of the *t* statistic and (2) adjust the degrees of freedom. The assumptions and formulae are given in panel D of Table 12–1. The panel designation is shaded because this application of the *t* test is common.

We see in Box 12–5 that both rules-of-thumb are violated. We (1) use the separate sample variances in the denominator of the *t* statistic and (2) adjust the degrees of freedom. Note that we round the adjusted degrees *down* to the nearest whole value. This adjusted value (df_{Adj} = 67 in this example) is used to determine the critical value of *t* for a two-tailed test with α = 0.05. The critical value is ±1.9958, based on interpolation, from Table A–2 in the appendix of statistical tables. Because the calculated value of *t* is 6.77, we reject the null hypothesis of no difference. We conclude that mean patient satisfaction differs significantly between MSG and HMO patients (*p*-value < 0.001).

Box 12–5. Testing the null hypothesis of equal overall satisfaction with care in two groups of patients.

1. *State the Scientific Hypothesis*
The mean level of overall satisfaction with care received by MSG patients in the 12 months prior to the study differs from that of HMO patients.

2. *Formulate the Statistical Hypotheses*
$H_0 : \mu_{MSG} - \mu_{HMO} = 0$
$H_A : \mu_{MSG} - \mu_{HMO} \neq 0$

3. *Determine the Decision Rules*
    a. Student's *t* statistic for the difference between two independent means
    b. Sampling distribution of the difference between two independent means
    c. α = 0.05
    d. t_{crit} = ±1.9958 (based on interpolation) for $df_{Adjusted}$ = 67 (see below)

4. *Analyze the Data*

Group 1: MSG Patients	Group 2: HMO Patients
$\overline{X}_{MSG}$ = 80	$\overline{X}_{HMO}$ = 63
s_{MSG} = 6	s_{HMO} = 15
n_{MSG} = 20	n_{HMO} = 50

Check the variance rule-of-thumb:

$$\left(\frac{15^2}{6^2} \right) = 6.25 > 4 \text{ (Not satisfied)}$$

Check sample size rule-of-thumb:

$$\frac{50}{20} = 2.5 > 2 \text{ (Not satisfied)}$$

Use the separate sample variances to calculate the denominator of *t* statistic:

$$s_{\overline{x}_1 - \overline{x}_2} = \sqrt{\frac{s^2_{MSG}}{n_{MSG}} + \frac{s^2_{HMO}}{n_{HMO}}}$$

$$= \sqrt{\frac{6^2}{20} + \frac{15^2}{50}}$$

$$= \sqrt{6.3}$$

$$= 2.51$$

Determine the adjusted degrees of freedom:

$$df_{Adjusted} = \frac{\left[\left(\frac{s^2_1}{n_1} \right) + \left(\frac{s^2_2}{n_2} \right) \right]^2}{\left[\frac{(s^2_1/n_1)^2}{(n_1 - 1)} \right] + \left[\frac{(s^2_2/n_2)^2}{(n_2 - 1)} \right]}$$

$$df_{Adjusted} = \frac{\left[\frac{6^2}{20} + \frac{15^2}{50} \right]^2}{\left[\frac{\left(\frac{6^2}{20} \right)^2}{(20 - 1)} + \frac{\left(\frac{15^2}{50} \right)^2}{(50 - 1)} \right]} = 67.9866$$

$df_{Adjusted} = 67$ **(round *down* to the nearest integer)**

Use 67 degrees of freedom to obtain the critical value of t ($t_{crit} = \pm 1.9958$ for $\alpha = 0.05$)
Calculate the t statistic:

$$t = \frac{80 - 63}{2.51} = 6.77$$

5. *Evaluate the Statistics*
Reject the null hypothesis.

6. *Interpret the Statistics*
In two groups of patients, a significant difference exists in mean patient satisfaction with care received during the 12 months prior to the study; MSG patients express a higher level of overall satisfaction than HMO patients (80 versus 63, respectively; $t_{calc} = 6.77$, $t_{crit} = \pm 1.9958$, $df_{Adj} = 67$, p-value < 0.001).

The significance test result is confirmed by the 95% two-sided confidence interval. Calculations appear in Box 12–6. Zero, the difference given in the null hypothesis, is not captured in this interval. Therefore, the null hypothesis is rejected. A significant difference exists between the overall mean satisfaction of MSG and HMO patients. Further, we are 95% confident that the mean difference is between 12 and 23 points, when it is represented as $(\overline{X}_{MSG} - \overline{X}_{HMO})$. Because it appears that MSG patients are more satisfied with overall care received during the 12 months prior to the study, clinicians and administrators may want to identify the sources of lower satisfaction in HMO patients.

Box 12–6. Two-sided confidence 95% interval to test null hypothesis of equal mean overall patient satisfaction with care in two groups of patients.

Write the Statistical Hypotheses
$H_0 : \mu_{MSG} - \mu_{HMO} = 0$
$H_A : \mu_{MSG} - \mu_{HMO} \neq 0$
Construct the 95% Two-sided Interval

$$(\overline{X}_{MSG} - \overline{X}_{HMO}) \pm t_{\alpha/2} \left(\sqrt{\frac{s_1^2}{n_1} + \frac{s_2^2}{n_2}} \right)$$

$(80 - 63) \pm 1.9958 \, (2.51) = (80 - 63) \pm 5.0095 = (11.9905, 22.0095)$

Interpret the Statistics
Reject the null hypothesis of no difference. A significant difference exists between MSG and HMO patients in mean overall satisfaction with care in the 12 months prior to the study. Further, we are 95% confident that the difference between the two means is between approximately 12 and 23 points, when the difference is constructed as $(\overline{X}_{MSG} - \overline{X}_{HMO})$.

Nonnormally Distributed Populations

In the three preceding examples, we assume that the populations are distributed normally or approximately normally. As with problems involving one mean, the Student's t statistic does not apply when the population distributions are nonnormal. Instead, the z statistic is used. If the population variances are known, the z statistic and relevant two-sided confidence interval are expressed as

$$z = \frac{\overline{X}_1 - \overline{X}_2}{\sqrt{\frac{\sigma_1^2}{n_1} + \frac{\sigma_2^2}{n_2}}} \qquad\qquad 12.10$$

$$(\overline{X}_1 - \overline{X}_2) \pm z_{\alpha/2} \sqrt{\frac{\sigma_1^2}{n_1} + \frac{\sigma_2^2}{n_2}}. \qquad\qquad 12.11$$

These formulas and the corresponding assumptions appear in panel E of Table 12–1. No example is presented to highlight their application, because population variances are typically unknown. Instead, we use sample values to estimate these variances. When populations are distributed nonnormally or their shape is unknown, the Central Limit Theorem applies. If samples are large, the sampling distribution of the difference between two independent means will tend to follow a normal curve. The rule-of-thumb for "large" is $n_1 \geq 30 \ and \ n_2 \geq 30$. If this guideline is satisfied, the z statistic and two-sided confidence interval are modified, as follows:

$$z = \frac{\overline{X}_1 - \overline{X}_2}{\sqrt{\frac{s_1^2}{n_1} + \frac{s_2^2}{n_2}}}$$

12.12

$$(\overline{X}_1 - \overline{X}_2) \pm z_{\alpha/2} \sqrt{\frac{s_1^2}{n_1} + \frac{s_2^2}{n_2}} .$$

12.13

Note that assumptions about equality of population variances are not required. The assumptions required to use Formulas 12.11 and 12.12, as well as the formulae, appear in panel F in Table 12–1. The panel designator is shaded because these procedures are used commonly. The following clinical example highlights their use.

Clinical Problem: Atherectomy Versus Balloon Angioplasty

> Nonnormally distributed populations
> Unknown population variances
> Large sample sizes

> Mean time to coronary artery renarrowing is compared in two groups of randomly selected patients who undergo surgery for a blocked coronary artery. One group ($n_{Ath} = 54$) has atherectomy to open the clogged artery; the other group ($n_{Angio} = 48$) has balloon angioplasty. Mean time to renarrowing of the affected artery is 6 months in patients who had atherectomy ($s_{Ath} = 2.3$) and 5.3 months ($s_{Angio} = 2.1$) in patients who had angioplasty. Assume time to renarrowing is distributed nonnormally in both treatment populations.

Is there a difference in mean time to artery renarrowing in these two groups of patients? The answer appears in Boxes 12–7 (significance test) and 12–8 (confidence interval).

Even though the populations are nonnormal, the Central Limit Theorem applies because n_1 and $n_2 \geq 30$. We compute the z statistic with sample variances in this denominator. The obtained value of z is approximately 1.61; we compare it to the critical value of ± 1.96 for a two-tailed test with $\alpha = 0.05$. We retain the null hypothesis of no difference between the means. Although patients having atherectomy experience a slightly longer time to artery renarrowing than patients having angioplasty, we conclude that no significant difference exists (p-value ≈ 0.11). Recall that the p-value corresponds to the two-tailed area for $z = 1.61$ because H_A is nondirectional.

The 95% two-sided confidence interval in Box 12–8 leads to the same conclusion. The confidence interval extends from approximately -0.15 to 1.55 and includes zero. Therefore, no significant difference exists between these two groups in mean time to artery renarrowing.

In summary, to select the appropriate test statistic or confidence interval for inference about the difference between two independent means, we must first determine whether the populations are distributed normally or nonnormally. If populations are distributed normally and population variances are unknown, as is frequently the case, the Student's t statistic is employed. In addition to normality, equal population variances are assumed. Routine testing for homogeneity of population variances is not recommended, in part, because the t test is robust with respect to moderate departures from equality of variance, when sample sizes are relatively equal. If population variances appear relatively equal, the t statistic is calculated with a pooled estimate of the population standard deviation in its denominator and

Box 12–7. Testing the null hypothesis of equal mean time to coronary artery renarrowing in two groups of patients.

1. *State the Scientific Hypothesis*
Mean time to coronary artery renarrowing (months) differs in patients having atherectomy to open a clogged coronary artery, versus those undergoing balloon angioplasty.

2. *Formulate the Statistical Hypotheses*
$H_0 : \mu_{Ath} - \mu_{Angio} = 0$
$H_A : \mu_{Ath} - \mu_{Angio} \neq 0$

3. *Determine the Decision Rules*
   a. z statistic for the difference between two independent means
      Population variances are unknown, populations are nonnormal; n_1 and $n_2 \geq 30$.
   b. Sampling distribution of the difference between two independent means
   c. $\alpha = 0.05$
   d. $z_{crit} = \pm 1.96$

4. *Analysis*

   Atherectomy | Balloon Angioplasty
   $\overline{X}_{Ath} = 6$ months | $\overline{X}_{Angio} = 5.3$ months
   $s_{Ath} = 2.3$ months | $s_{Angio} = 2.1$ months
   $n_{Ath} = 54$ | $n_{Angio} = 48$

   Calculate the standard error of the difference for denominator of z statistic:

   $$s_{\overline{x}_1 - \overline{x}_2} = \sqrt{\frac{s_{Ath}^2}{n_{Ath}} + \frac{s_{Angio}^2}{n_{Angio}}}$$

   $$= \sqrt{\frac{2.3^2}{54} + \frac{2.1^2}{48}} = 0.4357$$

   Calculate the z statistic:

   $$z = \frac{6 - 5.3}{0.4357} = 1.6066$$

5. *Evaluate the Statistics*
Retain the null hypothesis.

6. *Interpret the Statistics*
No significant difference exists in mean time to artery renarrowing in patients undergoing atherectomy to open a clogged coronary artery and in those having balloon angioplasty ($z_{calc} = 1.6066$, $z_{crit} = \pm 1.96$, p-value = 0.1074).

$df = n_1 + n_2 - 2$ (Table 12–1, panel B). If the populations variances are unequal and samples sizes are relatively equal, the t test applies as just described (Table 12–1, panel C). If variances *and* sample sizes differ considerably, two adjustments are made. First, the denominator of the t statistic is computed from the separate sample variances. Second, the degrees of freedom are adjusted downward (Table 12–1, panel D).

The Student's t statistic cannot be used if the populations are nonnormal. Instead, the z statistic is employed. If the population variances are unknown, as often occurs, and sample

Box 12–8. Two-sided confidence 95% interval to test null hypothesis of equal time to recurrence in two groups of patients undergoing a procedure to open a clogged coronary artery.

Write the Statistical Hypotheses
$H_0 : \mu_{Ath} - \mu_{Angio} = 0$
$H_A : \mu_{Ath} - \mu_{Angio} \neq 0$
Construct the 95% Two-sided Interval

$$(\overline{X}_1 - \overline{X}_2) \pm z_{\alpha/2} \sqrt{\frac{s_1^2}{n_1} + \frac{s_2^2}{n_2}}$$

$(6 - 5.3) \pm 1.96\,(0.4357) = (6.0 - 5.3) \pm 0.8540 = (-0.1540, 1.5540)$

Conclusion
Retain the null hypothesis. No significant difference exists in mean time to coronary artery renarrowing in patients undergoing atherectomy and in those having balloon angioplasty to open a clogged coronary artery.

sizes are sufficiently large (n_1 and $n_2 \geq 30$), we use the z statistic with sample variances in the denominator (Table 12–1, panel F).

Whether t or z is used to construct a confidence interval, we reject the null hypothesis of no difference between means if the interval does not include zero. We retain the null hypothesis if the interval captures zero.

INFERENCES FROM DEPENDENT GROUPS DESIGNS

As noted earlier in this chapter, investigators use dependent groups designs to control extraneous sources of variation by creating pairs of subjects; the members of a pair are as similar as possible with regard to these extraneous factors. Dependent groups designs, typically referred to as matched/paired designs, are created in one of three ways: within-subject, naturally occurring pairs, and investigator-created pairs.

In the analysis of matched/paired data, we focus on the *difference between pairs of observations,* rather than the individual observations. The analysis of matched/paired data is similar conceptually to problems involving one mean. The sampling distribution is the random sampling distribution of matched/paired differences. If sampling is from a normally distributed population of differences, the mean of the sampling distribution is μ_d, which equals $\mu_1 - \mu_2$. The standard error of the sampling distribution is the standard error of a matched/paired difference: $\sigma_{\bar{d}} = \frac{\sigma_d}{\sqrt{n}}$, where σ_d is the population standard deviation of the matched/paired differences and n is the number of pairs of observations. However, because the σ_d is usually unknown, the standard error is estimated from sample data; $\sigma_{\bar{d}}$ becomes $s_{\bar{d}} = \frac{s_d}{\sqrt{n}}$, where s_d is the sample standard deviation of the matched/paired differences.

The statistical hypotheses take one of the following forms:

$$H_0 : \mu_d = 0 \qquad H_0 : \mu_d = 0 \qquad H_0 : \mu_d = 0$$

$$H_A : \mu_d \neq 0 \qquad H_A : \mu_d > 0 \qquad H_A : \mu_d < 0$$

The null hypothesis indicates that the mean of the population of matched/paired differences is zero. This is equivalent to indicating no difference between treatments. The first alternative hypothesis indicates a difference between the treatments, but the direction is not specified. The second and third yield a directional or one-tailed test; one leads to a greater than and the other leads to a less than alternative hypothesis.

We employ the Student's t statistic to test hypotheses about the mean of the matched/paired differences if (1) sampling has been from a normally distributed population of differences and (2) the population variance of the matched/paired differences is unknown. The t statistic is

$$t = \frac{\bar{d} - \mu_d}{s_{\bar{d}}} \text{ with } df = n - 1 \qquad \qquad 12.14$$

where $\bar{d}$ is the mean of the sample of matched/paired differences; it equals $(\bar{X}_1 - \bar{X}_2)$;

   μ_d is the mean of the population of matched/paired differences; it equals $(\mu_1 - \mu_2) = 0$;

   $s_{\bar{d}}$ is the standard error of the sample of matched/paired differences; and

   n is the number of pairs.

The two-sided confidence interval, built from the t statistic, is

$$\bar{d} \pm t_{\alpha/2} s_{\bar{d}} \text{ , where} \qquad \qquad 12.15$$

$\bar{d}$ and $s_{\bar{d}}$ are as defined above and $t_{\alpha/2}$ is the critical value of t corresponding to a two-tailed test, α, and specified degrees of freedom. The assumptions and formulae are summarized in panel H of Table 12–1. The panel designator is shaded because this application is common.

The hypothetical Clinical Example 2 at the beginning of the chapter, repeated below, illustrates the analysis of matched/paired data.

Clinical Example: Over-the-Counter Cholesterol Test

The Food and Drug Administration evaluated an over-the-counter home cholesterol test in 10 randomly selected individuals. Patients fast for 12 hours, then measure their total cholesterol level using the home test. Total cholesterol level is then assessed in a certified clinical laboratory. Mean total cholesterol determined from the home test is 201.50 mg/dL. The mean level as measured in the laboratory is 200.6 mg/dL. Is the home test a viable tool to monitor total cholesterol? Assume the population distribution of differences is normal.

Note that the experimental design is within-subjects, because the total cholesterol of each participant is measured under two conditions (home test versus laboratory). Data from the 10 study participants are displayed in Table 12–2. A test of the null hypothesis is presented in Box 12–9; the confidence interval is summarized in Box 12–10.

The hypothesis test follows the conventional steps, beginning first with the scientific hypothesis. The statistical hypotheses are formulated next. The decision rules are specified, including the critical value of t for $\alpha = 0.05$. We begin the analysis by determining the difference between the laboratory-measured cholesterol level and the home test value for each pair of measurements. The mean difference, standard deviation of the matched/paired differences, and standard error are calculated. Finally, the t statistic is obtained. The calculated value of t is approximately -0.42; the critical value is ± 2.262 for $df = 9$ and $\alpha = 0.05$. Thus we retain the null hypothesis of no difference. We conclude that the two tests yield comparable mean measurements. By examining the differences, the reader can see quickly that no apparent consistent measurement error exists for the home test; its values are neither uniformly higher nor lower than those obtained by the clinical laboratory. Based on these limited data, it appears that the over-the-counter home test merits further evaluation in a large number of individuals.

The 95% two-sided confidence interval for the cholesterol data is presented in Box 12–10. The confidence interval extends from approximately -5.8 to 4.0. Because zero is included, we retain the null hypothesis of no mean difference.

In summary, the Student's t test is used for matched/paired data that result from within-subject designs, naturally occurring pairs, and investigator-constructed pairs. When we use the t statistic, we assume that the population distribution of differences is normal and that the population variance is unknown. If the assumption of normality is violated, a statistician should be consulted. Alternately, a confidence interval can be used to make a decision about the null hypothesis.

Table 12–2. Within-subject data to examine comparability of an over-the-counter home and a laboratory test to measure total cholesterol (mg/dL).

Study Participant	Laboratory Test Result	Home Test Result
1	200	208
2	153	147
3	147	156
4	175	169
5	182	191
6	246	252
7	194	187
8	355	357
9	161	155
10	193	193

Box 12–9. Student's *t* test to examine the null hypothesis of comparability of two methods of measuring total cholesterol in 10 individuals.

1. *State the Scientific Hypothesis*
A difference exists between the mean total cholesterol levels (mg/dL) determined in a certified clinical laboratory and from an over-the-counter home test.

2. *Formulate the Statistical Hypotheses*
$H_0 : \mu_d = 0$
$H_A : \mu_d \neq 0$

3. *Determine the Decision Rules*
   a. Student's *t* statistic for a matched/paired design
   b. Sampling distribution of matched/paired differences
   c. $\alpha = 0.05$
   d. $t_{crit} = \pm 2.262$ for $df = 10 - 1 = 9$

4. *Analyze the Data*

Determine the difference for each pair of observations:

Pair	(Lab − Home)	Difference
1	(200 − 208)	−8
2	(153 − 147)	+6
3	(147 − 156)	−9
4	(175 − 169)	+6
5	(182 − 191)	−9
6	(246 − 252)	−6
7	(194 − 187)	+7
8	(355 − 357)	−2
9	(161 − 155)	+6
10	(193 − 193)	0

Calculate the mean of the matched/paired differences

$$\bar{d} = \frac{\sum_{i=1}^{10} d_i}{n} = \frac{(d_1 + d_2 + \ldots + d_{10})}{n}$$

$$\sum_{i=1}^{10} d_i = -8 + 6 + (-9) + \ldots + 0 = -9.0$$

$$\bar{d} = \frac{-9}{10} = -0.90$$

Verify that $\bar{d} = (\bar{X}_{LAB} - \bar{X}_{HOME})$:

$$\bar{X}_{LAB} = \frac{200 + 153 + \ldots + 193}{10} = \frac{2006}{10} = 200.6$$

$$\bar{X}_{HOME} = \frac{208 + 147 + \ldots + 193}{10} = \frac{2015}{10} = 201.50$$

$$(\bar{X}_{LAB} - \bar{X}_{HOME}) = 200.6 - 201.50 = -0.90$$

The calculations check.

Calculate the standard deviation of the differences:

$$s_d^2 = \frac{\sum_{i=1}^{n} d_i^2 - \frac{\left(\sum_{i=1}^{n} d_i\right)^2}{n}}{n - 1}$$

$$\sum_{i=1}^{n} d_i^2 = (-8)^2 + 6^2 + \ldots + 0^2 = 423$$

$$s_d^2 = \frac{423 - \frac{(-9)^2}{10}}{10 - 1} = \frac{414.9}{9} = 46.10$$

$$s_d = \sqrt{s_d^2} = \sqrt{46.10} = 6.7897$$

Obtain the standard error of the difference (denominator of the *t* statistic):

$$s_{\bar{d}} = \frac{s_d}{\sqrt{n}} = \frac{6.7897}{\sqrt{10}} = 2.1471$$

Calculate the t statistic:

$$t = \frac{\bar{d} - \mu_d}{s_{\bar{d}}} = \frac{-0.90 - 0}{2.1471} = -0.4192$$

5. *Evaluate the Statistics*
Retain the null hypothesis.

6. *Interpret the Statistics*
No significant difference exists between the mean total cholesterol levels determined in a certified clinical laboratory and from an over-the-counter home cholesterol test ($t_{calc} = -0.42$, $t_{crit} = \pm 2.262$, $df = 9$, p-value > 0.10, $\alpha = 0.05$).

Box 12–10. Two-sided 95% confidence interval to examine the null hypothesis of no difference between two tests to measure total cholesterol.

Formulate the Statistical Hypotheses
$H_0 : \mu_d = 0$
$H_A : \mu_d \neq 0$
Construct the 95% Two-sided Confidence Interval

$\bar{d} \pm t_{\alpha/2} s_{\bar{d}}$

$-0.90 \pm 2.262 (2.1471) = -0.90 \pm 4.8567 = (-5.7567, 3.9567)$

Interpret the Statistics
Retain the null hypothesis. No significant difference exists in mean total cholesterol determined in a certified clinical laboratory and from an over-the-counter home cholesterol test.

SUMMARY

Figure 12–1 identifies necessary decisions for selecting the appropriate test statistic to examine hypotheses about the difference between two means. Choosing the appropriate test statistic or confidence interval requires that we determine first whether observations are from an independent groups or matched/paired design.

Analyses from an independent groups model involve determining whether the populations are distributed normally or nonnormally. The Student's t statistic is used if populations are distributed normally; population variances are unknown, but assumed equal. We use sample statistics to estimate these unknown population variances. Routine testing for equal population variances is no longer recommended, in part because the t test is robust with respect to moderate departures from equal population variances, *if sample sizes are relatively equal*. We use rules-of-thumb to examine the sample variances and sample sizes and determine if adjustments to the t statistic and its degrees of freedom are required.

The Student's t statistic cannot be used if the populations are nonnormal; the z statistic is employed instead. If the population variances are unknown, as is typically the case, and sample sizes are sufficiently large (n_1 *and* $n_2 \geq 30$), the z statistic is used with sample variances in the denominator.

The Student's t test for matched/paired data rests on the assumption that the population distribution of differences is normal and its variance is unknown. If the assumption of normality is violated, consult a statistician.

Regardless of the design (independent groups versus matched/paired model), a confidence interval can be used to make a decision about the null hypothesis. The null hypothesis is rejected if the difference given in the null hypothesis (typically zero) falls outside the interval. Many journals require that confidence intervals supplement significance tests, particularly when the null hypothesis is rejected. Although many statisticians recommend eliminating conventional significance tests in favor of confidence intervals, the use of significance tests is so ingrained that this recommendation has not been widely adopted.

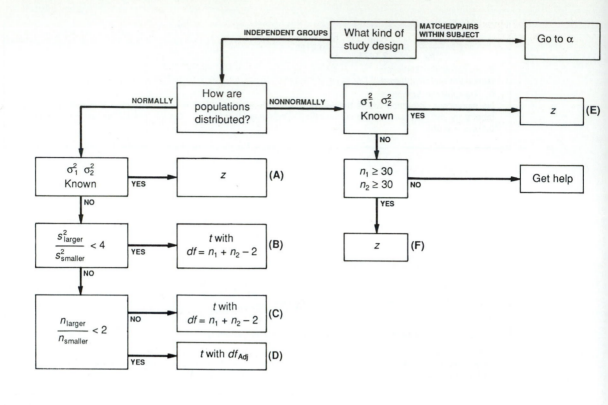

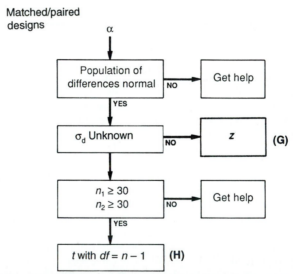

Figure 12–1. Flowchart for the analysis of two means. (Letters in brackets refer to the lettered panel in Table 12–1 in which inference about two means is summarized.)

REFERENCES

Daniel W: *Biostatistics: A Foundation for Analysis in the Health Sciences,* 5th ed. Wiley, 1991.

Dawson-Saunders B, Trapp R: *Basic and Clinical Biostatistics,* 2nd ed. Appleton & Lange, 1994.

Hays W: *Statistics,* 3rd ed. Holt, Rinehart and Winston, 1981.
Potter S et al: Influences of infant feeding method on maternal post-partum weight loss. *J Am Dietetic Assoc* 1991;**91**:441.
Rosner B: *Fundamentals of Biostatistics,* 2nd ed. Duxbury Press, 1986.
Winer BJ: *Statistical Principles in Experimental Design,* 2nd ed. McGraw-Hill, 1971.

Self-study Questions

Part I: Definitions

Define each of the following terms.

Dependent groups design (matched/paired design)
Independent groups design
Homogeneity or equality of variance

Part II: Brief Answer Questions

1. Explain why a matched/paired study design is used.
2. Explain the difference between a within-subject study design and one in which investigator-created pairs are used.
3. Compare the *statistical* hypotheses for independent and matched/paired study designs.
4. List the questions that should be answered to select the appropriate test statistic (including its denominator and degrees of freedom) for the analysis of the difference between two independent means.
5. Summarize how the assumption of equal population variances affects selection of the test statistic to examine the difference between two independent means.
6. Explain the effect of adjusting the degrees of freedom on the critical value of t.
7. Identify the factors to consider when selecting a test to analyze the mean difference in a matched/paired study.

Part III: Analysis Identification

Read the following problems and determine if two mean analysis techniques are appropriate. Justify your response.

1. Physicians from the World Health Organization (WHO) travel to Bangladesh to study resistance to nalidixic acid, an antibiotic used to treat *Shigella dysenteriae*. Based on case reports, WHO officials suspect an increase in the number of patients who have contracted resistant strains. It was well established in 1985 that 30% of patients with this disease developed a strain that was resistant to nalidixic acid. In a 1994 survey of 10 consecutive admissions to a hospital in Bangladesh, 9 patients presented with a strain of *Shigella dysenteriae* that was resistant to nalidixic acid.
2. A cardiologist studies the effectiveness of vitamin D to control high blood pressure in 15 patients with intermittent hypercalcemia. Mean systolic blood pressure at the beginning of the trial is 162.4 mm Hg; it is 146.8 mm Hg at the end of 6 months ($s_d = 15.86$).

Part IV: Problems and Analysis

Read each problem and analyze the data as indicated. If an hypothesis is to be tested, identify the scientific and statistical hypotheses, state the decision rules, do the analysis, make a decision about the null hypothesis, and interpret the results. Set $\alpha = 0.05$ in all problems.

1. A radiologist assesses the viability of carotid B-mode ultrasonography to evaluate artherosclerosis in 20 randomly selected patients. Two tests are conducted, 48 hours apart. The same technician performs all tests. The space between the carotid lesions, known as the minimum residual lumen (MRL), is measured by the same radiologist who was unaware of the purpose of the study. The difference between measurements is computed by subtracting the smaller MRL reading from the larger one. The mean difference is 0.65 mm ($s_d = 0.43$). Construct the 95% confidence interval about the mean difference and use it to test the null hypothesis of no mean difference. Assume the relevant population distribution(s) is (are) normal.

2. Diabetics often have an abnormality of the capillary basal lamina (basement membrane) characterized by added layers and increased thickness of the lamina, which are detected easily in the major capillary beds of skin and skeletal muscle. A preliminary clinical trial was conducted to determine the effectiveness of an experimental drug to treat this abnormality in randomly sampled diabetics. Forty diabetics were treated with the drug for 2 years; the mean thickness of the capillary basal lamina at the end of the treatment period was 161.0 mm ($s = 10.2$). Thirty-four diabetics received an apparently-identical placebo for 2 years; for the placebo group, the mean thickness was 170.9 mm ($s = 14.7$) at the end of two years. Do these means differ significantly? Assume the population distributions are normal.

3. In their first investigation, two clinicians compared 11 different tests of tobacco smoke intake to detect smoking. They found that measuring the level of carbon monoxide in an individual's breath was inexpensive and reproducible. Their objective in a second study was to determine if smokers have a higher level of carbon monoxide in their breath than nonsmokers. The mean level of expired carbon monoxide in 25 randomly selected non-smokers was 7.5 ppm ($s = 4.3$); it was 21.3 ppm ($s = 10.2$) in 10 randomly chosen cigarette smokers. Assume normality of relevant distributions.

4. Three psychiatrists hypothesize that the psychological well-being of families with a child who has a chronic physical illness will be significantly lower than that of families with a healthy child. Parental education (both parents having at least a BA or BS degree), family income (gross $100,000 or greater), number of children (only one), and family type (married, both parents living in the family home) are controlled for by sampling families with similar characteristics. The mean well-being of families with a chronically ill child is 50.6 ($s = 7.9$, $n = 37$) and that of families with a healthy child is 61.5 ($s = 3.1$, $n = 50$). Assume that relevant population(s) is (are) distributed nonnormally.

Part V: Interpretation

Read the following problem. Was the conclusion determined appropriately? Why or why not?

In 1959, three clinicians studied the cholesterol level of two groups of healthy men, age 19 to 23 years, with and without a family history of coronary heart disease. The mean cholesterol of the 70 young men with a positive family history was 263 mg/dL ($s = 70$). The mean cholesterol of the 61 young men with a negative family history was 220 mg/dL ($s = 55$). The researchers constructed a two-sided 95% confidence interval about the mean of 263 and found it did not include 220: 95% CI = ($250 \leq \mu \leq 276$). They concluded that a significant difference exists between these two groups of men with respect to mean cholesterol levels.

Solutions

Part III: Analysis Identification

1. *Shigella dysenteriae*
   The dependent variable is *qualitative* and, in particular, binomial. A patient either has or does not have a strain of *Shigella dysenteriae* that is resistant to nalidixic acid. Analyses of one and two means require that the dependent variable be *quantitative*. Therefore, nei-

ther a one-mean nor a two-mean analysis is appropriate. Instead, we should employ an analysis that will allow us to test an hypothesis about one proportion.

2. *Vitamin D and High Blood Pressure*
   A pre-post design was used to assess the effectiveness of vitamin D to control high blood pressure. If the population distribution for the differences is normal, the Student's *t* test for matched/paired data is used.

Part IV: Problems and Analysis

1. *Carotid B-mode Ultrasonography*
   State the Scientific Hypothesis:
   A difference exists between the mean width of the minimum residual lumen measured on two different occasions in the same group of patients.
   Formulate the Statistical Hypotheses:

$$H_0 : \mu_d = 0$$

$$H_A : \mu_d \neq 0$$

If carotid B-mode ultrasonography is used to evaluate the space between carotid lesions and to assess the degree of artherosclerosis, the procedure should yield highly consistent results, if tests are repeated on the same patient within a relatively short period of time. Therefore, the radiologist hopes to retain the null hypothesis of no difference.

Determine the Decision Rules:
a. Student's *t* statistic for a matched/paired design (within-subjects).
b. Sampling distribution of matched/paired differences.
c. $\alpha = 0.05$.
d. $t_{crit} = \pm 2.093$, $df = 20 - 1 = 19$.

Analyze the Data:
Givens:

$$\bar{d} = 0.65 \ mm$$

$$s_d = 0.43$$

$$n = 20$$

Calculate the standard error of a matched/paired difference:

$$s_{\bar{d}} = \frac{0.43}{\sqrt{20}} = 0.0962$$

Construct the 95% two-sided confidence interval:

$$0.65 \pm (2.093)\ (0.0962) = 0.65 \pm 0.2013 = (0.4487, 0.8513)$$

Evaluate the Statistics:
Reject the null hypothesis of no difference.

Interpret the Statistics:
The two-sided 95% confidence interval extends from a mean difference of approximately 0.45 to 0.85 mm. Therefore, a significant mean difference exists in the MRL measurements from two separate carotid B-mode ultrasonographic procedures, done within 48 hours of each other on the same patients. Factors contributing to this difference should be explored and eliminated before considering the use of this procedure to evaluate artherosclerosis (eg, the skill level of the technician). In addition, the magni-

tude of the differences in results should be evaluated to determine if they are clinically significant.

2. *Thickness of the Basement Membrane in Diabetics*

State the Scientific Hypothesis:

A difference exists at the end of 2 years in the mean thickness of the capillary basal lamina in diabetics who receive an experimental drug versus diabetics who receive an identically-appearing placebo.

Formulate the Statistical Hypotheses:

$$H_0 : \mu_{DRUG} - \mu_{PLACEBO} = 0$$

$$H_A : \mu_{DRUG} - \mu_{PLACEBO} \neq 0$$

Decision Rules:

a. Student's t statistic for the difference between two independent means.
b. Random sampling distribution of the difference between two independent means.
c. $\alpha = 0.05$.
d. $t_{crit} = \pm 1.996$ (based on interpolation), $df = 40 + 34 - 2 = 72$.

See below for verification of rules-of-thumb.

Analysis:

(D = Drug, P = Placebo.)

$\bar{X}_D = 161.0$ $\bar{X}_P = 170.9$
$s_D = 10.2$ $s_P = 14.7$
$n_D = 40$ $n_P = 34$

Check the variance rule-of-thumb:

$$\left(\frac{14.7^2}{10.2^2} \right) = 2.077 < 4 \text{ (Satisfied)}$$

Because the variance rule-of-thumb is satisfied, we proceed with the analysis. We use a pooled estimate of the common population standard deviation in the denominator of the t statistic, and evaluate it with $df = n_D + n_P - 2$.

Calculate the pooled estimate of the common population standard deviation:

$$s^2_{pooled} = \frac{(40 - 1)\, 10.2^2 + (34 - 1)\, 14.7^2}{40 + 34 - 2} = 155.3963$$

$$s_{pooled} = 12.4658$$

Calculate the standard error of the difference for the denominator of the t test:

$$s_p \sqrt{\frac{1}{n_D} + \frac{1}{n_P}} = 12.4658 \sqrt{\frac{1}{40} + \frac{1}{34}} = 2.9078$$

Calculate t:

$$t = \frac{161 - 170.9}{2.9078} = -3.4046$$

Evaluate the Statistics:

We reject the null hypothesis of no difference.

Interpret the Statistics:

A significant difference exists between the mean thickness of the capillary basal lamina in diabetic patients who took an experimental drug for 2 years and those who received an identical-appearing placebo ($t_{crit} = -3.4046$, $t_{crit} = \pm1.996$, $df = 72$, p-value < 0.001). Mean thickness of this membrane was less in patients who took the drug ($\overline{X} = 161.0$ mm) than in diabetic individuals who received the placebo ($\overline{X} = 170.9$ mm).

3. *Expired Carbon Monoxide Levels in Smokers and Nonsmokers*

State the Scientific Hypothesis:

The mean level of expired carbon monoxide is higher in the breath of a smoker than in a nonsmoker.

Formulate the Statistical Hypotheses:

$$H_0 : \mu_S - \mu_{NS} = 0$$

$$H_A : \mu_S - \mu_{NS} > 0$$

Decision Rules:

a. Student's t statistic for the difference between two independent means.

b. Random sampling distribution of the difference between two independent means.

c. $\alpha = 0.05$.

d. $t_{crit} = 1.812$, $df_{Adj} = 10$ (see below).

Analysis:

(S = Smoker, NS = Nonsmoker.)

$\overline{X}_S = 21.3$ ppm $\overline{X}_{NS} = 7.5$ ppm

$s_S = 10.2$ $s_{NS} = 4.3$

$n_S = 10$ $n_{NS} = 25$

Check the variance rule-of-thumb:

$$\left(\frac{10.2^2}{4.3^2} \right) = 5.63 > 4 \text{ (Not satisfied)}$$

Because the variance rule-of-thumb is not satisfied, we check the sample size rule-of-thumb. If it is violated, we use the separate sample variances to determine the standard error. We then adjust the degrees of freedom.

Check the sample size rule-of-thumb:

$$\frac{25}{10} = 2.5 \text{ (Not satisfied)}$$

Compute the standard error of the difference (use separate sample variances):

$$\sqrt{\frac{s_S^2}{n_S} + \frac{s_{NS}^2}{n_{NS}}} = \sqrt{\frac{10.2^2}{10} + \frac{4.3^2}{25}} = 3.3382$$

Adjust the degrees of freedom (use the adjusted value to identify the critical value of t for $\alpha = 0.05$ and a one-tailed *greater than* test):

$$df_{Adj} = \frac{\left[\left(\frac{10.2^2}{10} \right) + \left(\frac{4.3^2}{25} \right) \right]^2}{\dfrac{\left(\frac{10.2^2}{10} \right)^2}{(10-1)} + \dfrac{\left(\frac{4.3^2}{25} \right)^2}{(25-1)}} = 10.3055 = 10$$

Calculate the t statistic:

$$t = \frac{21.3 - 7.5}{3.3382} = 4.1340$$

Evaluate the Statistics:
We reject the null hypothesis.

Interpret the Statistics:
The mean level of expired carbon monoxide is significantly higher in smokers ($\bar{X}$ = 21.3 ppm) than nonsmokers ($\bar{X}$ = 7.5 ppm; t_{calc} = 4.1340, t_{crit} = 1.812, df_{Adj} = 10, p-value < 0.005).

4. *Family Well-being*

State the Scientific Hypothesis:
The well-being of families with a child who has a chronic physical illness is significantly lower than that of families with a healthy child.

Formulate the statistical hypotheses:

$$H_0 : \mu_I - \mu_H = 0$$

$$H_A : \mu_I - \mu_H < 0$$

Decision Rules:
a. z statistic, because populations are distributed nonnormally and n_1 and $n_2 \geq 30$.
b. Random sampling distribution of the difference between two independent means. The standard normal curve will be used to evaluate the z statistic.
c. $\alpha = 0.05$.
d. $z = -1.645$ (Note that the direction is a function of how we set up H_A).

Analysis:

(I = Ill, H = Healthy.)

$\bar{X}_I = 50.6$ $\bar{X}_H = 61.5$
$s_I = 7.9$ $s_H = 3.1$
$n_I = 37$ $n_H = 50$

Calculate the standard error of the difference:

$$\sqrt{\frac{7.9^2}{37} + \frac{3.1^2}{50}} = 1.3708$$

Determine the value of z:

$$z = \frac{50.6 - 61.5}{1.3703} = -7.9518$$

Evaluate the Statistics:
We reject the null hypothesis.

Interpret the Statistics:
Families with a child who has a chronic physical illness function at a level of psychological well-being significantly below that of families with a healthy child (p-value < 0.0005). We note, however, that these findings may be limited to one-child families in which both parents are married and live in the family home; both parents have at least a bachelor's degree; and the family has a yearly minimum gross income of $100,000.

Part V: Interpretation

These clinicians committed a common error. They have constructed a confidence interval about one sample mean, and used the interval to answer a question about the *difference between two means*. No conclusion is justified until the data are analyzed appropriately.

Testing Hypotheses About a Proportion   13

Clinical Example: Migraine Headache

Ergotamine tartrate was compared to standard aspirin to determine which is more effective in providing relief after the onset of migraine headache. It is well documented that 20% of migraine patients experience relief if they take aspirin immediately following the onset of headache. Ten randomly chosen migraine sufferers took an appropriate oral dose of ergotamine tartrate immediately after migraine headache onset; four experienced relief. If taken immediately after onset of headache, is ergotamine tartrate more effective than standard aspirin in relieving migraine pain?

To answer research questions about means in the three previous chapters, we computed means, standard deviations, and standard errors; we also used the Student's *t* test and *z* statistic. In contrast, the outcome of interest in the current chapter is binomial, such as relief (yes/no), survival (yes/no), or remission (yes/no), rather than quantitative (eg, total cholesterol in mg/dL, or blood pressure in mm Hg). Research questions for which the outcome is binomial involve examining frequencies and proportions. In this chapter, we discuss the binomial exact test and the normal approximation to the binomial.

OBJECTIVES

When you complete this chapter, you should be able to:

- Select between the binomial exact test and normal approximation to the binomial to test a hypothesis about one proportion.
- Conduct a test of a null hypothesis about one proportion by utilizing the appropriate test statistic or confidence interval.
- Translate the findings from a test of a null hypothesis about one proportion into non-statistical language.

SINGLE-GROUP STUDIES

Single-group investigations may be used to estimate a population parameter or to pilot an experimental treatment, procedure, or diagnostic test; the outcome in the group is then compared to (1) a well-established value that is treated as a population parameter or (2) a response under a well-accepted treatment regime.

Consider the following examples. Suppose that 23% of men diagnosed in 1974 with stage D prostate cancer survived 5 years with conventional treatment. In 1987, 100 randomly selected men newly diagnosed with stage D prostate cancer received an experimental treatment; 30% survived 5 years. Was there a significant increase in 5-year survival among the affected men who received the experimental treatment in 1987 versus the men who received conventional treatment in 1974?

Fifty percent of patients diagnosed with congestive heart failure (CHF) in 1948 survived 2 to 3 years after diagnosis. Among 250 randomly selected men diagnosed in 1988 with CHF, 130 or 52% survived 2 to 3 years after diagnosis. Has a significant increase occurred over the last 40 years in the proportion of men who survive 2 to 3 years following a diagnosis of CHF?

The binomial distribution, introduced in Chapter 8, can be used to answer these questions. The binomial model applies when there are n independent trials, with the number of trials (n) specified in advance. Two outcomes are possible; only one will be observed on any given trial. The probability of a given outcome is constant over all trials. The sample proportion is p and equals X/n, where X is the count of the number of occurrences of the outcome of interest. We use sample data to estimate the population proportion or to test the null hypothesis. The statistical hypotheses may take one of the following forms, where π is the population proportion and π_0 is its specific value:

$$H_0 : \pi = \pi_0 \qquad H_0 : \pi = \pi_0 \qquad H_0 : \pi = \pi_0$$

$$H_A : \pi \neq \pi_0 \qquad H_A : \pi < \pi_0 \qquad H_A : \pi > \pi_0$$

The first set of hypotheses produces a nondirectional or two-tailed test. The second and third set yield directional or one-tailed tests: one produces a *less than* and the other a *greater than* test.

BINOMIAL EXACT TEST

The *binomial exact test* employs the binomial formula to compute the one- or two-tailed probability of X occurrences of the outcome of interest in n independent trials. In this chapter, the binomial formula, introduced in Chapter 8 (Formula 8.1), is modified slightly in order to test a hypothesis about the population proportion, π. The modified formula is

$$\frac{n!}{X!(n-X)!} \pi^x (1 - \pi)^{n-X} \qquad \textbf{13.1}$$

Pi (π) is the value of the population proportion in the null hypothesis; $(1 - \pi)$ is its complement. X is the count of the number of occurrences (frequency) of the outcome of interest in n independent trials. In the previous examples, each patient was treated as if he or she constituted a trial.

The test of the null hypothesis is referred to as the "exact" test because the probabilities associated with the outcome of interest are computed directly from the formula (13.1) that describes the binomial probability distribution. Before we discuss the exact test in greater detail, we describe a binomial population and the sampling distribution generated from this population.

Binomial Population and Sampling Distribution of a Sample Proportion

Consider a large population of binomial events, with one outcome designated arbitrarily as a "success" and assigned a value of 1. The other outcome is identified as a "failure" and assigned a value of 0. The mean of this binomial population equals the population proportion of successes, that is, $\mu = \pi$. The standard deviation of this population is $\sigma = \sqrt{\pi(1 - \pi)}$. We create the sampling distribution by taking repeated random samples of size n, computing the proportion of 1s in each sample, and casting these sample proportions into a relative frequency distribution. The result is the sampling distribution of the sample proportion. This distribution, with a mean of π and standard error of $\sqrt{[\pi(1 - \pi)]/n}$ is bell-shaped when π equals 0.50. For values of π other than 0.50, however, the sampling distribution approaches a Gaussian (normal, bell-shaped) distribution, as sample size increases (Colton, 1974, pp 153–155). Because the binomial exact test is applied generally to relatively small samples and because π seldom equals 0.50, the sampling distribution is skewed. Therefore, the probability for a two-tailed test is not a simple doubling of the probability in one tail. Examples of research involving one- and two-tailed binomial exact tests appear below.

Testing a Directional Hypothesis: Ergotamine Tartrate Revisited

Recall the hypothetical clinical example at the beginning of the chapter. The statistical question to be answered is: "If ergotamine tartrate has the same chance of yielding relief as aspirin, how likely is it that *four or more* patients will experience relief after taking ergotamine tartrate?" Box 13–1 contains the answer to this question.

The one-tailed binomial exact test requires that we compute the probability of all events *as extreme or more extreme* than the sample result in the direction consistent with the alternative hypothesis. We compute $pr(X \geq 4)$ in this example, because the alternative hypothesis is a *greater than* statement. We can follow two approaches to calculate the desired probability, also known as the obtained probability or p-value. We could determine $pr(X = 4)$, $pr(X = 5)$, $pr(X = 6)$, $pr(X = 7)$, $pr(X = 8)$, $pr(X = 9)$, and $pr(X = 10)$ and add them together. We could also recognize that

$$pr(X \geq 4) = 1 - [pr(X = 0) + pr(X = 1) + pr(X = 2) + pr(X = 3)].$$

Box 13–1. Testing the effectiveness of ergotamine tartrate compared to standard aspirin.

1. *State the Scientific Hypothesis*
A larger proportion of migraine headache sufferers will experience relief after taking ergotamine tartrate than standard aspirin immediately after migraine onset.

2. *Formulate the Statistical Hypotheses*
$H_0 : \pi = 0.20$
$H_A : \pi > 0.20$

3. *Determine the Decision Rules*
   a. Binomial exact test.
   b. Sampling distribution for a sample proportion.
   c. $\alpha = 0.05$.

4. *Analyze the Data*
$X = 4$ (number of patients experiencing relief after taking ergotamine tartrate)
$n = 10$ (total number of patients in the study)

   Although the sample proportion is not required, it typically is reported:

   $$p = \frac{X}{n} = \frac{4}{10} = 0.40$$

   Compute the probability of all events *as extreme or more extreme* than the sample result:
   $$pr(X \geq 4) = pr(X = 4) + pr(X = 5) + \ldots + pr(X = 10)$$
   Computational effort can be reduced if we recognize that:
   $$pr(X \geq 4) = 1 - [pr(X = 0) + pr(X = 1) + pr(X = 2) + pr(X = 3)]$$
   $$pr(X = 0) = \frac{10!}{0!(10 - 0)!} \cdot 20^0(1 - 0.20)^{10-0} = (1)(1)0.80^{10} = 0.1074$$
   $$pr(X = 1) = \frac{10!}{1!(10 - 1)!} \cdot 20^1(1 - 0.20)^{10-1} = (10)(0.20^1)(0.80^9) = 0.2684$$
   $$pr(X = 2) = \frac{10!}{2!(10 - 2)!} \cdot 20^2(1 - 0.20)^{10-2} = (45)(0.20^2)(0.80^8) = 0.3020$$
   $$pr(X = 3) = \frac{10!}{3!(10 - 3)!} \cdot 20^3(1 - 0.20)^{10-3} = (120)(0.20^3)(0.80^7) = 0.2013$$
   $$pr(X \geq 4) = 1 - [0.1074 + 0.2684 + 0.3020 + 0.2013] = 0.1209$$

5. *Evaluate the Statistics*
Because the obtained probability (0.1209) is greater than $\alpha = 0.05$, the null hypothesis is retained.

6. *Interpret the Statistics*
Although 40% of 10 migraine patients experienced relief after taking ergotamine tartrate, the data do not support a claim that ergotamine tartrate, taken immediately after headache onset, is *significantly* more effective than standard aspirin in relieving migraine headaches (p-value = 0.12, $\alpha = 0.05$).

The *p*-value, as seen in Box 13–1, is approximately 0.12. If the *p*-value is greater than α, we retain the null hypothesis; if the *p*-value is less than or equal to α, we reject the null hypothesis:

Retain H_0 if *p*-value $> α$
Reject H_0 if *p*-value $\leq α$.

This *p*-value leads to the retention of the null hypothesis (*p*-value $> α$: $0.12 > 0.05$). The sample proportion of 0.40 is compatible with a population of binomial events in which 0.20 of patients experience migraine headache relief after taking standard aspirin. Recall that at least two competing explanations may account for this finding. First, the null hypothesis may be "true" and ergotamine tartrate and standard aspirin may be equally effective. Second, ergotamine tartrate may be more effective than standard aspirin (the alternative hypothesis), but the sample size may have been too small to permit the statistical detection of its effectiveness. Thus, if the investigators wish to repeat the study, they should increase the sample size.

Testing a Nondirectional Hypothesis

Clinical Example: Mycosis Fungoides

An uncommon form of lymphoma, mycosis fungoides initially manifests in the skin. Disease progression leads to dissemination to the lymph nodes, spleen, and internal organs. Conventional therapy for disease limited to the skin includes topical chemotherapy. This therapy offers the opportunity for clinical clearing and variable periods of remission. Treatment continues until the skin clears. After clearance, maintenance therapy is administered for 6 to 24 months (Abel et al, 1993, pp 93–115). Suppose that 20% of patients with advanced disease limited to the skin experience a 12-month disease-free interval with conventional therapy, after skin clearance.

In a study, 13 patients with advanced disease limited to the skin underwent PUVA photochemotherapy. Patients ingested 8-methoxypsoralen, a photosensitizing drug, followed by exposure to high-intensity longwave (UVA) irradiation. Five patients experienced a 12-month disease-free interval after skin clearance.

In this hypothetical example, does a difference exist between conventional therapy and PUVA photochemotherapy in the proportion of patients with advanced mycosis fungoides who experience a 12-month disease-free interval after treatment? A nondirectional question is formulated because the study is a pilot investigation and outcomes in both the *less than* and *greater than* direction would have clinical significance. The calculations for this example appear in Box 13–2.

To answer the statistical question posed earlier, follow these steps:

Write the hypotheses (steps 1 and 2).
Formulate the decision rules (step 3).
Compute the probability in the upper tail (step 4, part 1). In this case, the upper tail (the *greater than* direction) contains the sample outcome and all events that are as extreme or more extreme than the sample outcome. The upper tail contains counts of 5, 6, 7, 8, 9, 10, 11, 12, and 13. The probability is

$$pr(X \geq 5) = pr(X = 5) + pr(X = 6) + \ldots + pr(X = 13)$$

Because the sum of all mutually exclusive events is 1.00, we may utilize the following relationship to reduce computational labor:

$$pr(X \geq 5) = 1 - [pr(X = 0) + pr(X = 1) + \ldots + pr(X = 4)]$$

The probability of $X \geq 5$ is 0.0991 from Box 13–2. At this point, we know that we will retain the null hypothesis because the computed probability exceeds α. We continue the computations to illustrate how to figure the lower-tail probability.

Box 13–2. Examining PUVA photochemotherapy for the treatment of advanced mycosis fungoides.

1. *State the Scientific Hypothesis*
In the proportion of patients with advanced mycosis fungoides who experience a 12-month disease-free interval after treatment with maintenance, a difference will exist between those who receive conventional chemotherapy and those who receive PUVA photochemotherapy.

2. *Formulate the Statistical Hypotheses*
$H_0 : \pi = 0.20$
$H_A : \pi \neq 0.20$

3. *Determine the Decision Rules*
   a. Binomial exact test.
   b. Sampling distribution of a sample proportion.
   c. $\alpha = 0.05$.

4. *Analyze the Data*
$X = 5$ (number of patients experiencing a 12-month disease-free interval after PUVA therapy)
$n = 13$ (total number of patients in the study)

Although the sample proportion is not required, it should be computed:

$$p = \frac{X}{n} = \frac{5}{13} = 0.3846$$

Part 1: Compute the probability in the upper tail: The upper tail contains all events as extreme or more extreme in the greater than direction than the sample result.

$pr(X \geq 5) = pr(X = 5) + pr(X = 6) + \ldots + pr(X = 13)$

Computational effort can be reduced if we use the following relationship:

$pr(X \geq 5) = 1 - [pr(X = 0) + pr(X = 1) + \ldots + pr(X = 4)]$

$$pr(X = 0) = \frac{13!}{0!(13 - 0)!} \cdot 20^0(1 - 0.20)^{13-0} = (1)(1)0.80^{13} = 0.0550$$

$$pr(X = 1) = \frac{13!}{1!(13 - 1)!} \cdot 20^1(1 - 0.20)^{13-1} = (13)(0.20^1)(0.80^{12}) = 0.1787$$

$$pr(X = 2) = \frac{13!}{2!(13 - 2)!} \cdot 20^2(1 - 0.20)^{13-2} = (78)(0.20^2)(0.80^{11}) = 0.2680$$

$$pr(X = 3) = \frac{13!}{3!(13 - 3)!} \cdot 20^3(1 - 0.20)^{13-3} = (286)(0.20^3)(0.80^{10}) = 0.2457$$

$$pr(X = 4) = \frac{13!}{4!(13 - 4)!} \cdot 20^4(1 - 0.20)^{13-4} = (715)(0.20^4)(0.80^9) = 0.1535$$

$pr(X \geq 5) = 1 - [0.0550 + 0.1787 + 0.2680 + 0.2457 + 0.1535] = 0.0991$

Part 2: Compute the probability in the lower tail: The lower tail includes all counts in the opposite direction that are less likely to occur than the sample result.

Compute the probability of the sample result:

$$pr(X = 5) = \frac{13!}{5!(13 - 5)!} 0.20^5(1 - 0.20)^{13-5} = 1287(0.20^5)(0.20^8) = 0.0691$$

Select the most extreme count in the opposite direction, compute its probability, compare it to $pr(X = 5)$; the most extreme count in the opposite direction is $X = 0$:

$$pr(X = 0) = \frac{13!}{0!(13 - 0)!} 0.20^0(1 - 0.20)^{13-0} = 1(1)(0.80^{13}) = 0.0550$$

Include $X = 0$ in the lower tail if $pr(X = 0) < pr(X = 5)$: $0.0550 < 0.0691$.

Select the next most extreme count in the opposite direction and compute its probability:

$$pr(X = 1) = \frac{13!}{1!(13 - 1)!} 0.20^1(1 - 0.20)^{13-1} = (13)(0.20^1)(0.80^{12}) = 0.1787$$

Include $X = 1$ in the lower tail if $pr(X = 1) < pr(X = 5)$: $0.1785 > 0.691$. Thus, the lower tail includes only $X = 0$. Note that no other count in the opposite direction qualifies for inclusion in the lower tail: $pr(X = 2) = 0.2680$; $pr(X = 3) = 0.2457$; $pr(X = 4) = 0.1535$.

Part 3: Add the probabilities obtained in steps 1 and 2 to obtain the two-tailed p-value

p-value $= pr(X = 0) + pr(X \geq 5) = 0.0550 + 0.0991 = 0.1541$

5. *Evaluate the Statistics*
Because the obtained probability (0.1541) exceeds $\alpha = 0.05$, the null hypothesis is retained.

6. *Interpret the Statistics*
Approximately 38% of patients with advanced mycosis fungoides experienced a 12-month disease-free interval following PUVA photochemotherapy with maintenance, compared to 20% of patients who undergo conventional chemotherapy. However, no significant difference existed in the proportion of individuals experiencing a 12-month disease-free interval in patients who received PUVA regime and those who underwent conventional chemotherapy (p-value = 0.1541, $\alpha = 0.05$).

The lower tail contains counts in the opposite direction *that are individually less likely than the sample result* (step 4, part 2). Compute the probability of the sample result first: $pr(X = 5) = 0.0691$. Therefore, a count must have a probability less than 0.0691 to be included in the lower tail. Select the most extreme count in the opposite direction and compute its probability. The $pr(X = 0)$ is 0.0550; thus, $X = 0$ is captured in the lower tail. Now compute the probability of the next most extreme count in the direction opposite the sample result: $pr(X = 1) = 0.1787$. Because 0.1787 is greater than 0.0691, $X = 1$ is not included in the lower tail. Note also that no other count in the direction opposite the sample result qualifies for inclusion in the lower tail. Therefore, the lower tail includes only $X = 0$. The two-tailed p-value is obtained by adding the upper- and lower-tail probabilities:

$$p - value = pr(X = 0) + pr(X \geq 5) = 0.0550 + 0.0991 = 0.1541.$$

The null hypothesis is retained because this p-value is greater than α. Thus, a significant difference does not exist between PUVA photochemotherapy and conventional chemotherapy in the proportion of patients with advanced mycosis fungoides who experience a 12-month disease-free interval following therapy.

Performing the binomial exact test becomes arduous as sample size increases, unless calculations are done on a computer. As mentioned earlier, the sampling distribution formed from a binomial population is skewed unless $\pi = 0.50$ or the sample size is relatively large. When the sample size is relatively large, the sampling distribution approaches a normal curve; and an approximation to the binomial exact test can be used.

Normal Approximation to the Binomial Exact Test

As sample size increases, the sampling distribution of a sample proportion approaches the normal probability distribution and tabled values of the normal curve can be used as *estimates* of the exact probabilities computed from the binomial exact test. Colton (1974, pp 153–155) demonstrates that the sampling distribution of a sample proportion approximates a Gaussian distribution as sample size increases. The rule-of-thumb for determining whether the normal distribution can be used as an approximation to the binomial is: $n\pi \geq 5$ and $n(1 - \pi) \geq 5$ (Colton, 1974, p 155). Note that the normal approximation to the binomial is a variation of the z statistic:

$$z = \frac{p - \pi}{\sqrt{\dfrac{\pi(1 - \pi)}{n}}} \qquad\qquad \textbf{13.2}$$

where p is the sample proportion computed as $\frac{X}{n}$ and π is the population proportion specified in the null hypothesis. The two-sided confidence interval based on the normal approximation is

$$p \pm z_{\alpha/2} \sqrt{\frac{\pi(1 - \pi)}{n}} . \qquad\qquad \textbf{13.3}$$

The following, hypothetical clinical example illustrates the use of the normal approximation.

Clinical Example: Embolism After Heart Valve Replacement

Major systemic embolism is an important complication in patients who undergo heart valve replacement. Consider that 12% of patients suffer a major systemic embolism within 4 years after valve replacement surgery. Three clinicians want to determine if aspirin use affects the percentage of patients experiencing embolic complications. Following heart valve replacement surgery, 186 randomly chosen patients are maintained on 100 mg aspirin daily throughout the 4-year follow-up period. Thirteen patients experience a major systemic embolism during the follow-up period.

In this hypothetical example, although the clinicians hope the antithrombotic effects of aspirin will produce a decrease in the percentage of patients with embolic complications following heart valve replacement surgery, the researchers opt for a nondirectional test because they believe outcomes in both directions will be clinically significant. The use of the normal approximation to test the null hypothesis and to compute a two-sided confidence interval appears in Box 13–3.

After writing the scientific and statistical hypotheses (steps 1 and 2), we formulate the decision rules that govern the statistical test (step 3). We must decide whether to apply the binomial exact test or the normal approximation to the binomial. We use the normal approximation because both rule-of-thumb criteria are satisfied. Alpha and the critical value of z are identified ($\alpha = 0.05$ and $z_{crit} = \pm 1.96$, two-tailed test). The sample proportion is computed ($p = 0.0699$). After the calculated value of z is determined ($z_{calc} = -2.11$) and compared to the critical value ($z_{crit} = \pm 1.96$), we reject the null hypothesis. The 95% two-sided confidence interval is constructed (0.0233, 0.1165) and used to interpret the findings.

Recall that we could have used a two-sided confidence interval to test the null hypothesis. Note that the value of π (0.12) is not captured in the interval. With respect to the proportion

Box 13–3. Studying the effectiveness of aspirin following heart valve replacement surgery.

1. *State the Scientific Hypothesis*
Among patients who have surgery alone and those who have surgery and take 100 mg of aspirin daily, a difference exists in the proportion experiencing major embolic complications within 4 years following heart valve replacement surgery.

2. *Formulate the Statistical Hypotheses*
$H_0 : \pi = 0.12$
$H_A : \pi \neq 0.12$

3. *Determine the Decision Rules*
   a. Check the rule of thumb to determine if the normal approximation can be used.

   $n\pi = 186(0.12) = 22.32 > 5$

   $n(1 - \pi) = 186(1 - 0.12) = 186(0.88) = 163.68 > 5$

   Use the normal approximation to the binomial exact test.
   b. Sampling distribution for a sample proportion.
   c. $\alpha = 0.05$.
   d. $z_{crit} = \pm 1.96$.

4. *Analyze the Data*
$X = 13$ (number of patients experiencing embolic complications during follow-up)
$n = 186$ (total number of patients having valve replacement who received aspirin)
   Compute the sample proportion:

   $p = \dfrac{X}{n} = \dfrac{13}{186} = 0.06989247 = 0.0699$ *(avoid carrying too few decimal places)*

   Calculate the value of z:

   $z = \dfrac{0.0699 - 0.12}{\sqrt{\dfrac{0.12(1 - 0.12)}{186}}} = \dfrac{-0.0501}{0.0238} = -2.1050 = -2.11$

   Construct the two-sided interval:

   $p \pm z_{\alpha/2} \sqrt{\dfrac{\pi(1 - \pi)}{n}} = 0.0699 \pm 1.96(0.0238) = 0.0699 \pm 0.046648 = (0.0233, 0.1165)$

5. *Evaluate the Statistics*
The null hypothesis is rejected ($z_{calc} = -2.11$ versus $z_{crit} = \pm 1.96$).

6. *Interpret the Statistics*
With respect to the proportion who experience embolic complications within 4 years of surgery, a significant difference exists between heart valve replacement patients who have surgery alone and those who have surgery and take 100 mg of aspirin daily (p-value = 0.0348, $\alpha = 0.05$). The two-sided 95% confidence interval about the sample proportion indicates that between approximately 2.33% and 11.65% of heart valve replacement patients taking 100 mg of aspirin daily will experience embolic complications throughout the 4-year follow-up period.

who experience embolic complications within 4 years of surgery, a significant difference exists between heart valve replacement patients who have surgery only, and those who have surgery and take 100 mg of aspirin daily (p-value $= 0.0348$, $\alpha = 0.05$). The two-sided 95% confidence interval indicates that between approximately 2.33% and 11.65% of heart valve replacement patients taking 100 mg daily of aspirin throughout a 4-year follow-up period will experience embolic complications.

SUMMARY

Testing hypotheses and/or constructing confidence intervals about a binomial outcome, such as relief (yes/no), survived (yes/no), or disease status (in remission/active), involves selecting between the binomial exact test and the normal approximation. The binomial exact test uses the formula for the binomial probability distribution to compute the probabilities associated with the frequency of occurrence of the outcome of interest. Because the binomial exact test usually is applied to relatively small samples and π (pi) seldom equals 0.50, the sampling distribution of the sample proportion is typically skewed. Therefore, the probability for a two-tailed test is not obtained by doubling the probability in one tail. The probabilities in each tail are computed separately and added together to obtain the two-tailed p-value.

We use the normal approximation to the binomial when two rule-of-thumb criteria are satisfied: $n\pi \geq 5$ and $n(1 - \pi) \geq 5$. If both criteria are met, a variation of the z statistic is employed. To determine the status of the null hypothesis, we compare the computed value of z to tabled values of the normal curve. (Refer to Table A–1 in the appendix of statistical tables.) Table 13–1 summarizes the assumptions and tests used to examine a sample proportion. A flowchart to illustrate the selection of the appropriate test appears in Fig 13–1.

Table 13–1. Summary of testing and estimating a sample proportion.

Hypothesis	Assumptions	Test Statistic	Tables
$H_0 : \pi = \pi_0$	Dependent variable is binomial	Binomial exact test $$\frac{n!}{X!(n - X)!} \pi^X (1 - \pi)^{n-X}$$	None is required because the exact probability is obtained from the formula
$H_0 : \pi = \pi_0$	Dependent variable is binomial $n\pi \geq 5$ and $n(1 - \pi) \geq 5$	Normal approximation to the binomial $$z = \frac{p - \pi}{\sqrt{\dfrac{\pi(1 - \pi)}{n}}}$$	Normal curve
100 $(1 - \alpha)$% two-sided interval	Dependent variable is binomial. $n\pi \geq 5$ and $n(1 - \pi) \geq 5$	Normal approximation to the binomial $$p \pm z_{\alpha/2} \sqrt{\frac{\pi(-\pi)}{n}}$$	Normal curve

REFERENCES

Abel E, Wood G, Hoppe R: Mycosis fungoides: Clinical and histologic features, staging, evaluation, and approach to treatment. *CA* 1993;**43**:93.

Colton T: *Statistics in Medicine.* Little, Brown, 1974.

Daniel W: *Biostatistics: A Foundation for Analysis in the Health Sciences,* 5th ed. Wiley, 1991.

Dawson-Saunders B, Trapp R: *Basic and Clinical Biostatistics*. Appleton & Lange, 1991.
Rosner B: *Fundamentals of Biostatistics,* 2nd ed. Duxbury, 1986.

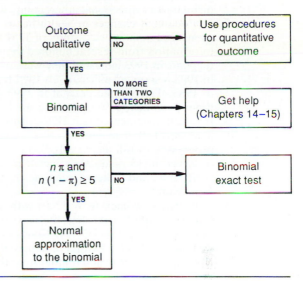

Figure 13–1. Flowchart for testing and estimating one proportion.

Self-study Questions

Part I: Outcome Identification

Indicate for each of the following whether the outcome is qualitative or quantitative; if it is qualitative, determine whether it is binomial.

1. Weight (under-, within normal, over-).
2. Amylase (U/dL).
3. Prostate-specific antigen (within-normal, elevated).
4. Satisfaction with medicine as a career choice (satisfied, dissatisfied, very dissatisfied).
5. Class of high blood pressure drugs (vasodilators, ACE inhibitors).
6. Breast cancer history in maternal grandmother, mother, or sister (absent, present, unknown).
7. Diabetic status (noninsulin-dependent, insulin-dependent).
8. Folic acid level (ng/mL).
9. Personality type (type A, type B).
10. Surgical procedure to open clogged coronary artery (balloon angioplasty, directional atherectomy, rotoblator).

Part II: Analysis Identification

Read each of the following and identify the correct analysis. Choices include analyses for one mean, two means, and one proportion.

1. At a prominent medical center, the costs of directional atherectomy and balloon angioplasty to open clogged coronary arteries were compared to determine if the two procedures (a) have similar costs and (b) are equally effective. Eighty-four men in good health except for clogged coronary arteries were matched on stenotic severity, age, and

smoking status. For each matched pair, one man was assigned randomly to undergo directional atherectomy; the other had balloon angioplasty. Effectiveness data are not given here. The mean cost of balloon angioplasty was $11,023.87 ($s$ = $3496.54); the mean cost of directional atherectomy was $13,633.91 ($s$ = $3523.86).

2. To document changes in health habits over the previous 10 years, *Prevention* magazine sponsored a nationwide study of 1251 adults in 1993; these data were compared to 1983 information from several hundred thousand adults. Investigators found that 66% of participants in 1993 indicated they were overweight, compared to 58% in 1983. Fifty percent in 1993 responded affirmatively to "I try hard to control my fat intake," compared to 57% in 1983. Thirty-three percent in 1993 reported they exercise strenuously three or more times per week; 34% responded similarly in 1983.

3. It is well documented that HIV-positive patients who receive conventional treatment live a mean of 18.9 months, with a standard deviation of 6.2 months, after their disease progresses to full-blown AIDS. In a recent trial, a mean survival of 19.3 months was observed in 15 randomly selected volunteers who received three drugs simultaneously: AZT, ddI, and either pyridinone or nevirapine. Is the increase in survival statistically significant?

4. Cancer-free women (n = 1200) with a mother or sister affected by breast cancer were followed for 12 years, and the occurrence of breast cancer was charted. Breast cancer developed in 208 (17.33%). Consider that it is well established that 6.9% of women without an affected mother or sister will develop breast cancer over a 12-year period. Are women with an affected mother or sister at greater risk?

5. For recurrent leukemia after a bone marrow transplant, conventional treatment produces a 12-month disease-free interval in 20% of patients. The experimental drug, filgrastim, was given to seven randomly selected volunteers with leukemia who suffered a relapse following a bone marrow transplant. Three of seven remain in remission for at least 12 months after treatment. Does the use of filgrastim increase the proportion of patients who remain in remission for at least 12 months following treatment for leukemia?

Part III: Problems and Analysis

Read each problem and analyze the data as indicated. If a hypothesis is to be tested, identify the scientific and statistical hypotheses, state the decision rules, perform the analysis, make a decision about the null hypothesis, and interpret the results. Set α = 0.05 in all problems.

1. Investigators at the Children's Defense Fund believe that the rapid progress in maternal and child health in the 1960s, 1970s, and through the mid-1980s has "been brought to a screeching halt." In 1970, 7% of infants were low-birthweight babies. It is hypothesized that an increase will be observed in 1993, compared to 1970, in the proportion of babies with low birthweights. In a random sample of 20 newborns at a large metropolitan midwestern hospital, 5 were identified as low-birthweight infants.

2. To assess the occurrence of restenosis following balloon angioplasty to open clogged coronary arteries, investigators conducted a multicenter, follow-up study involving several thousand patients. The researchers found that 6 months after balloon angioplasty, 80% of patients had stenosis limited to 50% or less of baseline. A relatively new procedure, directional atherectomy, is used sometimes to excise atherosclerotic plaque from coronary arteries. In a random sample of 100 patients who underwent directional atherectomy, 89 had stenosis limited to 50% or less of baseline 6 months after surgery. Based on these data, how does directional atherectomy compare with balloon angioplasty with respect to the proportion of patients who have restenosis?

3. Suppose that it is well documented that 70% of renal transplant patients treated with cyclosporine and prednisolone experience no acute episodes of transplant rejection within 12 months following surgery. Clinicians are interested in examining the effects of dietary fish oil on transplant rejection. Dietary fish oil affects renal hemodynamics in ways that may help to reduce acute episodes of transplant rejection. Thirteen randomly selected patients participated in a pilot study in which they received cyclosporine, prednisolone, and 6 g of dietary fish oil daily for the first postoperative year; 12 experienced no acute episodes of rejection. Both a decrease and an increase in the number of transplant

patients who experience an acute episode of rejection are significant clinically. What can be concluded about the benefits of dietary fish oil in these patients?

4. It has been well established in numerous studies that 26% of infants born to HIV-positive women test positive for the virus at, or shortly after, birth. Researchers believe, however, that the risk that a pregnant woman who is HIV-positive will infect her baby is associated directly with the mother's infection status. In a random sample of 150 babies born to women with high viral levels that suggest advanced infection, 107 infants were HIV-positive. Do these data support the expectation that a greater proportion of babies born to HIV-positive mothers with advanced infection were HIV-positive?

Solutions

Part I: Outcome Identification

1. Qualitative, with three categories.
2. Quantitative.
3. Qualitative, binomial.
4. Qualitative, with three categories.
5. Qualitative, binomial.
6. Qualitative, with three classes or categories.
7. Qualitative, binomial.
8. Quantitative.
9. Qualitative, binomial.
10. Qualitative, three classes or types of procedures.

Part II: Analysis Identification

1. *Study type:* matched pairs; *outcome:* cost treated as a quantitative variable; *analysis:* Student's *t* test for a paired difference.
2. *Study type:* single group; *outcomes:* three dependent variables, with each treated as a binomial outcome (yes/no); *analysis:* normal approximation to the binomial exact test.
3. *Study type:* single group; *outcome:* survival in months treated as a quantitative variable; *analysis:* z test for one mean (because the given standard deviation is treated as a population parameter).
4. *Study type:* single group; *outcome:* breast cancer development (yes/no), treated as a binomial variable; *analysis:* normal approximation to the binomial.
5. *Study type:* single group; *outcome:* 12-month remission (yes/no), treated as a binomial variable; *analysis:* binomial exact test [because $n\pi = 7(0.20) = 1.4 < 5$; $n(1 - \pi) = 7(0.80) = 5.6$; both criteria must be satisfied (≥ 5) to utilize the normal approximation].

Part III: Problems and Analysis

1. *Child Health*
   State the Scientific Hypothesis:
   An increase will be observed in 1993, compared to 1970, in the proportion of babies with low birthweights.
   Formulate the Statistical Hypotheses:

$$H_0 : \pi = 0.07$$

$$H_A : \pi > 0.07$$

Determine the Decision Rules:
a. Binomial exact test: $n\pi = 20 \ (0.07) = 1.4 < 5$.
   There is no need to examine $n(1 - \pi)$ because both criteria must ≥ 5.
b. Sampling distribution of a sample proportion.
c. $\alpha = 0.05$, one-tailed test in the *greater than* direction.

Analyze the Data:
Givens: $X = 5$, $n = 20$
Calculate p (for reporting purposes):

$$p = \frac{5}{20} = 0.25$$

Calculate the probability in the upper tail:

$$pr(X \geq 5) = pr(X = 5) + \ldots + pr(X = 20) = 1 - [pr(X = 0) + \ldots + pr(X = 4)]$$

$$pr(X = 0) = \frac{20!}{0!(20 - 0)!} \ 0.07^0 0.93^{20} = (1)(1)0.93^{20} = 0.2342$$

$$pr(X = 1) = \frac{20!}{1!(20 - 1!)} \ 0.07^1 0.93^{19} = (20)(0.07)0.93^{19} = 0.3526$$

$$pr(X = 2) = \frac{20!}{2!(20 - 2!)} \ 0.07^2 0.93^{18} = (190)(0.07^2)0.93^{18} = 0.252$$

$$pr(X = 3) = \frac{20!}{3!(20 - 3!)} \ 0.07^3 0.93^{17} = (1140)(0.07^3)0.93^{17} = 0.1139$$

$$pr(X = 4) = \frac{20!}{4!(20 - 4!)} \ 0.07^4 0.93^{16} = (4845)(0.07^4)0.93^{16} = 0.0364$$

$$pr(X \geq 5) = 1 - [0.2342 + 0.3256 + 0.2521 + 0.1139 + 0.0364] = 0.0180$$

Evaluate the Statistics:
The null hypothesis is rejected.

Interpret the Statistics:
Compared to 1970, a significant increase has occurred in 1993 with respect to the proportion of infants with low birthweights (1993: $p = 0.25$, 1970: $\pi = 0.07$, *p*-value $= 0.0378$, $\alpha = 0.05$).

2. *Coronary Revascularization*

State the Scientific Hypothesis:
Six months after surgery, a difference will exist between balloon angioplasty and directional atherectomy with respect to the proportion of patients who maintain a reduction in stenosis of 50% or less of baseline in the affected coronary arteries.

Formulate the Statistical Hypotheses:

$$H_0 : \pi = 0.80$$

$$H_A : \pi \neq 0.80$$

Determine the Decision Rules:
a. Normal approximation to the binomial:

$$n\pi = 100\,(0.80) = 80 > 5$$

$$n(1 - \pi) = 100\,(1 - 0.80) = 20 > 5$$

b. Sampling distribution of a sample proportion.
c. $\alpha = 0.05$, two-tailed test.
d. $z_{crit} = \pm 1.96$.

Analyze the data:
Givens: $X = 89$, $n = 100$
Calculate p:

$$p = \frac{89}{100} = 0.89$$

Calculate z:

$$z = \frac{0.89 - 0.80}{\sqrt{\dfrac{0.80(1 - 0.80)}{100}}} = \frac{0.09}{0.04} = 2.25$$

Evaluate the Statistics:
Reject the null hypothesis.

Interpret the Statistics:
Six months after surgery, a significant difference exists in patients who underwent balloon angioplasty versus those who had directional atherectomy, with respect to the proportion with stenosis of 50% or less of baseline (0.80 and 0.89, respectively; p-value = 0.0244; $\alpha = 0.05$).

3. *Dietary Fish Oil and Renal Transplants*

State the Scientific Hypothesis:
A difference exists between two groups of renal transplant patients with respect to the proportion who experience no acute episodes of transplant rejection within 12 months after surgery. One group of patients receives cyclosporine and prednisolone; the other group receives these drugs plus 6 g daily of dietary fish oil.

Formulate the Statistical Hypotheses:

$$H_0 : \pi = 0.70$$

$$H_A : \pi \neq 0.70$$

Determine the Decision Rules:
a. Binomial exact test:

$$n\pi = 13(0.70) = 9.1$$

$$n(1 - \pi) = 13(1 - 0.70) = 3.9 < 5$$

b. Sampling distribution of a sample proportion.
c. $\alpha = 0.05$, two-tailed test.

Analyze the Data:
Givens: $X = 12$, $n = 13$
Calculate p (for reporting purposes):

$$p = \frac{12}{13} = 0.9231$$

Calculate the probability in the upper tail (eight decimal places are carried, because some of the calculated probabilities will be quite small):

$$pr(X \geq 12) = pr(X = 12) + pr(X = 13)$$

$$pr(X = 12) = \frac{13!}{12!(13 - 12!)} \, 0.70^{12} 0.30^{13-12} = (13)(0.70^{12})0.30^1 = 0.05398102$$

$$pr(X = 13) = \frac{13!}{13!(13 - 13!)} \, 0.70^{13} 0.30^{13-13} = (1)(0.70^{13})(1) = 0.00968890$$

Add together $pr(X = 12)$ and $pr(X = 13)$ to obtain the upper-tail probability:

$$pr(X = 12) + pr(X = 13) = 0.05398102 + 0.00968890 = 0.06366992$$

We knew even before we calculated $pr(X = 13)$ that the null hypothesis is retained because $pr(X = 12) = 0.05398102 > \alpha = 0.05$. We continue calculations to illustrate computation of the lower-tail probability and to obtain the two-tailed p-value.

Obtain the lower-tail probability: Recall that the tail contains all events that are less likely to occur than the sample result $[pr(X = 12) = 0.05398102]$.

$$pr(X = 0) = \frac{13!}{0!(13 - 0!)} \, 0.70^0 0.30^{13} = (1)(1)0.30^{13} = 0.00000016$$

$$pr(X = 1) = \frac{13!}{1!(13 - 1!)} \, 0.70^1 0.30^{13-1} = (13)(0.70)0.30^{12} = 0.00000484$$

$$pr(X = 2) = \frac{13!}{2!(13 - 2!)} \, 0.70^2 0.30^{13-2} = (78)(0.70^2)0.30^{11} = 0.00006771$$

$$pr(X = 3) = \frac{13!}{3!(13 - 3!)} \, 0.70^3 0.30^{13-3} = (286)(0.70^3)0.30^{10} = 0.00057926$$

$$pr(X = 4) = \frac{13!}{4!(13 - 4!)} \, 0.70^4 0.30^{13-4} = (715)(0.70^4)0.30^9 = 0.00337901$$

$$pr(X = 5) = \frac{13!}{5!(13 - 5!)} \, 0.70^5 0.30^{13-5} = (1287)(0.70^5)0.30^8 = 0.01419184$$

$$pr(X = 6) = \frac{13!}{6!(13 - 6!)} \, 0.70^6 0.30^{13-6} = (1716)(0.70^6)0.30^7 = 0.04415240$$

$$pr(X = 7) = \frac{13!}{7!(13 - 7!)} \, 0.70^7 0.30^{13-7} = (1716)(0.70^7)0.30^6 = 0.10302226$$

Observe that $pr(X = 7) = 0.1030 > pr(X = 12) = 0.05398$. Therefore, the lower tail includes $X = 0$, $X = 1$, $X = 2$, $X = 3$, $X = 4$, $X = 5$, and $X = 6$. Add together these probabilities to determine the lower-tail probability:

$$pr(X = 0 \text{ or } X = 1 \text{ or } X = 2 \text{ or } \ldots \text{ or } X = 6) = 0.06237522$$

Compute the two-tailed p-value:

$$pr(X = 0 \text{ or } \ldots \text{ or } X = 6 \text{ or } X = 12 \text{ or } X = 13) = 0.12604514 \cong 0.126$$

Evaluate the statistics:
Reject the null hypothesis.

Interpret the statistics:
Although approximately 93% (12 of 13 patients) who received dietary fish oil daily, plus treatment with cyclosporine and prednisolone, experienced no acute transplant rejection in the year following surgery, a significant difference was not detected. With conventional treatment of cyclosporine and prednisolone alone during the first postoperative year, 80% experienced no acute rejection episodes (*p*-value $\approx$ 0.126, α = 0.05). If other indicators of renal function favor the fish-oil group, the investigators may wish to repeat their investigation and increase the sample size to permit the detection of significant differences, if they exist.

4. *Mother-to-Newborn HIV Transmission*

State the Scientific Hypothesis:
Among infants born to HIV-positive women with advanced infection, the proportion of infants who test positive for HIV at, or shortly after, birth will be greater than 0.26.

Formulate the Statistical Hypotheses:

$$H_0 : \pi = 0.26$$

$$H_A : \pi > 0.26$$

Determine the Decision Rules:
a. Normal approximation to the binomial:

$$n\pi = (150)(0.26) = 39 > 5$$

$$n(1 - \pi) = 150(1 - 0.26) = 111 > 5$$

b. Sampling distribution of a sample proportion.
c. α = 0.05, one-tailed test, greater than direction.
d. z_{crit} = 1.645.

Analyze the Data:
Givens: $X = 107$, $n = 150$

Calculate p:

$$p = \frac{107}{150} = 0.7133$$

Calculate z

$$z = \frac{0.7133 - 0.26}{\sqrt{\dfrac{0.26(1 - 0.26)}{150}}} = \frac{0.4533}{0.0358} = 12.66$$

Evaluate the statistics:
Reject the null hypothesis.

Interpret the Statistics:
Approximately 71% (107 of 150 infants) born to HIV-positive women with advanced infection were HIV positive at, or shortly after, birth compared to 26% of infants born to HIV-positive women without regard to the mother's infection status. The proportion of babies infected when the mother's HIV infection is advanced (0.7133) is significantly greater than the overall population proportion (0.26) (z_{calc} = 12.66, z_{crit} = 1.645, *p*-value = 0.000032, α = 0.05).

14 Testing Hypotheses About Two Proportions

Clinical Example: Environmental Exposure to Tobacco Smoke

The association between environmental exposure to tobacco smoke is examined in two groups of children with clinically diagnosed asthma. It is hypothesized that a greater proportion of asthmatic children with no or minimal exposure to environmental tobacco smoke will experience two or fewer exacerbations of their asthma during a 12-month period, compared to similar patients who are exposed to tobacco smoke.

Participants are selected randomly from children with asthma who are seen in the Department of Pediatrics at a multispecialty clinic located in a midwestern community with a population of approximately 175,000. As reported by parents, 121 children with asthma have no or very little exposure to tobacco smoke; 93 children are exposed to environmental tobacco smoke in the home and elsewhere. The mean age at time of enrollment in the study is 7.4 (SD = 2.8) years for exposed and 7.3 (SD = 2.9 years) for nonexposed children. The mean age at diagnosis of asthma is 4.1 (SD = 2.7) years in exposed and 4.0 (SD = 2.6) years in nonexposed children. Among the 121 asthmatic children with no or minimal exposure to environmental tobacco smoke, 73 have two or fewer acute exacerbations of asthma during the 12-month period beginning January 1, 1992. Among the 93 exposed children with asthma, 30 have two or fewer acute exacerbations during the same 12-month period.

To examine the hypothesis in this hypothetical study, we must look at the difference between two proportions. As with the analysis of the difference between two means (Chapter 12), we must determine whether the groups were formed independently or whether a matching/pairing process was used. In this chapter, we present procedures often used to test hypotheses about two proportions.

OBJECTIVES

When you complete this chapter, you should be able to:

- Identify the appropriate statistical procedure to test an hypothesis about two proportions.
- Conduct a test of a null hypothesis about two proportions by using the appropriate test statistic and/or confidence interval.
- Translate the findings from a test of a null hypothesis about two proportions into non-statistical language.

INDEPENDENT GROUPS DESIGNS

An independent groups design involves random selection and, if the independent variable is manipulated by the investigator, random assignment of study participants to groups. In the above example, children were selected randomly from two populations. Because the independent variable (exposure to environmental tobacco smoke) was not manipulated by the investigators, however, no random assignment to exposed/nonexposed groups occurred.

The proportion in the first population is π_1; the proportion in the second population is π_2. The statistical hypotheses take one of the following forms:

$$H_0: \pi_1 - \pi_2 = 0 \qquad H_0: \pi_1 - \pi_2 = 0 \qquad H_0: \pi_1 - \pi_2 = 0$$

$$H_A: \pi_1 - \pi_2 \neq 0 \qquad H_A: \pi_1 - \pi_2 > 0 \qquad H_A: \pi_1 - \pi_2 < 0$$

Although we may specify a difference other than zero, we restrict our study to the commonly encountered situation in which zero is used. The first set of hypotheses produces a non-directional or two-tailed test. The second and third set yield a directional or one-tailed test.

In the next section, we briefly discuss the random sampling distribution of the difference between two independent proportions, before considering statistical tests and confidence intervals.

Random Sampling Distribution of the Difference Between Two Independent Proportions

The random sampling distribution of the difference between two proportions is a relative frequency distribution of the difference between all possible pairs of proportion, calculated from independent random samples, each of size n, from two binomial populations. If sample sizes are sufficiently large, this distribution approximates a normal curve with mean and standard error $\pi_1 - \pi_2$ and $\sqrt{\dfrac{\pi_1(1 - \pi_1)}{n_1} + \dfrac{\pi_2(1 - \pi_2)}{n_2}}$, respectively (Rosner, 1986, p 304).

Techniques for the analysis of two independent proportions, like those for one proportion, include an exact test, known as Fisher's exact test, and a normal approximation. The normal approximation is described in this chapter; readers who are interested in the exact test are referred to other sources (Kanji, 1993, p 71; Rosner, 1986, pp 326–339).

Normal Approximation to the Exact Test

As sample sizes increase, the sampling distribution of the difference between two independent proportions approaches a normal probability distribution and tabled values of the normal curve are used to estimate the binomial probabilities. The normal approximation is another variation of the z statistic:

$$z = \frac{p_1 - p_2 - (\pi_1 - \pi_2)}{SE_{p_1-p_2}} \qquad 14.1$$

where $p_1 = \dfrac{X_1}{n_1}$, $p_2 = \dfrac{X_2}{n_2}$, and $SE_{p_1-p_2}$ is the standard error of the difference between two independent proportions. X_1 is the number of occurrences of the outcome of interest in the first sample; n_1 is the size of the first sample; p_1 is the proportion in sample one; π_1 is the population proportion in the first population; X_2, n_2, p_2, and π_2 are defined similarly for the second population.

The standard error, as noted above, is

$$SE_{p_1-p_2} = \sqrt{\frac{\pi_1(1 - \pi_1)}{n_1} + \frac{\pi_2(1 - \pi_2)}{n_2}} \qquad 14.2$$

Because the null hypothesis is one of equivalence of two proportions, $\pi_1 = \pi_2 = \pi$; here π is referred to as the *common population proportion*. If we rewrite the formula for the standard error to include the common population proportion and then simplify it, we obtain

$$SE_{p_1-p_2} = \sqrt{\frac{\pi_1(1-\pi_1)}{n_1} + \frac{\pi_2(1-\pi_2)}{n_2}}$$

$$= \sqrt{\frac{\pi(1-\pi)}{n_1} + \frac{\pi(1-\pi)}{n_2}}$$

$$= \sqrt{\pi(1-\pi)\left[\frac{1}{n_1} + \frac{1}{n_2}\right]}. \qquad \textbf{14.3}$$

In most situations, however, π_1 and π_2 are unknown; therefore, π is unknown. Consequently, we use sample data to estimate the common population proportion, π. The best estimate of π is a weighted combination of p_1 and p_2, with weights proportional to the number of observations in each sample (Colton, 1974, p 164). The common estimate of π, referred to as a *pooled estimate*, is expressed as

$$p = \frac{n_1 p_1 + n_2 p_2}{n_1 + n_2}. \qquad \textbf{14.4a}$$

We can simplify the above formula by recognizing that $p_1 = \dfrac{X_1}{n_1}$ and $p_2 = \dfrac{X_2}{n_2}$:

$$p = \frac{n_1 p_1 + n_2 p_2}{n_1 + n_2}$$

$$= \frac{n_1\left(\dfrac{X_1}{n_1}\right) + n_2\left(\dfrac{X_2}{n_2}\right)}{n_1 + n_2}$$

$$= \frac{X_1 + X_2}{n_1 + n_2} \qquad \textbf{14.4b}$$

If the pooled estimate (p) replaces the unknown common population proportion, π, in Formula 14.3, the standard error of the difference is

$$SE_{p_1-p_2} = \sqrt{p(1-p)\left[\frac{1}{n_1} + \frac{1}{n_2}\right]}. \qquad \textbf{14.5}$$

The z statistic can be rewritten as

$$z = \frac{p_1 - p_2 - (\pi_1 - \pi_2)}{\sqrt{p(1-p)\left[\dfrac{1}{n_1} + \dfrac{1}{n_2}\right]}}. \qquad \textbf{14.6}$$

Because $\pi_1 - \pi_2 = 0$ in our examples, the right-hand component of the numerator can be omitted. We use the z statistic when four criteria are met. These are described in the next section. If the z statistic is appropriate, the two-sided confidence interval is

$$(p_1 - p_2) \pm z_{\alpha/2} \sqrt{p(1-p)\left[\frac{1}{n_1} + \frac{1}{n_2}\right]} \qquad \textbf{14.7}$$

where $z_{\alpha/2}$ is the critical value of z corresponding to a two-tailed test with specified α; we define p, p_1, p_2, n_1, and n_2 as we did earlier.

Rule-of-Thumb Criteria for the Normal Approximation

We employ the normal approximation to the exact test when four criteria are satisfied (Colton, 1974, p 165):

$n_1 p \geq 5$
$n_2 p \geq 5$
$n_1(1 - p) \geq 5$
$n_2(1 - p) \geq 5$

Note that similar criteria are employed to determine if the normal approximation for one proportion can replace the binomial exact test (ie, $n\pi \geq 5$ and $n(1 - \pi) \geq 5$). Because two independent populations are sampled, the rule-of-thumb criteria must be satisfied in each sample—hence, four conditions exist. The advice of a statistician should be obtained if *all* criteria are not satisfied.

Normal Approximation to the Exact Test

The hypothetical research discussed at the beginning of the chapter illustrates the use of the normal approximation for the analysis of two independent proportions. In this example, the association between environmental tobacco smoke and asthma is investigated. The independent variable is exposure to environmental smoke. The dependent variable is binomial: two or fewer acute exacerbations of asthma in a 12-month period (yes/no). Let's review the step-by-step analysis presented in Box 14–1.

First, we write the hypotheses (steps 1 and 2). Then we detail the decision rules (step 3). Next, the pooled estimate of π is computed to determine whether the rule-of-thumb criteria are satisfied. Observe that the normal approximation is appropriate because each criterion is met. The data are analyzed in step 4. The proportion of children experiencing two or fewer acute exacerbations of asthma in a 12-month period is obtained for each sample; the standard error is calculated; z is computed (step 5). We reject the null hypothesis because the calculated value of z (4.07) falls in the region of rejection ($z_{crit} = 1.645$). Observe also that the p-value (p-value < 0.000032) is less than α ($=0.05$). We conclude that a significantly greater proportion of asthmatic children not exposed to environmental tobacco have two or fewer acute exacerbations of asthma during a 12-month period, compared to asthmatic exposed to environmental tobacco smoke (approximately 60% versus 32%, respectively).

As with the analysis of proportions from an independent groups design, two statistical tests exist when proportions from a matched/paired design are examined: an exact test and a normal approximation. These analyses, called tests for correlated proportions, are described next.

MATCHED/PAIRED DESIGNS

The analysis of matched/paired data requires that we array the data in a 2×2 table and examine particular cells of the table, as we did in Chapter 7. Based on the sample data, we then determine whether the exact test or a normal approximation is appropriate. The following hypothetical research illustrates this point.

Box 14–1. Exposure to environmental tobacco smoke and acute exacerbations of asthma in children with asthma.

1. *State the Scientific Hypothesis*

During a 12-month period, a greater proportion of asthmatic children with no or minimal exposure to environmental tobacco smoke will experience two or fewer exacerbations of their asthma compared to asthmatic children exposed to tobacco smoke.

2. *Formulate the Statistical Hypotheses*

H_0: $\pi_{NOT\ EXPOSED} - \pi_{EXPOSED} = 0$
H_A: $\pi_{NOT\ EXPOSED} - \pi_{EXPOSED} > 0$

3. *Determine the Decision Rules*

  a. Determine whether the normal approximation can be employed.

    Compute the pooled estimate, *p:*

    Let NE represent not exposed and EXP designate exposed:

    $X_{NE} = 73$ and $n_{NE} = 121$
    $X_{EXP} = 30$ and $n_{EXP} = 93$

$$p = \frac{X_{NE} + X_{EXP}}{n_{NE} + n_{EXP}} = \frac{73 + 30}{121 + 93} = 0.4813$$

    Check the rules of thumb:

    $n_{NE}p = 121(0.4813) = 58.2373 \geq 5$
    $n_{EXP}p = 93(0.4813) = 44.7609 \geq 5$
    $n_{NE}(1 - p) = 121(1 - 0.4813) = 62.7627 \geq 5$
    $n_{EXP}(1 - p) = 93(1 - 0.4813) = 48.2391 \geq 5$

    The rules-of-thumb are satisfied; use the normal approximation.

  b. The normal probability distribution is used to approximate the binomial distribution.

  c. $\alpha = 0.05$.

  d. $z_{crit} = +1.645$ (one-tailed test).

4. *Analyze the Data*

Use sample data to compute the sample proportions and standard error of the difference.
Sample proportions: (NE = not exposed, EXP = exposed)

$X_{NE} = 73$ and $n_{NE} = 121$
$X_{EXP} = 30$ and $n_{EXP} = 93$

$$p_{NE} = \frac{73}{121} = 0.6033 \text{ (Approximately 60\% had 2 or fewer exacerbations)}$$

$$p_{EXP} = \frac{30}{93} = 0.3226 \text{ (Approximately 32\% had 2 or fewer exacerbations)}$$

Standard error of the difference:

$$SE_{p_{NE} - p_{EXP}} = \sqrt{p(1 - p)\left[\frac{1}{n_{NE}} + \frac{1}{n_{EXP}}\right]}$$

$$= \sqrt{0.4813(1 - 0.4813)\left[\frac{1}{121} + \frac{1}{93}\right]}$$

$$= \sqrt{0.0047} = 0.0689$$

Compute the *z* statistic:

$$z = \frac{0.6033 - 0.3226}{0.0689} = 4.07$$

5. *Evaluate the Statistics*
Reject the null hypothesis.

6. *Interpret the Statistics*
A significantly greater proportion of children with asthma who were not exposed to environmental tobacco smoke experienced two or fewer acute exacerbations of asthma in a 12-month period, compared to those who were exposed (approximately 60% and 32%, respectively; $z_{calc} = 4.07$, $z_{crit} = 1.645$, *p*-value ≈ 0.000032, $\alpha = 0.05$).

The 2 × 2 Contingency Table for Matched/Paired Data

Clinical Example: Osteoarthritis of the Knee

The effectiveness of acetaminophen versus ibuprofen was compared in patients with osteoarthritis of the knee. A total of 130 men with osteoarthritis of the knee were selected randomly; 65 pairs were formed by matching according to age and severity of disease. One member of each pair was assigned randomly to receive appropriate daily doses of acetaminophen; the other member of the pair was given appropriate daily doses of ibuprofen. Each participant indicated after 3 months of treatment whether he experienced symptomatic improvement (yes/no). The research question asks: "In men with osteoarthritis of the knee, is acetaminophen more or less effective in providing symptomatic improvement compared to ibuprofen?"

The data for this hypothetical study appear in Table 14–1. The analysis requires that we (1) treat the matched pair as the basic unit of observation and (2) classify pairs according to whether or not each treatment was effective for members of that pair (Colton, 1974, p 171; Rosner, 1986, p 333). We see from Table 14–1 that there are

23 pairs in which the member improved while taking acetaminophen and his pairmate also improved while receiving ibuprofen (cell 1,1—intersection of row 1 and column 1).

17 pairs in which the man receiving ibuprofen improved, but his pairmate who received acetaminophen did not (cell 2,1—intersection of row 2 and column 1).

12 pairs in which the patient receiving acetaminophen improved, but his pairmate receiving ibuprofen did not (cell 1,2—intersection of row 1 and column two).

13 pairs in which neither participant improved (cell 2,2—intersection of row 2 and column 2).

Pairs in which the outcomes are the same for each member are *tied or concordant pairs* (cells 1,1 and 2,2). Pairs in which the outcomes differ for each member are *untied or discordant pairs* (Rosner, 1986, p 334). The cells in which the untied or discordant pairs occur in Table 14–1 are shaded. The tied or concordant pairs provide no information about differences between treatments; therefore, they are not used in the analysis. The analysis, then, focuses on the untied pairs. Two types of untied or discordant pairs exist. In a *type A discordant pair*, the participant receiving acetaminophen improves and the pairmate receiving ibuprofen does not (cell 1,2). In a *type B discordant pair,* the patient receiving ibuprofen improves and the pairmate receiving acetaminophen does not (cell 2,1). Table 14–1 contains 12 type A discordant pairs and 17 type B discordant pairs.

If acetaminophen and ibuprofen are equally effective, we would expect an equal number of type A and type B discordant pairs. Therefore, under the null hypothesis of equal effectiveness, an equal number of untied pairs should occur in cells (1,2) and (2,1). Thus, the analysis

Table 14–1. Effectiveness of acetaminophen versus ibuprofen in providing symptomatic improvement in men with osteoarthritis of the knee.[a]

Acetaminophen	Ibuprofen		Total
	Improvement: Yes	*Improvement: No*	
Improvement: Yes	23	12	35
Improvement: No	17	13	30
Total	40	25	65

[a]Shaded cells represent the untied or discordant pairs.

of matched/paired data reduces to a test of the null hypothesis that $\pi = 0.50$ (Colton, 1974, p 172; Rosner, 1986, p 334). For the osteoarthritis example, the statistical hypotheses are

$$H_0: \pi = 0.50$$

$$H_A: \pi \neq 0.50$$

Although in this example the alternative hypothesis is nondirectional, it may be one-tailed in other situations that justify a directional test. After formulating the hypotheses, we determine whether the normal approximation or the binomial exact test is appropriate. In this example, we use the normal approximation to analyze the data in Table 14–1.

Normal Approximation for Matched/Paired Data

In the analysis of matched/paired data, the unit of analysis is the pair; X is the number of pairs in which one member of the pair evidences the outcome of interest and his or her pairmate does not; n is the number of untied or discordant pairs; π equals 0.50, under the null hypothesis of equal treatment effectiveness.

The normal approximation for matched/paired data is

$$z = \frac{p - \pi}{\sigma_p} = \frac{p - \pi}{\sqrt{\dfrac{\pi(1 - \pi)}{n}}}, \qquad 14.8$$

where $p = \dfrac{X}{n}$ and we retain the earlier definitions of X, n, and π. Thus, the analysis of matched/paired data is similar to the analysis of one proportion in which the type A discordant pair is analogous flipping a fair coin and obtaining a head; the type B discordant pair is like observing a tail. If the rule-of-thumb criteria are met, the normal approximation to the exact test applies. The rule-of-thumb criteria are: $n\pi \geq 5$ and $n(1 - \pi) \geq 5$, where $\pi = 0.50$ and n is the number of untied or discordant pairs. Because $\pi = 0.50$, $n\pi = n(1 - \pi)$. Thus if one criterion is satisfied, the other criterion is met.

Let's return to the question of interest: "In men with osteoarthritis of the knee, is acetaminophen more or less effective than ibuprofen in providing symptomatic improvement?" A nondirectional question is formulated, because an increase or decrease in the proportion experiencing relief would be important clinically. The analysis appears in Box 14–2.

The scientific hypothesis and statistical hypotheses are stated in steps 1 and 2, respectively. The decision rules are formulated in step 3. To determine if the normal approximation is appropriate, we calculate $n\pi$ and $n(1 - \pi)$ and check that the rule-of-thumb criteria are satisfied. (When they are not satisfied, the researcher should consult a statistician for an alternative test.) In this example, the normal approximation applies. Thus, the normal probability distribution replaces the binomial distribution; the critical value of $z = \pm 1.96$ for a two-tailed test with $\alpha = 0.05$.

The sample proportion, p, is computed; recall that p represents the proportion of *pairs* in which the participant taking acetaminophen improved and the pairmate receiving ibuprofen did not ($p = 0.5862$). The standard error is calculated ($\sigma_p = 0.0928$) and used in the denominator of the z statistic. The value of z is determined ($z_{calc} = 0.93$) and compared to the critical value ($z_{crit} = \pm 1.96$). The null hypothesis is retained (step 5). We conclude that among pairmates who respond differently to therapy for osteoarthritis of the knee, the patient taking daily doses of acetaminophen is neither more nor less likely to experience symptomatic relief than the pairmate taking ibuprofen (p-value ≈ 0.35, $\alpha = 0.05$).

As described above, the normal approximation is employed when $n\pi$ and $n(1 - \pi) \geq 5$. When the rule-of-thumb is not satisfied, the exact test must be used. Another commonly encountered test is the McNemar test, which utilizes the chi-square distribution (χ^2) rather

Box 14–2. Analysis of effectiveness of acetaminophen versus ibuprofen in providing symptomatic improvement in men with osteoarthritis of the knee.

1. *State the Scientific Hypothesis*
   The proportion of men with osteoarthritis of the knee who improve after three months of therapy will differ, depending upon therapy with acetaminophen or ibuprofen.

2. *Formulate the Statistical Hypotheses*
   H_0: $\pi = 0.50$
   H_A: $\pi \neq 0.50$

3. *Determine the Decision Rules*
   a. Determine if the normal approximation is appropriate. Define X as equal to the number of pairs in which the participant taking acetaminophen improves and the pairmate receiving ibuprofen does not; n equals the number of untied pairs.

   $X = 17$

   $n = 29$

   $n\pi = 29(0.50) = 14.5 \geq 5$

   $n(1 - \pi) = 29(1 - 0.50) = 14.5 \geq 5$

   Use the normal approximation to the exact test.
   b. Sampling distribution is binomial with $\pi = 0.50$.
   c. $\alpha = 0.05$.
   d. $z = \pm 1.96$.

4. *Analyze the Data*
   $X = 17$ (number of pairs in which participant receiving acetaminophen improves; pairmate receiving ibuprofen does not)
   $n = 29$ (number of untied pairs)
   Compute p:

   $$p = \frac{17}{29} = 0.5862$$

   Compute the standard error of the paired difference:

   $$\sigma_p = \sqrt{\frac{\pi(1 - \pi)}{n}} = \sqrt{\frac{0.50(1 - 0.50)}{29}} = 0.0928$$

   Calculate z:

   $$z = \frac{p - \pi}{\sigma_p} = \frac{0.5862 - 0.50}{0.0928} = 0.9289$$

5. *Evaluate the Statistics*
   Retain the null hypothesis.

6. *Interpret the Statistics*
   In pairs of men with osteoarthritis of the knee who responded differently to the two drugs, no significant difference in effectiveness was noted between acetaminophen and ibuprofen (p-value ≈ 0.35, $\alpha = 0.05$). The member of the pair taking daily doses of acetaminophen for 3 months is neither more nor less likely to experience symptomatic relief than the member of the pair taking ibuprofen ($z_{calc} = 0.93$, $z_{crit} = \pm 1.96$).

than the normal curve as a surrogate for the binomial probability distribution. Because of the mathematical relationship between z and χ^2 in a 2 × 2 table, however, the two tests lead to similar conclusions. Individuals interested in reading about the McNemar test should consult other sources, such as Dawson-Saunders and Trapp (1994, pp 155–156) or Rosner (1986, p 335).

Binomial Exact Test for Matched/Paired Data

The binomial exact test for matched/paired data is identical mathematically to the binomial exact test for a single proportion (Chapter 13):

$$\frac{n!}{X!(n - X)!}\pi^X(1 - \pi)^{n-X} \qquad 14.8$$

where X is the number of pairs in which one member of the pair evidences the outcome of interest and the pairmate does not; n is the number of untied or discordant pairs; and π equals 0.50, under the null hypothesis of no difference. The following hypothetical example illustrates the use of the binomial exact test for matched/paired data.

Clinical Example: Comedonal Acne

A dermatologist wishes to compare the effectiveness of an experimental cream and a 2.5% benzoyl peroxide cream to treat comedonal acne. The 2.5% of benzoyl peroxide cream is used because (1) the 2.5% and 10% preparations have been shown to be equally effective and (2) the 2.5% strength cream is less irritating than its 10% counterpart (Goldstein and Odom, 1993, p 92).

Thirty-three pairs of participants are created by matching according to age, sex, and severity of comedonal acne. Participants are taught proper daily cleansing procedures and are provided identical cleansing agents. One member of the pair is assigned randomly to apply the experimental cream topically to affected facial areas; the other receives the benzoyl peroxide cream. Photographs of affected facial areas are taken at baseline and again after 2 months of treatment. A colleague unfamiliar with the purpose of the study then determines if each participant's acne has improved (yes/no).

In this hypothetical study of treatment for comedonal acne, does a significant difference in effectiveness exist between therapeutic creams? The data appear in Table 14–2. Observe that in 22 pairs, both patients improve; in 2 pairs, neither patient improves. Thus, twenty-four pairs are tied or concordant. There are 9 untied or discordant pairs; in 8 of these pairs, the participant receiving the experimental cream improves and the pairmate using benzoyl peroxide does not. Because the dermatologist is interested in the pairs in which the patient receiving the experimental cream improves and the pairmate applying the benzoyl peroxide cream does not, we define X as equal to 8. The task is to determine if the occurrence of 8 pairs in cell 2,1 and one pair in 1,2 is consistent with the null hypothesis, which states that the untied pairs distribute themselves evenly between these two cells, that is, H_0: $\pi = 0.50$.

The analysis is summarized in Box 14–3. The scientific and statistical hypotheses are specified (steps 1 and 2). The decision rules are outlined next (step 3); here we determine whether the binomial exact test or normal approximation for matched/paired data is appropriate. Because the rule-of-thumb criteria for applying the normal approximation are not satisfied, the binomial exact test must be employed.

The binomial exact test allows us to compute directly the two-tailed probability; this is done in step 4. The upper tail includes counts of 8 or 9. If the two creams are equally effective, the probability of eight outcomes of interest in nine pairs is 0.0176. The probability of $X = 9$ under the null hypothesis of $\pi = 0.50$ is 0.002. The probability in the upper tail is the sum of the probability of these two counts. Because the binomial sampling distribution is symmetric when π equals 0.50, the probability in the lower tail is the same as the upper-tail probability; the one-tailed probability, then, could be doubled to obtain the two-tailed p-value. Doubling the one-tailed probability produces the two-tailed p-value of approximately 0.0391. The probability in both tails is computed separately in Box 14–3, to illustrate the symmetry of the sampling distribution when $\pi = 0.50$.

Table 14–2. Effectiveness of benzoyl peroxide cream and an experimental cream for treating comedonal acne.[a]

Experimental Cream	Benzoyl Peroxide Cream (2.5%)		Total
	Improvement: Yes	Improvement: No	
Improvement: Yes	22	8	30
Improvement: No	1	2	3
Total	23	10	33

[a]Shaded cells represent the untied or discordant pairs.

Box 14–3. Testing the effectiveness of two creams for treating comedonal acne

1. *State the Scientific Hypothesis*
In the treatment of comedonal acne, a significant difference in effectiveness will exist between benzoyl peroxide cream and an experimental cream.

2. *Formulate the Statistical Hypotheses*

H_0: $\pi = 0.50$
H_A: $\pi \neq 0.50$

3. *Determine the decision rules*
   a. Use the binomial exact test if $n\pi$ and $n(1 - \pi) \geq 5$.

   $X = 8$

   $n = 9$ (number of untied pairs)

   $n\pi = 9(0.50) = 4.5$ and $n(1 - \pi) = 9(1 - 0.50) = 4.5 < 5$

   Apply the exact test.
   b. The sampling distribution is binomial.
   c. $\alpha = 0.05$.

4. *Analyze the Data*
Compute the upper tail probability:

$pr(X \geq 8) = pr(X = 8) + pr(X = 9)$

$pr(X = 8) = \dfrac{9!}{8!(9 - 8)!} \; 0.50^8(1 - 0.50)^{9-8} = 9(0.50^8)(0.50) = 0.01757813$

$pr(X = 9) = \dfrac{9!}{9!(9 - 9)!} \; 0.50^9(1 - 0.50)^{9-9} = 1(0.50^9)(1) = 0.00195313$

$pr(X \geq 8) = 0.01757813 + 0.00195313 = 0.01953126$

Compute the lower-tail probability. (We could simply double the upper tail probability to obtain the two-tailed *p*-value, because the binomial is symmetric when $\pi = 0.50$. The lower-tail probability is computed, however, to illustrate its determination.)
Select the most extreme observation in the opposite direction and obtain its probability:
The lower tail includes those counts whose probability is individually equal to or less likely than that of the observed count [$pr(X = 8) = 0.01757813$].

$pr(X = 0) = \dfrac{9!}{0!(9 - 0)!} \; 0.50^0(1 - 0.50)^{9-0} = 1(1)(0.50^9) = 0.00195313$

$pr(X = 1) = \dfrac{9!}{1!(9 - 1)!} \; 0.50^1(1 - 0.50)^{9-1} = 9(0.50)(0.50^8) = 0.01757813$

$pr(X = 2) = \dfrac{9!}{2!(9 - 2)!} \; 0.50^2(1 - 0.50)^{9-2} = 36(0.50^2)(0.50^7) = 0.07031250$

Thus the lower tail includes $X = 0$ and $X = 1$. Obtain the lower-tail probability by adding their probabilities (verify that the lower-tail probability is identical to the upper-tail probability):

$pr(X = 0) + pr(X = 1) = 0.00195313 + 0.01757813 = 0.01953126$

Calculate the two-tailed *p*-value:

$pr(X = 0 \text{ or } 1 \text{ or } 8 \text{ or } 9) = 0.01953126 + 0.01953126 = 0.03906252 = 0.0391$

5. *Evaluate the Statistics.*
The null hypothesis is rejected because the *p*-value is less than α (0.0391 < 0.05, respectively).

6. *Interpret the Statistics*
In pairs of individuals with comedonal acne who responded differently to the two creams, a significant difference was noted between the participant who used the experimental cream and the pairmate who used benzoyl peroxide cream (*p*-value = 0.0391, $\alpha = 0.05$). The participant who used the experimental cream was more likely to experience improvement in his or her comedonal acne after 2 months of treatment, versus the pairmate who applied benzoyl peroxide cream (2.5% concentration).

There are two ways to determine the counts to be included in the lower tail. The first method is to follow the procedure outlined in Chapter 13, that is, to include counts in the extreme opposite direction with a probability *equal to* or *less likely than* the observed count. The second involves relying on the symmetry of the sampling distribution; in this case, we reason that if the upper tail includes counts of 8 and 9, the lower tail must encompass the mirror image. Nine, for example, is all of the untied pairs; the comparable count in the opposite direction is zero. Eight untied pairs is one less than nine; therefore, its counterpart is one more than zero. We see, then, that the lower tail includes $X = 0$ and $X = 1$. Our reasoning is confirmed by calculation. We also find in step 4 that the two-tailed probability, derived by computing the upper- and lower-tail probabilities separately, equals the one-tailed probability multiplied by two.

We reject the null hypothesis because the two-tailed p-value is less than α (step 5). The conclusion: In pairs of individuals with comedonal acne who respond differently to the two creams, a significant difference exists in improvement between the patient using the experimental cream and the other member of the pair using the benzoyl peroxide cream (p-value $= 0.0391$, $\alpha = 0.05$). The participant using the experimental cream is more likely to improve than the pairmate who applies benzoyl peroxide. Thus, the experimental cream appears to warrant testing on a larger scale.

SUMMARY

The analysis of two proportions requires that we determine whether an independent or matched/paired design has been used. In testing hypotheses about two proportions from an independent groups design, the normal approximation to the exact test is employed, if four criteria are satisfied: $n_1 p \geq 5$, $n_2 p \geq 5$, $n_1(1 - p) \geq 5$, and $n_2(1 - p) \geq 5$, where p is the pooled estimate of π. The null hypothesis is $\pi_1 - \pi_2 = 0$. The normal approximation is a variation of the z statistic; to determine the status of the null hypothesis, the calculated value of z is compared to the critical value for specified α.

Tests for matched/paired designs are often called tests for correlated proportions. After

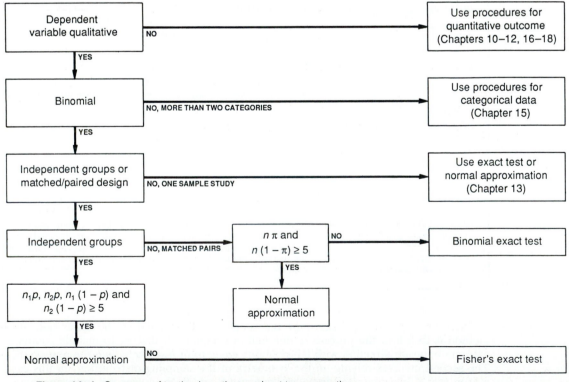

Figure 14–1. Summary of testing hypotheses about two proportions.

Table 14–3. Summary of testing hypotheses about two proportions.

Hypothesis	Assumptions	Test Statistic	Tables
$H_0: \pi_1 - \pi_2 = 0$	Independent groups design Dependent variable is binomial $n_1 p$, $n_2 p$, $n_1(1 - p)$, and $n_2(1 - p) \geq 5$	Normal approximation to the exact test for the difference between two independent proportions $$z = \dfrac{p_1 - p_2}{\sqrt{p(1 - p)\left[\dfrac{1}{n_1} + \dfrac{1}{n_2}\right]}}$$	Normal curve
$H_0: \pi = 0.50$	Matched/paired design Dependent variable is binomial $n\pi = n(1 - \pi) \geq 5$	Normal approximation to the binomial exact test for matched/paired design for correlated proportion $$z = \dfrac{p - \pi}{\sqrt{\dfrac{\pi(1 - \pi)}{n}}}$$	Normal curve
$H_0: \pi = 0.50$	Matched/paired design Dependent variable is binomial $n\pi = n(1 - \pi) < 5$	Binomial exact test for matched/paired data for correlated proportions $$\dfrac{n!}{X!(n - X)!}\,\pi^X(1 - \pi)^{n-x}$$	None because the probability is computed from the formula
$100(1 - \alpha)\%$ two-sided confidence interval	Independent groups design Dependent variable is binomial $n_1 p$, $n_2 p$, $n_1(1 - p)$, and $n_2(1 - p) \geq 5$	Normal approximation to the exact test for the difference between two independent proportions $$(p_1 - p_2) \pm z_{\alpha/2}\sqrt{p(1 - p)\left[\dfrac{1}{n_1} + \dfrac{1}{n_2}\right]}$$	Normal curve

casting the data into a 2×2 contingency table, we focus on the discordant or untied pairs. Under the null hypothesis of no difference, $\pi = 0.50$, we expect the discordant pairs to distribute themselves equally between two cells of the 2×2 table. The binomial exact test is identical mathematically to the exact test for a single proportion; for matched/paired data, X is the number of pairs in which one member of the pair evidences the outcome of interest and his or her pairmate does not; n is the number of untied or discordant pairs; and π equals 0.50 under the null hypothesis. The p-value is computed directly from the binomial formula and compared to α. The normal approximation is employed if $n\pi \geq 5$ and $n(1 - \pi) \geq 5$. A variant of the z statistic is used; the calculated value of z is compared to the critical value determined from the table of the standard normal curve.

The tests used in this chapter and their assumptions are summarized in Table 14–3; a flowchart test appears in Figure 14–1.

REFERENCES

Colton T: *Statistics in Medicine*. Little, Brown, 1974.

Dawson-Saunders B, Trapp R: *Basic and Clinical Biostatistics*, 2nd ed. Appleton & Lange, 1994.

Goldstein S, Odom R: Skin and Appendages. In Tierney S Jr, et al (editors): *Current Medical Diagnosis and Treatment*. Appleton & Lange, 1993.

Kanji G: *100 Statistical Tests*. Sage, 1993.

Rosner B: *Fundamentals of Biostatistics*, 2nd ed. Duxbury, 1986.

Self-study Questions

Part I: Review

1. Review the three ways in which dependent groups designs can be created.
2. Describe how randomization is used in matched/paired designs.
3. Explain how randomization is used in independent groups designs.

Part II: Analysis Identification

Read each of the following and identify the correct analysis. Choices include analyses for one mean, two means, one proportion, and two proportions.

1. The effectiveness of a new antibody treatment to shrink liver tumors too large for surgical removal was evaluated in 104 patients. After 10 weeks of treatment, liver tumors shrunk in 50 patients by at least 20%.
2. The Blood Pressure Control Task Force evaluated whether a direct relationship exists between maternal hypertension and systolic blood pressure in healthy female children, ages 8 to 12 years. Two groups of healthy female children, ages 8 to 12 years, were selected randomly; systolic blood pressure was measured. The mothers of the female children in group one have no history of hypertension; the mean systolic blood pressure of these girls was 102.5 mm Hg with a standard deviation of 11.4 mm Hg ($n_1 = 65$). The mean systolic blood pressure of girls with a hypertensive mother was 112.8 mm Hg with a standard deviation of 10.9 ($n_2 = 54$). Assume that at least one of the population distributions is nonnormal.
3. It is well documented that college graduates with a bachelor's degree (BA or BS) are more likely to stop smoking than individuals with fewer years of education. However, it is unknown whether graduate degree holders (MA, MS, or PhD) are more likely to stop smoking than individuals with a bachelor's degree but no graduate, degree. Among 52 randomly selected individuals who smoked while earning undergraduate degrees between 1980 and 1982, 31 currently were ex-smokers for at least 12 months. Among 50 graduate degree holders who smoked while earning undergraduate degrees between 1980 and 1982, 38 currently were ex-smokers for at least 12 months.
4. An orthopedist hypothesizes that men with an occupational back injury and men with a nonoccupational back injury differ with respect to the number of weeks on disability leave before returning to work ($\leq$ 12 weeks or $>$ 12 weeks). Fifteen pairs of men at an automotive manufacturing plant are matched retrospectively, according to severity of the back injury, then followed through treatment and eventual return to work. Data appear in Table 14–4.

Table 14–4. Type of back injury and length of disability leave.

	Occupational Injury		
Nonoccupational Injury	$\leq$ 12 weeks	$>$ 12 weeks	Total
$\leq$ 12 Weeks	3	7	10
$>$ 12 Weeks	2	3	5
Total	5	10	15

5. The association between the HLA-DR4 histocompatability antigen and rheumatoid arthritis is investigated in randomly selected patients with and without rheumatoid arthritis. It is postulated that a greater proportion of patients with rheumatoid arthritis will be HLA-DR4 positive compared to healthy patients without rheumatoid arthritis. In a sample of 103 patients with rheumatoid arthritis, 76 are HLA-DR4 positive, compared to 27 of 51 healthy patients without rheumatoid arthritis.

6. The effect of gastrointestinal malignancy on whole-body metabolism is studied in 10 patients with advanced gastric and colorectal cancer. It is hypothesized that gastrointestinal malignancy increases leucine metabolism. In a population of healthy patients, mean leucine flux is 1.71 (mL/kg/per day). The mean leucine flux of the study participants is 2.30 (mL/kg/per day) with a standard deviation of 0.32. Assume normality of the relevant population distribution.

Part IV: Problems and Analysis

Read each problem and analyze the data, as appropriate. If an hypothesis is to be tested, identify the scientific and statistical hypotheses, state the decision rules, perform the analysis, make a decision about the null hypothesis, and interpret the results. Allow $\alpha = 0.05$ in all problems.

1. Anecdotal reports indicate that foundry workers have higher blood pressure levels than nonfoundry workers. To determine whether an association exists between the heat and noise in a foundry (or some other occupational factor) and elevated blood pressure, investigators study two groups of randomly selected men, ages 24 to 34 years. Among 100 men who work in a foundry, 68 have high blood pressure; among 100 nonfoundry employees who work in a hot and noisy factory, 56 have high blood pressure.
2. The effectiveness of aspirin (500 mg) and acetaminophen and caffeine (325 mg and 35 mg, respectively), taken orally every 4 hours, is examined for the treatment of chronic, nonmigraine, headaches. It is hypothesized that the combination of acetaminophen and caffeine will provide relief to a greater proportion of patients than aspirin only. Forty pairs of patients are matched on age, sex, and clinical judgments about headache severity; each follows a medication regime for 4 weeks. At the end of the trial, each patient reports whether the medication generally relieves his or her headaches (yes/no). Data appear in Table 14–5.

Table 14–5. Aspirin and acetaminophen and caffeine to treat chronic headaches.

Aspirin	Acetaminophen and Caffeine		Total
	Headache Relief: Yes	Headache Relief: No	
Headache Relief: Yes	8	6	14
Headache Relief: No	16	10	26
Total	24	16	40

3. Staff in a clinical laboratory in a large metropolitan hospital perform 400 white blood cell counts per day with an electric counting device. Ten percent of these counts are abnormally high, on average, because the hospital serves a population with a wide spectrum of diseases, including some that cause elevated white blood cell counts. On a certain day, the laboratory performs white blood cell counts on 260 randomly selected samples; 35 have abnormally high white blood cell counts. Test the hypothesis that this proportion of abnormal white blood cell counts is greater than would be expected on a typical day.
4. In 1944, clinicians at a prominent medical center compared outcomes in two groups of skin graft patients: those who received intramuscular penicillin injections in conjunction with surgery and those who received standard treatment, which at the time did not include the use of an antibiotic. The goal is to determine if the use of penicillin increases the proportion of patients in whom a satisfactory skin graft take occurs. Patients with third-degree burns who were to receive a single skin graft were assigned randomly to one of two treatment conditions. Except for the use of penicillin, techniques for preparing the burn site, grafting the skin, and postgraft care were identical in the two groups. Fourteen of the 15 patients in the penicillin group had a satisfactory graft. Ten of the 30 patients in the other group had a satisfactory graft.

Table 14–6. The effectiveness of isosorbide nitrate (ISDN) and trinitroglycerine (TNG) to treat angina.

Trinitroglycerine	Isosorbide Nitrate		Total
	Improvement: Yes	*Improvement: No*	
Improvement: Yes	14	1	15
Improvement: No	8	2	10
Total	22	3	25

5. Isosorbide nitrate (ISDN) and trinitroglycerine (TNG), a relatively standard therapy, were compared for the treatment of angina. Because ISDN has a longer duration of action than TNG, it was hypothesized that a greater proportion of angina patients taking ISDN would improve, compared to those receiving TNG. Twenty-five pairs of men matched on angina severity participated in a double blind trial; one member of the pair was assigned randomly to receive ISDN and the other member to receive TNG. At the end of the trial, each patient was evaluated by a clinician unfamiliar with the purpose of the study to determine if the participant's angina improved. Data appear in Table 14–6.

Solutions

Part II: Analysis Identification

1. *Liver Tumors*
Data were gathered from a single sample of 104 patients. The outcome is binomial (tumor shrunk at least 25%: yes/no). No hypothesis is formulated. Consequently, the objective is to estimate the range within which the parameter, π, is likely to be captured. Because π is unknown, the best estimate is p, the sample proportion. Use p to determine if the rules-of-thumb have been satisfied. If they have, use the normal approximation to construct the 95% confidence interval: $p = (50/104) = 0.4808$; $np = 104(0.48) = 49.92$; $n(1 - p) = 104(1 - 0.48) = 54.08$. Both criteria are satisfied. The 95% confidence interval is $(p - z_{\alpha/2}\sigma_p \leq \pi \leq p + z_{\alpha/2}\sigma_p) = p \pm z_{\alpha/2}\sigma_p$, where p is the sample proportion, $z_{\alpha/2}$ is the two-tailed critical value, and σ_p is the standard error of the sample proportion.

2. *Maternal Hypertension*
Two independent groups were sampled. The dependent variable is systolic blood pressure; it is treated quantitatively. We are interested in the difference between two independent means. At least one population distribution is nonnormal. Both n_1 and n_2 are greater than or equal to 30. Use the z statistic for the difference between two independent means:

$$z = \frac{\overline{X}_1 - \overline{X}_2}{\sqrt{\dfrac{s_1^2}{n_1} + \dfrac{s_2^2}{n_2}}}.$$

3. *Smoking and Education*
Two independent groups were sampled. The dependent variable is binomial: Exsmoker for at least last 12 months: yes/no. Determine if the normal approximation for the difference between two independent proportions applies by computing p, the pooled estimate of π, and checking all four criteria.

Bachelor's Degree	MA, MS, or PhD
$X_1 = 31$	$X_2 = 38$
$n_1 = 52$	$n_2 = 50$

$$p = \frac{31 + 38}{52 + 50} = 0.6765$$

$n_1 p = 52(0.6765) = 35.18 \geq 5$ $n_2 p = 50(0.6765) = 33.82 \geq 5$
$n_1(1 - p) = 52(1 - 0.6765) = 16.82 \geq 5$ $n_2(1 - p) = 50(1 - 0.6765) = 16.18 \geq 5$

All four criteria are satisfied; use the normal approximation to the binomial for the difference between two independent proportions.

4. *Skin Grafts and Penicillin*
   Use a matched/paired design with a binomial, dependent variable: Length of disability leave: ≤ 12 weeks / > 12 weeks. Check $n\pi$ and $n(1 - \pi)$ to determine whether to employ the binomial exact test or the normal approximation for matched/paired data. Define X as the number of pairs in which the worker with an occupational injury was on leave for > 12 weeks and his pairmate was on leave for ≤ 12 weeks; $X = 7$, $n = 9$, and $\pi = 0.50$: $n\pi = n(1 - \pi) = 9(0.50) = 4.5 < 5$. Therefore, use the binomial exact test to examine the proportion from a matched/paired design.

5. *HLA-DR4 and Rheumatoid Arthritis*
   Two independent samples were studied. The dependent variable is binomial: HLA-DR4: positive/negative. Check the rule-of-thumb criteria to determine if the normal approximation applies.

Rheumatoid Arthritis	No Rheumatoid Arthritis
$X_1 = 76$	$X_2 = 27$
$n_1 = 103$	$n_2 = 51$

$$p = \frac{76 + 27}{103 + 51} = 0.6688$$

$n_1 p = 103(0.6688) = 68.89 \geq 5$ $n_2 p = 51(0.6688) = 34.11 \geq 5$

$n_1(1 - p) = 103(1 - 0.6688) = 34.11 \geq 5$ $n_2(1 - p) = 51(1 - 0.6688) = 16.89 \geq 5$

All four criteria are satisfied; use the normal approximation to the binomial for the difference between two independent proportions.

6. *Gastrointestinal Malignancy*
   A single group is sampled and the leucine flux of each patient is measured (mL/kg/per day). The dependent variable, leucine flux, is quantitative. The population standard deviation is unknown. The sampling distribution is assumed normal. Use the Student's t statistic for one mean: $t = \dfrac{\bar{X} - \mu}{s_{\bar{X}}}$ with $df = n - 1$.

Part III: Problems and Analysis

1. *Blood Pressure in Foundry and Nonfoundry Workers*
   State the Scientific Hypothesis:
   Men, ages 24 to 34 years, who work in a foundry and similarly aged men who work in a hot and noisy, nonfoundry setting will differ significantly with respect to the proportion who have high blood pressure.
   Formulate the statistical hypotheses:
   (F = Foundry Workers, NF = Workers in a Nonfoundry Environment)

$$H_0: \pi_F - \pi_{NF} = 0$$

$$H_A: \pi_F - \pi_{NF} \neq 0$$

Determine the decision rules:
a. Check the rules-of-thumb to determine if the normal approximation applies.

Compute the pooled estimate of π:

$$X_F = 68 \qquad X_{NF} = 56$$

$$n_F = 100 \qquad n_{NF} = 100$$

$$p = \frac{68 + 56}{100 + 100} = 0.62$$

$$n_F p = 100(0.62) = 62 \geq 5 \qquad\qquad n_{NF}p = 100(0.62) = 62 \geq 5$$

$$n_F(1 - p) = 100(1 - 0.62) = 38 \geq 5 \qquad n_{NF}(1 - p) = 100(1 - 0.62) = 38 \geq 5$$

Because all four criteria are satisfied, use the normal approximation to the exact test for the difference between two independent proportions.
b. Sampling distribution of the difference between two independent proportions.
c. $\alpha = 0.05$.
d. $z_{crit} = \pm1.96$.
Analyze the Data:

$$X_F = 68 \qquad X_{NF} = 56$$

$$n_F = 100 \qquad n_{NF} = 100$$

Compute each sample proportion:

$$p_F = \frac{68}{100} = 0.68$$

$$p_{NF} = \frac{56}{100} = 0.56$$

Calculate the standard error of the difference:

$$SE_{p_F - p_{NF}} = \sqrt{ p(1 - p) \left[\frac{1}{n_F} + \frac{1}{n_{NF}} \right] }$$

$$= \sqrt{ 0.62(1 - 0.62) \left[\frac{1}{100} + \frac{1}{100} \right] }$$

$$= \sqrt{0.0047} = 0.0686$$

Obtain the calculated value of z:

$$z = \frac{0.68 - 0.56}{0.0686} = 1.7493$$

Evaluate the Statistics:
The null hypothesis is retained ($z_{calc} = 1.7493 < z_{crit} = \pm 1.96$).
Interpret the Statistics:
Although the proportion of men, ages 24 to 34 years, who work in a foundry and have high blood pressure (0.62) is greater than similarly aged men who work in a hot, noisy non-foundry environment (0.56), no significant difference existed between these two proportions (p-value ≈ 0.08, $\alpha = 0.05$). Because the results are consistent with anecdotal reports, the investigators may wish to replicate the investigation and include additional occupational and health-related variables.

2. *Chronic Headaches*
State the Scientific Hypothesis:
A greater proportion of chronic, nonmigraine, headache-sufferers who take acetamino-phen and caffeine orally every 4 hours will experience headache relief, versus similar patients who take aspirin every 4 hours.
Formulate the Statistical Hypotheses:
Note that a matched/paired design was used and the outcome of interest is binomial: headache relief (yes/no). Therefore, it is hypothesized that the discordant pairs will distribute themselves equally between cells 2,1 and 1,2. Thus, half the discordant pairs will fall in cell 2,1 and the other half in cell 1,2.

$$H_0: \pi = 0.50$$

$$H_A: \pi > 0.50$$

Determine the Decision Rules:
a. Decide whether the exact test or a normal approximation is appropriate.

> $X = 16$ (number of pairs in which the individual taking acetaminophen and caffeine improved and the pairmate taking only aspirin did not improve)
> $n = 22$ (total number of discordant or untied pairs)
> $n\pi = n(1 - \pi) = 22(0.50) = 11 \geq 5$

Use the normal approximation for matched/paired data.
b. Sampling distribution is binomial; normal curve will serve as an approximation.
c. $\alpha = 0.05$.
d. $z_{crit} = 1.645$.
Analyze the Data:

$$X = 16$$

$$n = 22$$

Compute the proportion (where X = number of untied pairs in which the individual taking acetaminophen and caffeine improved and the pairmate taking aspirin did not improve):

$$p = \frac{16}{22} = 0.7273$$

Calculate the standard error:

$$\sigma_p = \sqrt{\frac{\pi(1 - \pi)}{n}} = \sqrt{\frac{0.50(1 - 0.50)}{22}} = 0.1066$$

Determine z:

$$z = \frac{0.7273 - 0.50}{0.1066} = 2.1323$$

Evaluate the Statistics:
The null hypothesis is rejected ($z_{calc} = 2.1323$, $z_{crit} = 1.645$).
Interpret the Statistics:
In pairs of individuals with chronic, nonmigraine, headaches that respond differently to the two drug regimens, the member of the pair taking acetaminophen and caffeine is significantly more likely to experience headache relief than the other member who uses aspirin only (p-value ≈ 0.0166, $\alpha = 0.05$).

3. *White Blood Cell Counts*
State the Scientific Hypothesis:
The proportion of abnormally high white blood cell counts is greater than 0.10, the proportion that would be expected during a typical day.
Formulate the Statistical Hypotheses:
Note that this is a single sample study.

$$H_0: \pi = 0.10$$

$$H_A: \pi > 0.10$$

Determine the Decision Rules:
a. Use the normal approximation for one proportion, if $n\pi$ and $n(1 - \pi) \geq 5$. $n\pi$ = 260(0.10) = 26 ≥ 5 and $n(1 - \pi)$ = 260(1 − 0.10) = 234 ≥ 5.
b. Sampling distribution for a sample proportion (normal approximation will be used as a stand-in for the binomial).
c. $\alpha = 0.05$.
d. $z_{crit} = 1.645$.
Analyze the Data:

$$X = 35 \text{ (number of white cell counts that are abnormally high)}$$

$$n = 260 \text{ (number of counts performed)}$$

Calculate the sample proportion:

$$p = \frac{35}{260} = 0.1346$$

Determine the standard error of the sample proportion:

$$\sigma_p = \sqrt{\frac{\pi(1 - \pi)}{n}} = \sqrt{\frac{0.10(1 - 0.10)}{260}} = 0.0186$$

Determine z:

$$z = \frac{0.1346 - 0.10}{0.0186} = 1.8602$$

Evaluate the Statistics:
The null hypothesis is rejected ($z_{calc} = 1.86$, $z_{crit} = +1.645$).
Interpret the Statistics:
A significant increase has been noted in the proportion of abnormally high white blood cell counts (0.1346), compared to white blood cell counts on a typical day (0.10) (z_{calc} = 1.86, z_{crit} = 1.645, p-value ≈ 0.0314, α = 0.05). The hospital may wish to evaluate potential explanations, such as the need to calibrate the electric counting device or the possibility that the finding is seasonal, that is, that an unexpectedly large number of individuals presented with illnesses that elevate the white blood cell count.
4. *Skin Grafts and Penicillin*
State the Scientific Hypothesis:
The use of intramuscular penicillin injections following skin graft surgery increases the proportion of patients in which a satisfactory take occurs, compared to standard treatment which does not include the use of an antibiotic.
Formulate the Statistical Hypotheses:
(P = penicillin, s = standard practice)

$$H_0: \pi_P - \pi_S = 0$$

$$H_A: \pi_P - \pi_S > 0$$

Determine the Decision Rules:
a. Decide whether the normal approximation to the exact test for the difference between two independent proportions applies.

$$X_P = 14 \qquad X_S = 10$$

$$n_P = 15 \qquad n_S = 30$$

Calculate p, the pooled estimate of π:

$$p = \frac{14 + 10}{15 + 30} = \frac{24}{45} = 0.5333$$

Check the rules-of-thumb:

$$n_P p = 15(0.5333) = 7.99 \geq 5$$

$$n_P(1 - p) = 15(1 - 0.5333) = 7.0 \geq 5$$

$$n_S p = 30(0.5333) = 15.99 \geq 5$$

$$n_S(1 - p) = 30(1 - 0.5333) = 14.00 \geq 5$$

Use the normal approximation to the exact test.
b. Sampling distribution of the difference between two independent proportions.
c. $\alpha = 0.05$.
d. $z_{\text{crit}} = 1.645$.
Analyze the Data:

$$X_P = 14 \qquad X_S = 10$$

$$n_P = 15 \qquad n_S = 30$$

Calculate the two sample proportions:

$$p_P = \frac{14}{15} = 0.9333$$

$$p_S = \frac{10}{30} = 0.3333$$

Obtain the standard error of the difference:

$$SE_{p_P - p_s} = \sqrt{p(1-p) \left[\frac{1}{n_p} + \frac{1}{n_s} \right]}$$

$$= \sqrt{0.5333(1 - 0.5333) \left[\frac{1}{15} + \frac{1}{30} \right]} = 0.1578$$

Compute the value of z:

$$z = \frac{0.9333 - 0.3333}{0.1578} = 3.8023$$

Evaluate the Statistics:
The null hypothesis is rejected ($z_{calc} = 3.80$, $z_{crit} = 1.645$).
Interpret the Statistics:
A significantly greater proportion of patients with third-degree burns who received intra-muscular penicillin injections following skin graft surgery had a satisfactory skin graft (14 of 15, or 93.33%) compared to similar patients who received standard treatment only, which did not include the use of an antibiotic (10 of 33, or 33.33%) (*p*-value < 0.000072, α = 0.05).

5. *ISDN and TNG for the Treatment of Angina*
   State the Scientific Hypothesis:
   A greater proportion of men with angina will improve while taking isosorbide nitrate, compared to those taking trinitroglycerine.
   Formulate the Statistical Hypotheses:

$$H_0: \pi = 0.50$$

$$H_A: \pi > 0.50$$

Determine the Decision Rules:
a. Decide whether the exact test or normal approximation applies.

$X = 8$ (number of pairs in which the individual taking ISDN improved and the pairmate taking TNG did not)
$n = 9$ (total number of discordant or untied pairs)
$n\pi = n(1 - \pi) = 9(0.50) = 4.5 < 5$

Use the exact test for matched/paired data.
b. Sampling distribution is binomial.
c. $\alpha = 0.05$.
Analyze the Data:

$$X = 8$$

$$n = 9$$

Compute the proportion for reporting purposes (where X = number of untied pairs in which the individual taking ISDN improved and the pairmate taking TNG did not):

$$p = \frac{8}{9} = 0.8889$$

Use the binomial formula to calculate the one-tailed probability:

$$pr(X = 8) = \frac{9!}{8!(9-8)!} \ 0.50^8(1-0.50)^{9-8} = 9(0.50^8)0.50 = 0.0176$$

$$pr(X = 9) = \frac{9!}{9!(9 - 9)!}0.50^9(1 - 0.50)^{9-9} = 1(0.50^9)(1) = 0.001953$$

Add the two probabilities together to obtain the *p*-value:

$$pr(X \geq 8) = 0.0176 + 0.001953 = 0.019553 = 0.0196$$

Evaluate the Statistics:
The null hypothesis is rejected.
Interpret the Statistics:
Among pairs of men with angina who responded differently to treatment, the member of the pair who took isosorbide nitrate was significantly more likely to experience improvement in his angina than the member of the pair who took trinitroglycerine (*p*-value = 0.0196, α = 0.05).

Testing Hypotheses About Frequencies and Proportions

15

Clinical Example: Racial Differences in Cardiac Arrest

> In a large midwestern city, the association between racial differences in the incidence of cardiac arrest and subsequent survival was studied in 6117 cases of nontraumatic, out-of-hospital cardiac arrest. During a 12-month period, fewer than 1% of African-Americans survived an arrest to hospital discharge (24 of 2910), compared to 2.6% of Caucasians (84 of 3207; Becker et al, 1993, pp 600–606).

This example focuses on the relationship between two nominal or qualitative variables. These variables are referred to as classification criteria, because each individual is cross-classified according to his or her race (African-American/Caucasian) and survival status (yes/no). We use a statistic known as chi-square (χ^2) to examine the frequency in each cross-classified category and to determine whether the criteria are independent. This application of chi-square is referred to as *testing for independence.* In addition to its use in assessing independence between two classification criteria, chi-square is used to test hypotheses about differences between two or more independent proportions from two or more populations. This second application is called *testing for equality or homogeneity of proportions.* Both applications are addressed in this chapter.

Readers who are interested in a third application, *testing for goodness-of-fit,* are referred to other sources (for example, Daniel, 1993, pp 531–542). Briefly, testing for goodness-of-fit compares a distribution of observed frequencies to a hypothesized distribution, to determine whether the two distributions are compatible. Let's illustrate this with a hypothetical problem (adapted from Daniel, 1991, p 539, with permission of John Wiley & Sons, Inc). Suppose research suggests that a particular human trait is inherited according to the ratio of 1:4:1 for homozygous dominant, heterozygous, and homozygous recessive. Suppose also that the trait is distributed the following way in a random sampling of 1000 individuals: homozygous dominant, 215; heterozygous, 650; and homozygous recessive, 135. In such a case, the investigators may choose to test the *goodness-of-fit* of the data by comparing the observed distribution to the hypothesized distribution. Based on the result, the researchers might retain or reject the hypothesis that the trait is distributed on a 1:4:1 basis.

OBJECTIVES

When you complete this chapter, you should be able to:

- Differentiate hypotheses about independence of two classification criteria from those about homogeneity of proportions.
- Conduct a chi-square test.
- Translate the findings from a chi-square test into nonstatistical language.

TESTING INDEPENDENCE

Chi-square (χ^2) is used frequently to test for independence of two nominal criteria applied to a sample of observations (Daniel, 1991, p 542). The null hypothesis states that the two criteria

Table 15-1. Two-way classification of n independent observations.

First Classification Criterion	Second Classification Criterion				Marginal Total
	Category 1	*Category 2*	...	*Category c*	
Category 1	O_{11}	O_{12}	...	O_{1c}	$n_{1.}$
.	.	.	.	.	.
.	.	.	.	.	.
.	.	.	.	.	.
Category r	O_{r1}	O_{r2}	...	O_{rc}	$n_{r.}$
Marginal total	$n_{.1}$	$n_{.2}$		n_{rc}	$n_{..}$

are independent; the alternative hypothesis indicates that the criteria are not independent but associated. Two criteria are independent if the "distribution of one criterion is the same no matter what the distribution of the other criterion" (Daniel, 1991, p 542). For example, if the incidence of breast cancer and family history of breast cancer are independent, we would expect the same relative frequency of women with and without breast cancer to have a positive family history.

To study the independence of two qualitative variables, we begin by obtaining a random sample of n independent observations. The observations are independent because the selection of one observation does not influence the selection of any other. Observations are classified subsequently according to the cells formed by the intersection of the rows and columns of a contingency table, as illustrated in Table 15-1. The rows, symbolized by r, consist of the mutually exclusive categories of one criterion; the columns, designated by c, comprise the mutually exclusive categories of the other criterion. The frequency of observations in each cell is determined along with the marginal totals. These observed frequencies are identified by O and subscripted to indicate the row and column. The first subscript marks the row; the second subscript designates the column. For example, O_{11} is the number of observations in the intersection of the first row and column; O_{12} is the number of observations in the intersection of the first row and second column. Represented by n with appropriate subscripts, the marginal totals reflect the number of observations in each row or column. The dot notation on these totals (.) indicates that summation has taken place over rows or columns, depending on the position of the dot. For example, $n_{1.}$ is the number of observations in the first row, where summation has occurred over columns: $n_{1.} = O_{11} + O_{12} + \ldots + O_{1c}$. The total number of observations is $n_{..}$, where summation has taken place over rows and columns. The two dots are omitted in the remainder of the chapter without loss of clarity; thus, n indicates total sample size.

Expected frequencies are computed for each cell under the null hypothesis of independence and compared to observed frequencies. If the difference between observed and expected frequencies is small, the calculated value of χ^2 is small and the null hypothesis is retained. If the difference between observed and expected frequencies is large, the calculated value of χ^2 is large. We reject the null hypothesis and conclude that the two criteria are not independent. The calculated value of χ^2 is compared to the critical value for specified degrees of freedom and level of significance, to determine if the differences between the observed and expected frequencies are large enough to lead us to reject the null hypothesis. If the calculated value of chi-square is equal to or greater than the critical value, the null hypothesis of independence is rejected:

$$\chi^2_{calc} \geq \chi^2_{crit} \Rightarrow \textbf{Reject H}_0$$

The chi-square statistic is

$$\chi^2 = \sum_{j=1}^{c} \sum_{i=1}^{r} \frac{(O_{ij} - E_{ij})^2}{E_{ij}} \text{ , with } df = (r-1)(c-1) \qquad \textbf{15.1}$$

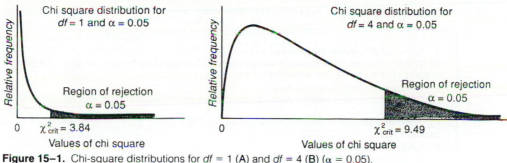

Figure 15–1. Chi-square distributions for $df = 1$ (A) and $df = 4$ (B) ($\alpha = 0.05$).

where O_{ij} is the observed frequency in cell i,j and E_{ij} is the expected frequency in cell i,j. The double summation operator indicates that summation is over all c columns, beginning with the first column, and r rows, beginning with the first row. Degrees of freedom is number of rows minus one times the number of columns minus one.

The chi-square distribution, like the Student's t distribution, is a family of probability distributions, each characterized by its degree of freedom. The mean of the distribution equals its degrees of freedom (df); the variance is twice the degrees of freedom ($2df$). Chi-square takes on values between zero and (positive) infinity. The distribution, skewed for small degrees of freedom, becomes more bell shaped as degrees of freedom increase. The region of rejection always appears in the upper tail of the distribution, because we square the differences between the observed and expected frequencies. Two chi-square distributions appear in Figure 15–1. Observe that the distributions for $df = 1$ and $df = 4$ differ considerably.

The survival data from the example at the beginning of the chapter are used to construct a 2 × 2 table, define expected frequencies, and calculate chi-square. Data appear in Table 15–2. Although χ^2 is determined in this example from a 2 × 2 table, χ^2 can also be determined from tables having more than two rows or columns. In this example, the rows define the two categories of race (Caucasian/African-American) and the columns consist of the categories of survival to discharge (yes/no). The *observed frequency* in each cell of the table is the number of cases occurring in the intersection of a particular row and column. For example, 24 African-Americans survived to hospital discharge. The *marginal totals* indicate the number of individuals in each row and column. For example, the sample consisted of 3207 Caucasians (row 1) and 2910 African-Americans (row 2); 108 individuals survived to hospital discharge (column 1) and 6009 died (column 2).

The analysis is summarized in Box 15–1. The scientific and statistical hypotheses are formulated in steps 1 and 2. The scientific and alternative hypotheses are *always nondirectional* in tests of independence. The null hypothesis postulates independence; the alternative hypothesis states simply that the two nominal variables are not independent. Decision

Table 15–2. Racial differences and survival in cases of nontraumatic, out-of-hospital cardiac arrest.

Race	Survival to Discharge		Total
	Yes	No	
Caucasian	84	3123	3207
African-American	24	2886	2910
Total	108	6009	6117

Adapted with permission from Becker L, et al: Racial differences in the incidence of cardiac arrest and subsequent survival. *N Engl J Med* 1993;**329**:600.

Box 15–1. Assessing the independence between race and survival in cases of nontraumatic out-of-hospital cardiac arrest.

1. *Develop the Scientific Hypothesis*
An association exists between race (African-American/Caucasian) and survival to hospital discharge (yes/no) in cases of nontraumatic out-of-hospital cardiac arrest.

2. *Formulate the Statistical Hypotheses*
H_0: Race and survival to hospital discharge are independent in cases of nontraumatic out-of-hospital cardiac arrest.
H_A: Race and survival to hospital discharge are *not* independent in cases of nontraumatic out-of-hospital cardiac arrest.

3. *Determine the decision rules*
   a. Chi-square statistic and distribution.
   b. $\alpha = 0.05$, $df = (2 - 1)(2 - 1) = 1$.
   c. $\chi^2_{crit} = 3.84$.

4. *Analyze the Data*
Calculate the expected frequency for each cell:

Cell 1,1 $\quad E_{11} = \dfrac{(3207)(108)}{6117} = 56.6219$

Cell 1,2 $\quad E_{12} = \dfrac{(3207)(6011)}{6117} = 3151.4267$

Cell 2,1 $\quad E_{21} = \dfrac{(2910)(108)}{6117} = 51.3781$

Cell 2,2 $\quad E_{22} = \dfrac{(2910)(6009)}{6117} = 2854.8161$

Check the rule-of-thumb for expected frequencies.
All expected frequencies are large; therefore, continue with the chi-square test.

Determine $\dfrac{(O_{ij} - E_{ij})^2}{E_{ij}}$ for each cell (these are referred to as the cell chi-square values):

Cell 1,1 $\quad \dfrac{(84 - 56.6219)^2}{56.6219} = 13.2380$

Cell 1,2 $\quad \dfrac{(3123 - 3151.4267)^2}{3151.4267} = 0.2564$

Cell 2,1 $\quad \dfrac{(24 - 51.3781)^2}{51.3781} = 14.5891$

Cell 2,2 $\quad \dfrac{(2886 - 2854.8161)^2}{2854.8161} = 0.3406$

Add the cell values together to obtain the calculated value of chi-square:
$\chi^2 = 13.2380 + 0.2564 + 14.5891 + 0.3406 = 28.4241$

5. *Evaluate the Statistics*
Compare the calculated value of chi-square to the critical value and make a decision about the null hypothesis:
$\chi^2_{calc} = 28.42 > \chi^2_{crit} = 3.84$
Reject H_0.

6. *Interpret the Statistics*
A significant association exists between race and survival to hospital discharge in cases of nontraumatic out-of-hospital cardiac arrest ($\chi^2_{calc} = 28.42$, $\chi^2_{crit} = 3.841$, $df = 1$, $\alpha = 0.05$, *p*-value < 0.005). The largest relative departures from expected were noted as follows: considerably more Caucasians than expected under the null hypothesis of independence survived to hospital discharge (observed frequency = 84, expected frequency = 56.62); fewer African-Americans than expected survived to discharge (observed frequency = 24, expected frequency = 71.38).

rules are specified in step 3. The chi-square distribution and statistic will be used; α is set at 0.05; the degrees of freedom equal one. The critical value of χ^2 is 3.84. The critical value is found in Table A-3 in the appendix of statistical tables.

Expected frequencies are calculated next. Let's briefly discuss the rationale for the calculation. Consider two categories, African-American (row 2) and survival to discharge (column 1). The probability that a study participant is African-American is (2910/6117) = 0.4757. The probability that an individual survives to discharge is (108/6117) = 0.0177. Next, consider the intersection of African-American and Survival to discharge (cell 2,1). If being an African-American and surviving to discharge are independent, as specified in the null hypothesis, the probability that a study participant will be African-American and survive to discharge is given by the multiplication rule for independent events (Formula 5.8, Chapter 5) and equals 0.0084:

$$pr(\text{African-American and survival to discharge}) = pr(\text{African-American})pr(\text{Survival to discharge})$$

$$= \left(\frac{2910}{6117} \right) \left(\frac{108}{6117} \right)$$

$$= 0.0084$$

The estimated probability associated with each of the remaining cells can be calculated similarly. When multiplied by the total number of observations (n), the estimated probabilities yield the *expected frequency* for each cell. For example, the *expected* number of study participants who are African-American and survive to discharge is

$$E_{21} = 0.0084(6117) = 51.3781$$

Thus we expect 51.3828 study participants to be African-American and survive to discharge, if race and survival are independent as postulated in the null hypothesis.

If the calculation for the expected frequency is written out, we find that it is (1) the product of the corresponding row and column marginal totals (2) divided by the total number of observations. For example:

Numerical Illustration

$$E_{11} = \left(\frac{3207}{6117} \right) \left(\frac{108}{6117} \right)(6117)$$

$$= \frac{(3207)(108)}{6117}$$

$$= 56.6219$$

$$= \frac{(\text{Row 1 Total})(\text{Column 1 Total})}{\text{Total Number of Observations}}$$

Symbolic Equivalent

$$E_{11} = \left(\frac{n_{1.}}{n} \right) \left(\frac{n_{.1}}{n} \right)(n)$$

$$= \frac{(n_{1.})(n_{.1})}{n}$$

$$= \frac{(\text{Row 1 Total})(\text{Column 1 Total})}{\text{Total Number of Observations}}$$

The expected frequencies for the remaining cells are calculated in Box 15–1. Note the discrepancies between the observed and expected frequencies. For example, the expected frequency for cell 1,1 (Caucasian and Survival to discharge) is 56.62 compared to the observed frequency of 84.

The expected frequencies are checked to determine if small expected frequencies occur. (Small expected frequencies are discussed in the next section.) In this case, all expected frequencies are acceptably large. Therefore, the cell chi-square values are computed and summed to obtain the overall value of 28.42. The null hypothesis is rejected, because this calculated value exceeds the critical value (3.84) for $df = 1$ and $\alpha = 0.05$ (step 5). We conclude that a significant association exists between race and survival to hospital discharge, in cases of nontraumatic out-of-hospital cardiac arrest (p-value < 0.0005; step 6). Interpretation of these findings is enhanced if we inspect the contribution of each cell to the total chi-square (Colton, 1971, p 181). The total chi-square derives primarily from cell 1,1 and 2,1, where we find that considerably more Caucasians than expected survived to discharge ($O = 84$, $E = 56.62$) and fewer African-Americans than expected survived to discharge ($O = 24$, $E = 71.38$).

Small Expected Frequencies

Like the normal approximation to the binomial exact test, the chi-square test is an approximate method. Theoretical chi-square distributions are smooth and continuous; however, chi-square statistics "have only discrete values and are discontinuous" with irregular, stepwise distributions (Minium et al, 1993, p 467). The chi-square statistics is not a valid approximation when expected frequencies are small. As with the normal approximation, rules-of-thumb guide us in determining whether chi-square should be used (Daniel, 1991, p 535, 547; Dawson-Saunders & Trapp, 1994, p 152; Rosner, 1986, p 340). Statisticians disagree about which rule-of-thumb applies. The following guidelines are recommended (Daniel, 1991, p 547; Dawson-Saunders & Trapp, 1994, p 152):

All expected frequencies should be equal to or greater than 2 (all $E_{ij} \geq 2$) and
No more than 20% of the cells should have expected frequencies of less than 5.

Two options exist if small expected frequencies are encountered. Fisher's exact test should be performed, if small expected frequencies exist in a 2×2 table. Adjacent categories may be combined in tables larger than 2×2 to achieve the minimum expected frequency—if doing so is clinically or biologically defensible. Consult a statistician if collapsing categories is not feasible or justifiable.

Expected Versus Observed Frequencies: A Source of Confusion

Many clinicians and researchers confuse expected and observed frequencies. Often research-ers incorrectly conclude that the chi-square statistic is inappropriate, if a zero or very small observed frequency appears in one or more cells. The rule-of-thumb focuses only on expected frequencies.

Yates' Correction for Continuity

Statisticians also disagree about the use of Yates' correction for continuity; readers of the literature will encounter older, as well as recent, articles that still employ the correction. Many statisticians have recommended that Yates' correction for continuity be used in 2×2 tables, to reduce the discrepancy between the calculated chi-square statistic and theoretical chi-square distribution. The correction involves subtracting 0.50 from the absolute value of the difference between the observed and expected frequency, before squaring:

$$\chi^2 = \sum_{j=1}^{c} \sum_{i=1}^{r} \frac{(| O_{ij} - E_{ij}| - 0.50)^2}{E_{ij}} .$$ **15.2**

Yates' correction reduces the calculated value of chi-square, thus making it somewhat more difficult to obtain a significant result (Minium et al, 1993, p 467). Statisticians have demon-strated that the uncorrected chi-square statistic is reasonably accurate when expected frequen-cies are as small as 2 (Minium et al, 1993, p 467). Therefore, most statisticians have discontin-ued using Yates' correction, because it causes a reduction of power.

TESTING EQUALITY OR HOMOGENEITY OF PROPORTIONS

In a chi-square test for independence, we examine the cross-classification of a *single sample* of observations on two qualitative variables, called a classification criteria. Chi-square applies also to problems involving *two or more independent populations,* where groups are compared according to the proportion having a particular qualitative outcome. This application of chi-square is called testing for *homogeneity or equality of proportions*. The following clinical example, in which four different thrombolytic treatments were compared, illustrates this application.

Clinical Example: Evolving Myocardial Infarction

> Patients with evolving myocardial infarction were assigned independently and randomly to one of four thrombolytic treatments, and then followed to determine 30-day mortality. The following 30-day mortality data were obtained: 705 of 9796 patients (7.2%) receiving streptokinase and subcutaneous heparin died; 768 of 10,377 patients (7.4%) receiving streptokinase and intravenous heparin died; 652 of 10,334 patients (6.3%) receiving accelerated tissue plasminogen activator (t-PA) died; and 723 of 10,328 patients (7.0%) receiving accelerated t-PA and streptokinase with intravenous heparin died. ("Accelerated" refers to the administration of t-PA over 90 minutes, with two thirds of the dose given in the first 30 minutes; t-PA is administered conventionally in 3 hours.) (GUSTO Investigators, 1993, pp 673–682)

Are these four treatment populations equal with respect to 30-day mortality? Data have been cast into a 2 × 4 contingency table (Table 15–3); the analysis is presented in Box 15–2. The columns define the four treatment conditions; rows represent the criteria used to categorize patients at the end of 30 days.

Hypotheses are written out in steps 1 and 2 in Box 15–2. As with problems of independence, the scientific and alternative hypotheses for problems of homogeneity of proportions are nondirectional. The null hypothesis indicates that the four treatment populations are homogeneous with respect to 30-day mortality. This hypothesis is equivalent to writing $\pi_1 = \pi_2 = \pi_3 = \pi_4$ for a binomial criterion, such as survival, in which there are only two mutually exclusive outcomes. The alternative hypothesis states that the populations are not homogeneous, that is, $\pi_1 \neq \pi_2 \neq \pi_3 \neq \pi_4$ for a binomial criterion. The decision rules are outlined in step 3. For example, the chi-square distribution and chi-square statistic are chosen. The critical value of chi-square is 7.81 for $df = 3$ and $\alpha = 0.05$.

Expected frequencies are calculated in step 4. Expected frequencies are computed under the null hypothesis of homogeneity. We see that the expected and observed frequencies are somewhat similar in all cells in row 1, and in two of the four cells in row 2 (2,1 and 2,2). We are interested in cell 2,3, accelerated t-PA and intravenous heparin, because in this cell it appears that considerably fewer patients than expected died within 30 days ($E_{23} \approx 721$, $O_{23} = 652$). Next, the rule-of-thumb is checked to determine if we can proceed with the calculations. All expected frequencies are large; none poses any problem. The cell chi-square values are computed and summed to obtain the overall chi-square value ($\chi^2_{calc} = 10.8537$). As anticipated, cell 2,3 has the largest cell chi-square value (6.65); this cell is the principal contributor to the magnitude of the overall chi-square statistic. We reject the null hypothesis (step 5). We conclude that the four thrombolytic treatment conditions are not equal with respect to 30-day mortality ($\chi^2_{calc} = 10.85$, $\chi^2_{crit} = 7.81$, $df = 3$, $\alpha = 0.05$, p-value < 0.025). We note also that the largest relative difference between observed and expected outcomes occurs in patients receiving accelerated t-PA and intravenous heparin, with fewer patients dying than expected ($E \approx 712$, $O = 652$).

Table 15–3. Four thrombolytic treatment strategies and 30-day mortality in patients with evolving myocardial infarction.

30-Day Outcome	Streptokinase and Subcutaneous Heparin	Streptokinase and Intravenous Heparin	Accelerated t-PA and Intravenous Heparin	Accelerated t-PA and Streptokinase with Intravenous Heparin	Total
Survived	9091	9609	9692	9605	37,997
Died	705	768	652	723	2848
Total	9796	10,377	10,344	10,328	40,845

Adapted with permission from GUSTO Investigators: An international randomized trial comparing four thrombolytic strategies for acute myocardial infarction. *N Engl J Med* 1993;**329**:673–682.

Box 15–2. Thirty-day mortality in four thrombolytic treatment groups of patients with evolving myocardial infarction.

1. *Develop the Scientific Hypothesis*
The four treatment populations are not homogeneous with respect to 30-day mortality.

2. *Formulate the Statistical Hypotheses*
H_0: The four treatment populations are homogeneous with respect to 30-day mortality.
H_A: The four treatment populations are not homogeneous with respect to 30-day mortality.

3. *Determine the Decision Rules*
   a. Chi-square statistic and distribution.
   b. $\alpha = 0.05$, $df = (2 - 1)(4 - 1) = 3$.
   c. $\chi^2_{crit} = 7.81$.

4. *Analyze the Data*
Calculate the expected frequency for each cell:

Cell 1,1 $E_{11} = \dfrac{(37,997)(9796)}{40,845} = 9112.9541$

Cell 1,2 $E_{12} = \dfrac{(37,997)(10,377)}{40,845} = 9653.4427$

Cell 1,3 $E_{13} = \dfrac{(37,997)(10,344)}{40,845} = 9622.7437$

Cell 1,4 $E_{14} = \dfrac{(37,997)(10,328)}{40,845} = 9607.8594$

Cell 2,1 $E_{21} = \dfrac{(2848)(9796)}{40,845} = 683.0459$

Cell 2,2 $E_{22} = \dfrac{(2848)(10,377)}{40,845} = 723.5573$

Cell 2,3 $E_{23} = \dfrac{(2848)(10,344)}{40,845} = 721.2563$

Cell 2,4 $E_{24} = \dfrac{(2848)(10,328)}{40,845} = 720.1406$

Check the rule-of-thumb for expected frequencies.
No expected frequency poses a problem; therefore, continue with the chi-square test.

Determine $\dfrac{(O_{ij} - E_{ij})^2}{E_{ij}}$ for each cell (these are referred to as the cell chi-square values):

Cell 1,1 $\dfrac{(9091 - 9112.9541)^2}{9112.9541} = 0.0529$

Cell 1,2 $\dfrac{(9609 - 9653.4427)^2}{9653.4427} = 0.2046$

Cell 1,3 $\dfrac{(9692 - 9622.7437)^2}{9622.7437} = 0.4984$

Cell 1,4 $\dfrac{(9605 - 9607.8594)^2}{9607.8594} = 0.0009$

Cell 2,1 $\dfrac{(705 - 683.0459)^2}{683.0459} = 0.7056$

Cell 2,2 $\dfrac{(768 - 723.5573)^2}{723.5573} = 2.7298$

Cell 2,3 $\dfrac{(652 - 721.2563)^2}{721.2563} = 6.6501$

Cell 2,4 $\dfrac{(723 - 720.1406)^2}{720.1405} = 0.0114$

Add the cell values together to obtain the calculated value of chi-square:
$\chi^2 = 0.0529 + 0.2046 + 0.4984 + 0.009 + 0.7056 + 2.7298 + 6.6501 + 0.0114 = 10.8537$

5. *Evaluation*
Compare the calculated value of chi-square to the critical value and make a decision about the null hypothesis:
$\chi^2_{calc} = 10.8537 > \chi^2_{crit} = 7.81$. Reject H_0.

6. *Interpretation*
The four thrombolytic treatment groups are not equal with respect to 30-day mortality ($\chi^2_{calc} = 10.85$, $\chi^2_{crit} = 7.81$, $df = 3$, $\alpha = 0.05$, p-value < 0.025). The largest relative departure from expected was noted in patients receiving accelerated t-PA and intravenous heparin, with fewer patients than expected dying. Under the null hypothesis of equality, approximately 721 patients were expected to die within 30 days; however, 652 died.

Small Expected Frequencies

The rules-of-thumb used to test independence apply also to homogeneity of proportions using chi-square. Thus, all expected frequencies should be equal to or greater than 2 (all $E_{ij} \geq 2$) and no more than 20% of the cells should have expected frequencies of less than 5.

Testing Equality in a 2 × 2 Table

Four treatment populations appear in the above example. However, clinicians and researchers may be interested in other situations where (1) two populations are sampled and (2) observations are grouped according to one classification criterion, with two mutually exclusive categories. For example, suppose that clinicians wish to evaluate 30-day mortality in two populations of patients with evolving myocardial infarction. Patients in the first group receive accelerated t-PA and intravenous heparin and patients in the second group receive conventionally-administered t-PA and intravenous heparin. Patients are followed and mortality status is assessed at the end of 30 days. The resulting contingency table has two rows (population 1 or 2), two columns (30-day mortality status: alive or dead), and one degree of freedom.

The null hypothesis of homogeneity in a 2 × 2 table states that the two treatment populations are homogeneous with respect to a binomial classification criterion. This is equivalent to $H_0: \pi_1 - \pi_2 = 0$. The alternative hypothesis is equivalent to $H_A: \pi_1 - \pi_2 \neq 0$. These hypotheses may be tested using chi-square for homogeneity *or* the normal approximation to the binomial for two independent proportions (assuming rules-of-thumb are satisfied). Conclusions derived from the two tests will be identical. *Interchangeable use of these two tests is appropriate only if the alternative hypothesis is nondirectional.*

Testing Equality in Matched/Paired Data

We noted in Chapter 14 that a test based on the chi-square distribution, referred to as the McNemar test, can be applied under certain conditions to matched/paired data arranged in a 2 × 2 table. Data from the osteoarthritis example in Chapter 14 are used to illustrate the McNemar test.

The McNemar Test is appropriate for matched/paired data for which the outcome is binomial and the alternative hypothesis is nondirectional. As shown in Table 15–4, data are arranged in a 2 × 2 table, with lettered cells. Tied pairs, which occur in cells a and d, are discarded; the number of observations in cells b and c, which contain the untied or discordant pairs, constitute the observed frequencies. We postulate that the discordant pairs are distributed equally in these two cells, under the null hypothesis. Thus, the expected

Table 15–4. Effectiveness of two treatments in providing symptomatic improvement in pairs of patients matched on severity of disease[a]

Treatment 1	Treatment 2		Total
	Improvement: Yes	*Improvement: No*	
Improvement: Yes	a	b	a + b
Improvement: No	c	d	c + d
Total	a + c	b + d	n = a + b + c + d

[a]Shaded cells represent the untied or discordant pairs.

frequency in each cell is the number of discordant pairs divided by two. The McNemar test statistic is

$$\chi^2 = \frac{(|b - c| - 1)^2}{b + c} \text{ with df} = 1 \text{ .}$$ 15.3

Box 15–3 contains the analysis of the osteoarthritis data originally presented in Table 14–1. The scientific and statistical hypotheses are written out in steps 1 and 2. Recall that the scientific and alternative hypotheses are nondirectional. The decision criteria are specified in step 3. In step 4, the number of discordant pairs is identified and the analysis is conducted. Rosner (1986, p 335) suggests that the test is valid if $\frac{n_{Discordant}}{4} \geq 5$. If this value is less than 5, use the binomial exact test for matched/paired data (refer to Chapter 14). In the osteoarthritis example, the test continues because the rule-of-thumb is met. The McNemar statistic is calculated and found to equal approximately 0.55. This calculated value is compared to the critical value ($\chi^2_{calc} = 0.55$, $\chi^2_{crit} = 3.84$) and the null hypothesis is rejected (step 5). We conclude that no *significant* difference exists between the proportion of pairs in which the only the patient taking acetaminophen improved (12/29 = 0.41) and the proportion in which only the patient taking ibuprofen improved (17/29 = 0.59; $\chi^2_{calc} = 0.5571 < \chi^2_{crit} = 3.84$, *p*-value > 0.10, $\alpha = 0.05$). This is the same conclusion we reached when we used the normal approximation to the binomial for these matched/paired data.

Box 15–3. McNemar test to examine the effectiveness of acetaminophen versus ibuprofen in providing symptomatic improvement of osteoarthritis of the knee in pairs of men (data presented originally in Table 14–1, Chapter 14).

1. *Develop the scientific hypothesis*
The proportion of (discordant) pairs in which only the patient taking acetaminophen experiences relief differs from the proportion in which only the patient taking ibuprofen experiences improvement.

2. *Formulate the statistical hypotheses*
H_0: No difference exists between the proportions.
H_A: A difference exists between the proportions.

3. *Determine the decision criteria*
   a. McNemar test for correlated proportions.
   b. Chi-square distribution.
   c. $\alpha = 0.05$ and *df* = 1.
   d. $\chi^2_{crit} = 3.84$.

4. *Analyze the data*
Identify the number of discordant pairs (cells b and c):
Cell b   12 Pairs in which the man taking acetaminophen experienced symptomatic improvement, but the pairmate taking ibuprofen did not.
Cell c   17 Pairs in which the man taking ibuprofen experienced symptomatic improvement, but the pairmate taking acetaminophen did not.
The number of discordant pairs, *n*, equals 29.
Check the rule-of-thumb:

$$\frac{n_{Discordant}}{4} \geq 5: \frac{29}{4} = 7.25$$

Proceed with the test.
Calculate the McNemar statistic:

$$\chi^2 = \frac{(|12 - 17| - 1)^2}{12 + 17} = 0.5517$$

5. *Evaluate the statistics*
Reject H_0: $\chi^2_{calc} = 0.5571 < \chi^2_{crit} = 3.84$

6. *Interpret the statistics*
No *significant* difference exists betwen the proportion of pairs in which only the patient taking acetaminophen experienced symptomatic improvement (12/29 = 0.41) and the proportion of pairs in which only the patient taking ibuprofen improved (17/29 = 0.59; $\chi^2_{calc} = 0.5571 < \chi^2_{crit} = 3.84$, *p*-value > 0.10, $\alpha = 0.05$).

NORMAL APPROXIMATION VERSUS THE MCNEMAR TEST
(for Matched/Paired Data)

Both tests are approximations to the binomial exact test; both are employed with matched/paired data. To use each test appropriately, a rule-of-thumb must first be met. The binomial exact test must be applied if the rule-of-thumb is not satisfied. Both tests focus on the discordant pairs. The normal approximation may be used when the alternative hypothesis is nondirectional or directional. The McNemar test, in contrast, is used only with nondirectional alternative hypotheses.

SUMMARY

Chi-square enjoys many uses in the medical literature, including testing for independence and homogeneity. However, the chi-square statistic, unlike z and Student's t, cannot be used to construct confidence intervals. The hypotheses and assumptions underlying tests of independence and homogeneity are summarized in Table 15–5. The chi-square statistic and its degrees of freedom are identical for both tests. Both rely on the same rules-of-thumb: that is, all expected frequencies should be equal to or greater than 2 and no more than 20% of the cells should have expected frequencies of less than 5. However, the two tests differ conceptually. The test for independence is based on a single sample of n independent observations. The observations are categorized according to two qualitative variables, also called classification criteria. The null hypothesis is one of independence between these two qualitative variables. The test for homogeneity for independent observations requires that two or more samples be obtained from two or more populations. The elements from each population are categorized on only one qualitative variable or classification criterion. The null hypothesis states that the populations are homogeneous with respect to the classification criterion.

In conclusion, the tests for independence and equality differ with regard to the (1) hypotheses examined, (2) number of populations sampled, (3) number of criteria on which observations are classified after sampling, and (4) conclusions derived from the analysis of data.

The McNemar test, based on the chi-square distribution with $df = 1$, is applied to matched/paired data for which the outcome is binomial. The test is sometimes referred to as a procedure for correlated proportions. Only discordant pairs are utilized in the analysis. The test is

Table 15–5. Chi-square for testing hypotheses of independence and equality.

	Independence	Equality
Hypotheses: H_0	Two classification criteria are independent.	Populations are homogenous with regard to one classification criterion.
H_A	The two classification criteria are not independent.	Populations are not homogeneous with regard to one classification criterion.
Requirements	One sample is selected randomly from a defined population.	Two or more samples are selected from two or more populations.
	Observations are cross-classified on two nominal criteria.	Observations are classified on one nominal criterion.
	Conclusions are phrased in terms of independence of the two classification criteria.	Conclusions are phrased with regard to homogeneity or equality of treatment populations.
Test statistic	$\chi^2 = \sum\limits_{j=1}^{c} \sum\limits_{i=1}^{r} \dfrac{(O_{ij} - E_{ij})^2}{E_{ij}}$, $df = (r-1)(c-1)$	$\chi^2 = \sum\limits_{j=1}^{c} \sum\limits_{i=1}^{r} \dfrac{(O_{ij} - E_{ij})^2}{E_{ij}}$, $df = (r-1)(c-1)$
Rules-of-thumb	All expected frequencies should be equal to or greater than 2 (all $E_{ij} \geq 2$) and *no more than 20%* of the cells should have expected frequencies of less than 5.	All expected frequencies should be equal to or greater than 2 (all $E_{ij} \geq 2$) and *no more than 20%* of the cells should have expected frequencies of less than 5.

an approximate method that is applied when the number of discordant pairs divided by four is equal to or greater than 5. The McNemar test is used to examine nondirectional alternative hypotheses. When a directional alternative hypothesis is formulated, the normal approximation to the binomial exact test for matched/paired data should be applied.

REFERENCES

Becker L et al: Racial differences in the incidence of cardiac arrest and subsequent survival. *N Engl J Med* 1993;**329**:600.

Colton T: *Statistics in Medicine.* Little, Brown, 1974.

Daniel W: *Biostatistics: A Foundation for Analysis in the Health Sciences,* 5th ed. Wiley, 1991.

Dawson-Saunders B, Trapp R: *Basic and Clinical Biostatistics,* 2nd ed. Appleton & Lange, 1994.

GUSTO Investigators: An international randomized trial comparing four thrombolytic strategies for acute myocardial infarction. *N Engl J Med* 1993;**329**:673–682.

Minium E, King B, Bear G: *Statistical Reasoning in Psychology and Education,* 3rd ed. Wiley, 1993.

Raz R, Stamm W: A controlled trial of intravaginal estriol in postmenopausal women with recurrent urinary tract infections. *N Engl J Med* 1993;**329**:753.

Rosner B: *Fundamentals of Biostatistics,* 2nd ed. Duxbury, 1986.

Self-study Questions

Part I: Review

1. Develop three examples of hypotheses of independence between two qualitative variables.
2. Develop three examples of hypotheses of homogeneity of proportions.
3. Identify similarities and differences between chi-square for independence and homogeneity.

Part II: Analysis Identification

1. Two pediatricians wish to test the effectiveness of an educational program that provides information to parents about the benefits of childhood immunizations. The researchers hypothesize that parents who participate in the program are more likely to have their children immunized, versus parents who do not participate. Two samples of parents and their children are formed randomly from records of a family practice clinic. One sample of parents participates in the program; the other sample does not. Of the 93 parents who participate in the program, 73 go on to obtain a full set of immunizations for their child. Of the 71 parents who do not participate in the program, 30 go on to obtain a complete set of immunizations for their child.

2. The association between the occurrence of bronchitis before age 2 years and subsequent development of bronchitis between ages 2 and 6 years is investigated in a sample of 55 children. Of the 27 children who had no bronchitic episodes before age 2 years, 4 had at least one bout of bronchitis between the ages of 2 and 6 years. Among 28 children who had bronchitis before age 2 years, 12 had at least one bout of bronchitis between the ages of 2 and 6 years.

3. The occurrence of dementia in patients, age 60 years and older, with idiopathic Parkinson's disease was investigated to determine if dementia occurs with greater frequency in this age than in the general population. Four percent of individuals in this age group in the general population have dementia. Two hundred seventy-two patients,

age 60 years and older, with idiopathic Parkinson's disease were examined; 36 exhibited dementia.

4. Irradiation to symptomatic areas, combined with intrathecal methotrexate, is the conventional treatment for neoplasms that metastasize to the leptomeninges. Long-term prognosis, however, is poor: only 10% of patients survive 12 months. In a South American clinic, 12 patients with carcinomatous meningitis receive an experimental treatment that couples irradiation and intrathecal methotrexate with dietary management and herbal remedies. The goal is to determine if the experimental regimen increases 12-month survival. Twelve months later, two patients who received the experimental treatment are alive.

5. Three populations of women in medicine are sampled to determine if differences exist with respect to satisfaction with medicine as a career choice (yes/no). Fifty-six of 100 first-year female medical students say they are satisfied with their choice of medicine as a career. Fifty-eight of 100 female residents express satisfaction. Thirty-eight of 100 practicing female clinicians, out of residency for at least 3 years, indicate satisfaction.

6. Postmenopausal women with a history of recurrent urinary tract infections are studied to determine if intravaginal administration of estriol cream decreases the incidence of recurrent urinary tract infections. Participants are assigned randomly to one of two treatment groups. Women in one group receive 0.5 mg of estriol in vaginal cream, according to a prescribed 8-month regimen ($n_{ESTRIOL} = 50$); the other group receives a similar looking placebo cream and follows the same regimen ($n_{PLACEBO} = 43$). Among the several findings are the following: the vaginal pH at the end of the trial is 3.6 (s = 7.08) in women in the estriol group and 6.1 (s = 13.12) in women in the placebo group (Raz & Stamm, 1993, p 756). Do these values differ significantly? Assume at least one pH distribution is nonnormal in the population.

Part III: Problems and Analysis

Read each problem and analyze the data, as appropriate. If an hypothesis is to be tested, identify the scientific and statistical hypotheses, state the decision rules, perform the analysis, make a decision about the null hypothesis, and interpret the results. Allow $\alpha = 0.05$ in all problems.

1. Investigators who examined postmenopausal women with a history of recurrent urinary tract infections (Part II, Problem 6) also evaluated whether differences exist in the proportion discontinuing treatment because of treatment side effects. Ten of the 50 women in the estriol group discontinued treatment, compared to 4 of 43 in the placebo group (Raz & Stamm, 1993, p 753).

2. In a clinic in a large city on the West Coast, men who are HIV positive, asymptomatic, and have CD4+ cell counts above $400/mL^3$ are chosen randomly to receive zidovudine or placebo for 36 months. Participants are followed (1) to monitor progression to group IV disease according to clinical criteria established by the Centers for Disease Control and Prevention (CDC) and (2) to determine if fewer patients receiving zidovudine experience disease progression. Seventy-eight of 300 men receiving zidovudine and 111 of 300 men receiving placebo experienced disease progression.

3. The association between the sex of teenage patients and their preference for having a nurse or parent present during physical examination of the genitals/rectum in males and breasts/genitals/rectum in females was studied in a midwestern family practice clinic. One hundred thirty-five teenage patients were sampled randomly and classified on sex (male/female) and preference (yes/no). Of the 50 males, 5 said they would like a parent or nurse to be present when the clinician examines their genitals/rectum. Of the 85 females, 45 said they would prefer that a parent or nurse be present when their breasts/genitals/rectum are examined.

4. Differences in the occurrence of gastrointestinal side effects associated with two forms of erythromycin are examined in age-matched, ambulatory patients who require antibiotic therapy and who have no history of gastrointestinal disease or disorders. Data appear in Table 15–6.

Table 15–6. Occurrence of gastrointestinal side effects of two forms of erythromycin in patients matched on age.

Erythromycin Ethylsuccinate	Particles-in-tablet Formulation		Total
	Side Effects: Yes	Side Effects: No	
Side Effects: Yes	7	15	22
Side Effects: No	5	23	28
Total	12	38	50

Part IV: Comment

For approximately 11 years following surgery, investigators studied outcomes in men who had surgery to replace an aortic or mitral valve. Men were assigned randomly before surgery to receive a mechanical or bioprosthetic valve. Of the 198 men who received a bioprosthesis, 30 experienced a valve failure during the 11 year follow-up period. In contrast, none of the 150 men who received a mechanical valve had valve failure. The investigators arrayed their data in a 2 × 2 table (valve type: mechanical or bioprosthesis; mechanical failure during follow-up: yes/no) and examined them using chi-square for homogeneity. A colleague commented that chi-square was inappropriate because one cell had a zero frequency. Evaluate this comment.

Solutions

Part II: Analysis Identification

The key elements of each problem are outlined below.

1. *Childhood Immunizations*
   Two samples are formed independently and randomly (93 and 71 participants, respectively).
   Outcome is binomial (obtained a complete set of immunizations: yes/no).
   Directional alternative hypothesis (rules out chi-square for homogeneity).
   Normal approximation to the binomial for two independent proportions.
   Check the rules-of-thumb:

$$p = \frac{75 + 30}{93 + 71} = 0.6402$$

$n_1 p = 93(0.6402) = 59.54$ $n_1(1 - p) = 93(1 - 0.6402) = 33.46$
$n_2 p = 71(0.6402) = 45.45$ $n_2(1 - p) = 71(1 - 0.6402) = 25.55$

All rules-of-thumb are satisfied. Normal approximation is appropriate.
2. *Bronchitis*
   One sample of 55 children.
   Children are categorized after sampling on two binomial variables (had bronchitis before age 2 years: yes/no; and had at least one bout of bronchitis between ages 2 and 6 years: yes/no).
   Nondirectional alternative hypothesis.
   Chi-square for independence.
   Cast the data into a 2 × 2 table (Table 15–7) and check the expected frequency rules-of-thumb:

Table 15–7. Occurrence of bronchitis before age 2 years and subsequent bouts between ages 2 and 6 years.

Bronchitis Before Age 2 Years	Bronchitis Between Ages 2 and 6 Years		Total
	Yes	No	
Yes	12	16	28
No	4	23	27
Total	16	39	55

$$\text{Cell 1,1} \quad E_{11} = \frac{28(16)}{55} = 8.15$$

$$\text{Cell 1,2} \quad E_{12} = \frac{28(39)}{55} = 19.85$$

$$\text{Cell 2,1} \quad E_{21} = \frac{27(16)}{55} = 7.85$$

$$\text{Cell 2,2} \quad E_{22} = \frac{27(39)}{55} = 19.15$$

All rules-of-thumb are satisfied. Chi-square for independence is appropriate.

3. *Dementia and Parkinson's Disease*
   One sample of (272) patients, age 60 years and older.
   Outcome is binomial (exhibited dementia: yes/no).
   Directional alternative hypothesis.
   Population proportion given ($\pi = 0.04$).
   Normal approximation to the binomial for one proportion.
   Check the rules-of-thumb:
   $n\pi = 272(0.04) = 10.88$
   $n(1 - \pi) = 272(1 - 0.04) = 261.12.$
   Both rules-of-thumb are satisfied. Normal approximation for one proportion is appropriate.

4. *Carcinomatous Meninges*
   One sample (12 patients).
   Outcome is binomial (12-month survival: yes/no).
   Directional alternative hypothesis.
   Population 12-month survival under conventional treatment is given ($\pi = 0.10$).
   Binomial exact test for one proportion ($n\pi = 12(0.10) = 1.2 < 5$).

5. *Medicine as a Career Choice*
   Three samples of women in medicine (each consisting of 100 participants).
   Outcome is binomial (career choice satisfaction: yes/no).
   Nondirectional alternative hypothesis.
   Chi-square for homogeneity.
   Array the data in a 2×3 table (or 3×2, depending on preference) and check the expected frequency rule-of-thumb; expected frequencies appear in each cell of Table 15–8, with the corresponding observed frequency.
   All expected frequencies are large. Chi-square for homogeneity is appropriate.

Table 15–8. Career choice satisfaction in three samples of women in medicine. (Expected frequencies in italics.)

Career Choice Satisfaction	Population Sampled			Total
	First-year Students	*Residents*	*Clinicians*	
Yes	$E = 50.67$ 56	$E = 50.67$ 58	$E = 50.67$ 38	152
No	$E = 49.33$ 44	$E = 49.33$ 42	$E = 49.33$ 62	148
Total	100	100	100	300

6. *Recurrent Urinary Tract Infections in Postmenopausal Women*
   Two samples formed independently (50 and 43 participants, respectively).
   Outcome is quantitative (vaginal pH after 8 months of treatment).
   Directional alternative hypothesis.
   The distribution of pH is assumed to be nonnormal in at least one of the populations sampled.
   z test for the difference between two independent means.
   Verify that both sample sizes are 30 or greater.
   The sample size rules-of-thumb are met. z test for the difference between two independent means is appropriate.

Part III: Problems and Analysis

1. *Recurrent Urinary Tract Infections in Postmenopausal Women*
   Scientific Hypothesis:
   With respect to the number of postmenopausal women with recurrent UTI who discontinue treatment because of side effects, a difference exists between patients who receive intravaginal estriol cream and those who receive placebo.
   Statistical Hypotheses:

$$H_0: \pi_{ESTRIOL} - \pi_{PLACEBO} = 0$$

$$H_A: \pi_{ESTRIOL} - \pi_{PLACEBO} \neq 0$$

Decision Rules:
a. The normal approximation for two independent proportions or chi-square for homogeneity may be used, if rules-of-thumb are satisfied. Chi-square will be employed to demonstrate its application.
b. Chi-square distribution with $df = 1$.
c. $\alpha = 0.05$.
d. $\chi^2_{crit} = 3.84$.
Analysis:
Construct a 2×2 table: Table 15–9 contains the data.

Table 15–9. Side effects causing treatment discontinuation in two groups of postmenopausal women.

Treatment Group	Discontinued Treatment		Total
	Yes	No	
Intravaginal Estriol	10	40	50
Placebo	4	39	43
Total	14	79	93

Calculate the expected frequencies, check the rule-of-thumb, and compute the cell chi-square value.

Cell	Observed	Expected	Cell Chi-square
1,1	10	$\frac{50(14)}{93} = 7.5269$	$\frac{(10 - 7.5269)^2}{7.5269} = 0.8126$
1,2	40	$\frac{50(79)}{93} = 42.4731$	$\frac{(40 - 42.4731)^2}{42.4731} = 0.1440$
2,1	4	$\frac{43(14)}{93} = 6.4731$	$\frac{(4 - 6.4731)^2}{6.4731} = 0.9449$
2,2	39	$\frac{43(79)}{93} = 36.5269$	$\frac{(39 - 36.5269)^2}{36.5269} = 0.1674$
		Sum of cell values	$\chi^2 = 2.0689$

No expected frequency poses a problem. The chi-square analysis is appropriate.
Evaluation:
The null hypothesis of homogeneity is retained ($\chi^2_{calc} = 2.07$, $\chi^2_{crit} = 3.84$).
Interpretation:
Twenty percent (10 of 50) of women who received estriol cream discontinued treatment compared to 9.3% (4 of 43) of women who used the placebo cream. However, the difference between these proportions was not significant statistically ($\chi^2_{calc} = 2.07$, $\chi^2_{crit} = 3.84$, *p*-value $\approx$ 70.10, $\alpha = 0.05$).

2. *Disease Progression in HIV-positive Men*
Scientific hypothesis:
Among men who are HIV positive, asymptomatic, and have CD4+ cell counts above 400/mL^3, a smaller proportion of men who receive zidovudine over 36 months will go on to develop CDC group IV disease, versus similar patients who receive a placebo over 36 months.
Statistical hypotheses:

$$H_0: \pi_{PLACEBO} - \pi_{ZIDOVUDINE} = 0$$

$$H_A: \pi_{PLACEBO} - \pi_{ZIDOVUDINE} > 0$$

Decision rules:
a. Normal approximation to the binomial for two independent proportions.
   Check the rules-of-thumb.
   Compute the pooled estimate of π:
   (Z = Zidovudine, P = Placebo)

$$X_Z = 78 \qquad X_P = 111$$

$$n_Z = 300 \qquad n_P = 300$$

$$p = \frac{78 + 111}{300 + 300} = 0.3150$$

$$n_Z p = 300(0.3150) = 94.5 > 5$$
$$n_Z(1 - p) = 300(1 - 0.3150) = 205.5 > 5$$

It is not necessary to compute these same criteria for the placebo group because both sample sizes are equal. It is appropriate to use the normal approximation.
b. The normal distribution will serve as an approximation to the binomial.
c. $\alpha = 0.05$.
d. $z_{crit} = 1.645$ (for a one-tailed greater-than test).
Analysis:
Compute each sample proportion:

$$p_Z = \frac{78}{300} = 0.26$$

$$p_P = \frac{111}{300} = 0.37$$

Calculate the standard error of the difference:

$$SE_{p_Z - p_P} = \sqrt{p(1 - p)\left[\frac{1}{n_Z} + \frac{1}{n_P}\right]}$$

$$= \sqrt{0.3150(1 - 0.3150)\left[\frac{1}{300} + \frac{1}{300}\right]}$$

$$= \sqrt{0.0014} = 0.0374$$

Obtain the calculated value of z:

$$z = \frac{0.37 - 0.26}{0.0374} = 2.9419$$

Evaluation:
The null hypothesis is rejected ($z_{calc} = 2.94$, $z_{crit} = 1.645$).
Interpretation:
In men who were HIV positive, asymptomatic, and had CD4+ cell counts above 400/mL^3, 26% (78 of 300) men who received zidovudine for 36 months progressed to CDC group IV disease compared to 37% (111 of 300) men who received a placebo. The proportion of men in the placebo group whose disease progressed is significantly greater than the proportion in the zidovudine group (p-value = 0.0016, $\alpha = 0.05$).

3. *Teenagers and Physician Examinations*
Scientific hypothesis:
An association exists between the sex of the teenage patient and his/her preference for having a nurse or parent present during physical examination of the genitals/rectum in males and breasts/genitals/rectum in females.
Statistical hypotheses:
H_0: The sex of the teenage patient and his or her preference are independent.
H_A: The sex of the teenage patient and his or her preference are not independent.
Decision rules:
a. Chi-square for independence; (expected frequency rule-of-thumb will be checked during the analysis).
b. Chi-square distribution with $df = 1$.
c. $\alpha = 0.05$.
d. $\chi^2_{crit} = 3.84$.
Analysis:
Construct a 2 × 2 table. (The data appear in Table 15–10.)

Table 15–10. Sex of teenage patient and his or her preference for having a parent or nurse present during the examination of genitals/rectum in males and breasts/genitals/rectum in females.

Preference: Nurse/ Parent Present	Patient Sex		Total
	Male	Female	
Yes	5	45	50
No	45	40	85
Total	50	85	135

Compute expected frequencies, check the rule-of-thumb, and obtain χ^2.

Cell	Observed	Expected	Cell Chi-square
1,1	5	$\frac{50(50)}{135} = 18.5185$	$\frac{(5 - 18.5185)^2}{18.5185} = 9.8685$
1,2	45	$\frac{50(85)}{135} = 31.4815$	$\frac{(45 - 31.4815)^2}{31.4815} = 5.8050$
2,1	45	$\frac{85(50)}{135} = 31.4815$	$\frac{(45 - 31.4815)^2}{31.4815} = 5.8050$
2,2	40	$\frac{85(85)}{135} = 53.5185$	$\frac{(40 - 53.5185)^2}{53.5185} = 3.4147$
		Sum of cell values	$\chi^2 = 24.8932$

Because all expected frequencies are large, the rule-of-thumb criteria are satisfied.
Evaluation:
The null hypothesis of independence is rejected ($\chi^2_{calc} = 24.98$, $\chi^2_{crit} = 3.84$).
Interpretation:
A significant association exists between the sex of the teenage patient and his or her preference for having a nurse or parent present during physical examination of the genitals/rectum in males and breasts/genitals/rectum in females (p-value < 0.005, $\alpha = 0.05$). Only 5 of 50 teenage males expressed a positive preference. This number was considerably less than expected ($O = 5$, $E = 18.52$). Teenage females were divided approximately equally in terms of their preference (positive preference, $O = 45$, negative preference, $O = 40$).

4. *Two Forms of Erythromycin and Gastrointestinal Side Effects*
Scientific hypothesis:
A difference will exist with respect to the occurrence of gastrointestinal side effects in pairs of patients in which one individual takes a particles-in-tablet formulation of erythromycin and the other member receives erythromycin ethylsuccinate.
Statistical hypotheses:
H_0: No difference will exist with respect to the occurrence of gastrointestinal side effects in pairs of patients taking two different formulations of erythromycin.
H_A: A difference will exist with respect to the occurrence of gastrointestinal side effects in pairs of patients taking two different formulations of erythromycin.
Decision rules:
a. Use the McNemar test if the rule-of-thumb is met.
   (Note: Normal approximation for matched/paired data could be used if the rules-of-thumb are met. The McNemar test is illustrated in this problem.)
b. Chi-square distribution with $df = 1$.
c. $\alpha = 0.05$.
d. $\chi^2_{crit} = 3.84$.
Analysis:
The data appear in Table 15–6.
Check the rule-of-thumb:

$$\frac{n_{Discordant}}{4} \geq 5$$

$$\frac{20}{4} = 5$$

Rule-of-thumb satisfied; proceed with the analysis.
Use the counts in the b and c cells to compute the McNemar test:

$$\chi^2 = \frac{(|b - c| - 1)^2}{b + c} = \frac{(|15 - 5| - 1)^2}{20} = 4.05$$

Evaluation:
Reject the null hypothesis ($\chi^2_{crit} = 4.05$, $\chi^2_{crit} = 3.84$).
Interpretation:
In pairs of individuals who took two different forms of erythromycin and responded differently with respect to the occurrence of gastrointestinal side effects, a significant difference exists with respect to (1) the proportion of pairs in which only the member who took the particles-in-tablet formulation experienced gastrointestinal side effects and (2) the proportion in which only the member who took erythromycin ethylsuccinate experienced gastrointestinal side effects (p-value < 0.005, $\alpha = 0.05$). In 15 of the 20 pairs in

which a differential response was noted, the member of the pair who took the particles-in-table formulation experienced gastrointestinal side effects.

Part IV: Comment

The individual who advised his/her colleagues not to use the chi-square statistic because a zero *observed* frequency occurred in one cell committed a common error. The rule-of-thumb focuses on *expected* and not observed frequencies.

16

Predicting the Value of One Variable From the Value of Another

Clinical Example: Asthma and Pulmonary Function

Asthma sufferers sometimes use bronchodilator drugs based on symptom intensity; symptom intensity, however, does not correlate well with clinical severity. Severe asthma requires measurement of arterial blood gas levels: normal or increased Pco_2 indicates moderate to severe asthma. Less severe asthma, however, is not reflected in arterial blood gas levels. In addition, frequent measurement of Pco_2 has obvious disadvantages, including cost and patient discomfort. Asthma severity is gauged also by the amount of airway obstruction, as reflected in increased airway resistance and reduced expiratory flow rates. A commonly accepted index of expiratory flow is FEV_1, the amount of air an individual can expel in one second. Many clinicians suggest initiating bronchodilator drugs when FEV_1 is less than 80% of the expected value, given the patient's age, height, race, and sex. Because it requires full expiration, the measurement of FEV_1 may provoke bronchoconstriction and increase symptoms. Further, FEV_1 measurements must be made by a qualified respiratory therapist on special equipment that must be calibrated frequently.

Although FEV_1 is considered the gold standard of expiratory flow rates, other indices are available. One such index, peak expiratory flow rate, can be obtained on a mini-Wright peak flow meter; this device is inexpensive, lightweight, accurate, compact, and easy to use, even by young patients. Measuring peak flow on the mini-Wright does not require full expiration; this reduces the likelihood of symptom exacerbation. Some clinicians suggest teaching asthmatic patients how to measure and use peak flow, in order to determine when to initiate bronchodilator treatment.

If patients and clinicians are to rely on peak flow to guide treatment decisions, peak flow must be shown to be a defensible substitute for FEV_1 measurements. Thus, it must be determined whether peak flow is a useful predictor of FEV_1. Moore and associates (1989) addressed this question in the pediatric patient with asthma. A portion of their data is used in the next three chapters to (1) illustrate how to develop an equation that predicts the value of one numerical variable from another (Chapter 16), (2) test the usefulness of this equation (Chapter 17), and (3) estimate the strength of the relationship between two variables (Chapter 18). To predict one variable from another, we rely upon statistical procedures known as *regression*. To determine the strength of the relationship between variables, we rely upon statistical procedures known as *correlation*. These techniques share many similarities.

Regression and correlation are employed in many studies. In 1983, Emerson and Colditz reported that these techniques had been used in 20% of articles in *The New England Journal of Medicine*. That percentage increased to 35% by 1991 (Altman, 1991). Unfortunately, regression and correlation are often abused and misinterpreted. For this reason, we emphasize the basic concepts, application, and interpretation of these techniques in the next four chapters.

OBJECTIVES

When you complete this chapter, you should be able to:

- Explain how to construct a scatter diagram.
- Inspect a scatter diagram and assess whether it is appropriate to develop a linear prediction equation.
- Understand and explain the basis for determining the line of best fit for predicting the value of one variable from another.
- Define the slope and intercept.
- Understand how to calculate and use a regression equation.

REGRESSION VERSUS CORRELATION

Although they share many similarities, regression and correlation have different objectives. **Regression** techniques are used to *predict* one quantitative variable from another quantitative variable. The independent variable, also called the **predictor** or **explanatory variable** is used to predict the other variable, known as the **dependent, response,** or **outcome variable.** An equation is developed that allows us to specify a particular value of the independent variable and to predict the corresponding value of the outcome variable. For example, "If an individual consumes 52% of total calories from fat, what low-density lipoprotein level (mg/dL) can we predict?"

In contrast, **correlation** analysis is performed when the goal is to develop an index that characterizes the *strength or magnitude of the relationship* between two numerical variables. For example, "What is the correlation between daily fat intake (expressed as a percentage of total calories) and low-density lipoprotein levels (mg/dL)?" "What is the correlation between average daily alcohol consumption (ounces) during the first trimester of pregnancy and infant birthweight (g)?"

In summary, the heart of regression is prediction. The focus of correlation is strength of the relationship.

SIMPLE VERSUS MULTIPLE REGRESSION

Simple regression involves using one explanatory variable to predict the outcome variable. Multiple regression involves using two or more explanatory variables to predict the outcome variable. This chapter focuses on **simple linear regression** in which an equation for a straight line is developed and used to predict the outcome variable from one explanatory variable.

SIMPLE LINEAR REGRESSION

The equation for a straight line in a population of observations is

$$Y = \beta X + \alpha + \varepsilon \qquad\qquad \textbf{16.1}$$

where β is the slope of the straight line, α is the intercept, and ε is the error term. An error term is included because the pairs of (X, Y) points do not fall typically on a straight line. The **slope** of the line reflects the amount of change in Y for each one unit change in X. A positive slope indicates that Y tends to increase as X increases, and vice-versa; a negative slope demonstrates that as X tends to increase, Y tends to decrease and vice-versa. The **intercept** is the point at which the line crosses the Y-axis. The corresponding equation for a sample of observations is:

$$Y = bX + \alpha \qquad\qquad \textbf{16.2}$$

where b is the sample estimate of the population slope and a is the sample estimate of the population intercept. *When the equation for the straight line is used for prediction,* we modify equation 16.2 to indicate that the outcome variable, Y, is predicted from the explanatory variable, X. This equation is the **regression equation** for Y-on-X. The line described by this equation is the regression line of Y-on-X. The regression equation for predicting Y from X in a *population* of (X, Y) observation is

$$\hat{Y}_i = \beta_{y.x} X_i + \alpha_{y.x} + \varepsilon \qquad\qquad \textbf{16.3}$$

where $\hat{Y}$ (read Y "hat") is the predicted value of Y for a given X_i; $\beta_{y.x}$ is the population slope (read beta "y dot x"), $\alpha_{y.x}$ is population intercept (read alpha "y dot x"), and ε (read as e or epsilon) is error. The subscript $y.x$ signifies that Y is predicted from X. When the regression equation is calculated from sample data, $b_{y.x}$ serves as the sample estimate of the population slope and $a_{y.x}$ functions as the estimate of the population intercept:

$$\hat{Y}_i = b_{y.x} X_i + a_{y.x} \qquad\qquad \textbf{16.4}$$

Suppose we collect three explanatory variables and designate them arbitrarily as X, W, and Z. We want to determine which provides the best prediction of Y. The equation for predicting Y from W (or Y-on-W) is

$$\hat{Y}_i = b_{y.w} W_i + a_{y.w}$$

The regression equation for predicting Y from Z is

$$\hat{Y}_i = b_{y.z} Z_i + a_{y.z}$$

The subscripts on b and a help to differentiate quickly between different regression equations and to identify the explanatory variable and the outcome. For example, the subscripts $y.z$ tell us that Y (outcome) is predicted from Z (explanatory variable). A regression equation for predicting Y-on-X is shown in Figure 16–1.

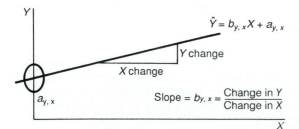

Figure 16–1. Slope and Intercept of the regression equation for predicting Y from X in a sample of (X, Y) observations.

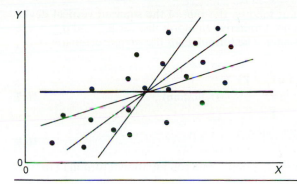

Figure 16-2. Pairs of (X,Y) points and four straight lines drawn through them.

Defining the Slope and Intercept

A hypothetical set of (X, Y) points is displayed in Fig 16-2. Each point represents one pair of (X, Y) values. An infinite number of straight lines could be drawn through these points; four lines are illustrated. Which of this infinite number of lines, however, best fits these points? This line is referred to as the **line-of-best fit.** A second hypothetical set of (X, Y) values is displayed in Figure 16-3. The line-of-best fit for Y-on-X is illustrated. The *predicted values* of Y, computed from the equation that describes this line, fall directly on the line. Note that the actual or observed values of Y for a given value of X differ from the predicted values. This difference between the predicted and observed values of Y is error, which is represented graphically as vertical scatter in Figure 16-3:

$$e_i = Y_{obs} - \hat{Y}_i \qquad\qquad 16.5$$

where e_i represents *error*, Y_{obs} is the actual or *observed* value of Y, and $\hat{Y}_i$ is the *predicted* value of Y for a given value of X.

The amount of error (vertical dispersion) is the criterion we use to judge the line that best fits the points. The line-of-best fit minimizes the sum of the squared vertical differences between the observed and predicted values of Y. Thus, the line of best fit is referred to as the **least squares line;** the criterion is known as the **Least Squares Criterion.** The line-of-best fit, then, is the "best" in the sense that it satisfies this criterion: The sum of the squared vertical deviations of the observed values of Y from the least squares line is smaller than the sum of squared vertical deviations of Y from any other line (Daniel, 1991, p 374). The Least Squares Criterion can be represented symbolically:

$$\sum_{i=1}^{n} (Y_{obs} - \hat{Y}_i)^2 \quad \text{is as small as possible} \qquad\qquad 16.6$$

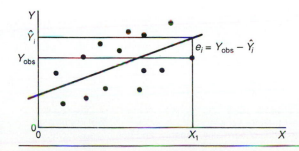

$$e_i = Y_{obs} - \hat{Y}_i$$

Figure 16-3. Graphic representation of error in predicting Y from X.

When the slope and intercept are defined as follows, the sum of the squared vertical deviations is minimized. Differential calculus is used to derive the formulae for $\beta_{y.x}$ and $\alpha_{y.x}$; these procedures are beyond the scope of this chapter. The formulae for the *sample* estimates of $\beta_{y.x}$ and $\alpha_{y.x}$ are, respectively

$$b_{y.x} = \frac{\sum_{i=1}^{n}(X_i - \overline{X})(Y_i - \overline{Y})}{\sum_{i=1}^{n}(X_i - \overline{X})^2} \quad \text{(Definition)} \qquad 16.7$$

$$a_{y.x} = \overline{Y} - b_{y.x}\overline{X} \qquad 16.8$$

Formula 16.7 is not convenient for computing the slope. The computational formula (16.9) is derived by performing the multiplication, distributing the summation operator, substituting the computational equivalents for $\overline{X}$ and $\overline{Y}$, and simplifying the formula; the super- and subscripts on the summation sign are omitted for convenience:

$$b_{y.x} = \frac{\sum X_i Y_i - \frac{(\sum X_i)(\sum Y_i)}{n}}{\sum X_i^2 - \frac{(\sum X_i)^2}{n}} \quad \text{(Computational form)} \qquad 16.9$$

Assumptions Underlying the Simple Linear Regression Model

Five assumptions underlie the development and use of a simple linear regression model: normality, linearity, homoscedasticity, independence, and random sampling. Normality, linearity, and homoscedasticity are depicted in Figure 16–4.

NORMALITY

For each value of X, there is a subpopulation of Y values which is distributed normally (Daniel, 1991, p 367). This assumption is important because it is the basis for inferential procedures used to test the predictive usefulness of the regression equation. Note that in Figure 16–4 three normal curves are turned on their side. The leftmost curve corresponds to

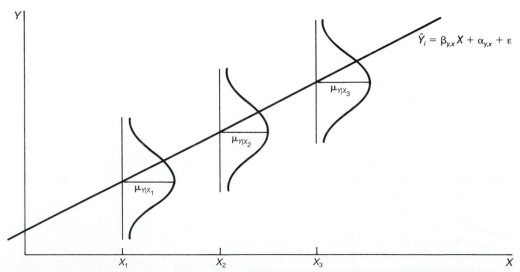

Figure 16–4. Graphic representation of the assumptions of normality, linearity, and homoscedasticity.

the normally distributed subpopulation of Y values for X_1; the middle curve represents the subpopulation of Y values given X_2; and the rightmost curve depicts the subpopulation of Y values for X_3. The mean of each subpopulation, $\beta_{y.x}X_i + \alpha_{y.x}$, can be represented symbolically as a conditional mean, $\mu_{y|x}$. The mean is conditional because it is the expected value of Y for a given value of X (Minium, 1993, p 176). For example, $\mu_{y|x_1}$ is the (conditional) mean of the subpopulation of Y values, given X_1. The standard deviation of each subpopulation of Y values, $\sigma_{y.x}$, is referred to as the standard error of estimate. We define the standard error of estimate later in Chapter 17. The population parameters are estimated by sample data: $\beta_{y.x}$ is estimated by $b_{y.x}$; $\alpha_{y.x}$ by $a_{y.x}$; $\mu_{y|x}$ by $\hat{Y}_i$ for given X_i; and $\sigma_{y.x}$ by $s_{y.x}$.

Normality is assumed by most investigators. We assume normality in our discussions of correlation and regression.

LINEARITY

The means of the subpopulation of Y values all lie on the same straight line (Daniel, 1991, p 368). Thus, the regression mean is a "running" mean or a series of means (Minium, 1993, p 176). The procedures of linear regression should not be used when data depart substantially from linearity. Although formal procedures exist to test linearity, we will rely on the "eyeball" method later in this chapter. If linearity is violated, a transformation may be applied, nonlinear regression models may be developed, or other statistical procedures may be employed.

HOMOSCEDASTICITY

"Homo" means like or same; "scedasticity" is synonymous with scatter or dispersion. **Homoscedasticity** means like or equal scatter. Therefore, the standard deviation of the subpopulation of Y values ($\sigma_{y.x}$) is equal, regardless of the value of X. Each normal curve in Figure 16–4, then, has the same standard deviation ($\sigma_{y.x}$). Homoscedasticity is equivalent to stating that the standard error of estimate of Y-on-X is constant throughout the range of X; or that the vertical dispersion about the line-of-best fit is the same for every value of X.

The advice of a statistician should be sought if the vertical dispersion of the Y observations about the regression line differs substantially for different values of X. He or she may recommend a suitable transformation or an alternate statistical technique.

INDEPENDENCE

The fourth assumption, **independence,** requires that the values of Y for given values of X are sampled independently, such that the values of Y for a specific value of X do not depend on the values of Y for any other value of X. Repeated measures designs violate this assumption. These designs involve obtaining two or more measurements on the same variable, for the same individuals, within the same study. A within-subjects (pre/post design) is the simplest repeated measures design. Within-subject designs were discussed in Chapter 12. The assumption of independence is violated in a repeated measures design, because the measurement made on an individual at one time is not independent from the measurement made on the same individual at another time. For example, the pretreatment systolic blood pressure of a hypertensive patient is not independent of this same patient's systolic blood pressure 6 weeks after taking medication to lower blood pressure. If a repeated measures design is chosen, a statistician should be asked to recommend techniques other than regression.

RANDOM SAMPLING

It is assumed that the (X, Y) observations are sampled randomly from the population of interest. Recall that **random sampling** has been assumed for all procedures covered in previous chapters. Regression analysis can still be conducted if sampling has not been random. Results, however, must be interpreted cautiously. They may not be generalizable beyond the subjects from whom data were collected.

Memory Aid

Daniel (1991, p 368) suggests using the acronym LINE to remember most of the assumptions used to develop a regression equation and to test its predictive utility: *L*inearity, *I*ndependence, *N*ormality, and *E*qual vertical dispersion (homoscedasticity).

Violating Assumptions

Because it is robust with respect to modest violations of assumptions, linear regression can be used in many situations if measurements are fairly reliable. Dawson-Saunders and Trapp (1994, p 174), note that "meeting the regression assumptions generally causes fewer problems in experiments or clinical trials than in observational studies because reliability of . . . measurements tends to be greater in experimental studies." Consult a statistician to assess the reliability of measurements and to answer questions about violations of assumptions.

Performing a Simple Linear Regression Analysis

The clinical example presented at the beginning of the chapter requires a simple linear regression analysis. The researchers who conducted the peak flow/FEV_1 study sought to determine if peak flow is a useful predictor of FEV_1 in the asthmatic pediatric patient. If the answer is yes, peak flow could be used as a surrogate for FEV_1 to help asthmatic pediatric patients determine when to begin bronchodilator treatment. To answer the question, follow these steps:

1. Construct a scatter diagram; examine it to determine if assumptions underlying the regression analysis are satisfied reasonably.

2. Determine the regression line from sample data.

3. Evaluate the regression line to determine its predictive utility.

4. Use the regression equation for prediction, if it has predictive utility.

Steps 1 and 2 are presented in this chapter; steps 3 and 4 are highlighted in Chapter 17.

STEP 1: CONSTRUCT AND EXAMINE THE SCATTER DIAGRAM

A **scatter diagram,** also called a scatter gram or scatter plot, is a "pattern of points that results from plotting two [numerical] variables on a graph" (Vogt, 1993, p 203). Each point is plotted at the intersection of the values of the two variables. We examine the scatter diagram for (1) obvious violations of the assumption of linearity and homoscedasticity and (2) the basic nature of the relationship between X and Y (eg, does Y tend to increase as X increases?). Figure 16–5 contains three scatter diagrams in which the assumptions of linearity and homoscedasticity are reasonably satisfied. In diagram A, as X increases, Y tends to decrease, and vice-versa. Thus, the slope of the line-of-best fit is negative. The slope, however, is positive in diagrams B and C, because Y tends to increase as X increases, and vice-versa. Figure 16–6 includes three scatter diagrams in which linearity is violated. If a straight line were fitted to these data, it would be parallel to the X axis and have a slope that approaches zero. Three diagrams are displayed in Figure 16–7 in which the assumption of linearity is reasonably satisfied, but the pairs of points are not homoscedastic. If a straight line were fitted to these points, the slope of the line would be positive in diagrams A and C and negative in diagram B.

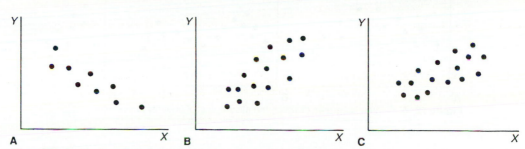

Figure 16–5. Scatter diagrams in which the assumptions of linearity and homoscedasticity are satisfied.

The peak flow/FEV$_1$ data appear in Table 16–1. These data were collected from 97 ambulatory pediatric patients selected randomly by a pediatrician who specializes in breathing-related problems like asthma. Patients range in age from 6 to 18 years, with a mean age of 11.47 years (SD = 3.46 years). The mean height is 146.83 cm (SD = 20.94 cm). Peak flow and FEV$_1$ measurements, standardized for age, sex, height, and race, are expressed as a percentage of what would be expected for a patient of a given age, height, sex, and race. Therefore, by standardizing these expiratory flow rates, a reading of 82 (%) has the same meaning for every

Table 16–1. Peak flow and FEV$_1$ standardized for age, race, sex, and height (expressed as a percentage).

Patient	Peak Flow	FEV$_1$		Patient	Peak Flow	FEV$_1$		Patient	Peak Flow	FEV$_1$
1	74	83		41	109	102		81	73	75
2	84	78		42	103	104		82	91	83
3	91	68		43	87	98		83	89	81
4	84	82		44	41	29		84	93	108
5	72	92		45	57	63		85	83	79
6	151	132		46	83	80		86	112	100
7	78	79		47	87	73		87	118	101
8	76	114		48	93	74		88	110	101
9	88	96		49	57	79		89	100	100
10	87	106		50	119	119		90	62	96
11	121	95		51	65	88		91	62	41
12	97	88		52	84	90		92	90	96
13	63	64		53	97	105		93	55	67
14	79	100		54	77	73		94	81	88
15	68	92		55	108	113		95	80	105
16	90	90		56	42	59		96	87	111
17	78	101		57	42	59		97	73	103
18	38	52		58	114	89				
19	78	91		59	62	47				
20	94	106		60	102	127				
21	90	92		61	88	110				
22	89	92		62	93	80				
23	110	122		63	87	52				
24	53	54		64	59	101				
25	63	59		65	63	82				
26	79	68		66	71	71				
27	106	108		67	79	82				
28	107	113		68	93	65				
29	46	40		69	46	93				
30	65	62		70	107	89				
31	90	73		71	93	108				
32	89	79		72	49	65				
33	110	82		73	114	82				
34	53	65		74	87	89				
35	63	89		75	79	109				
36	79	89		76	92	55				
37	106	88		77	59	70				
38	107	79		78	124	95				
39	46	60		79	105	94				
40	65	102		80	86	90				

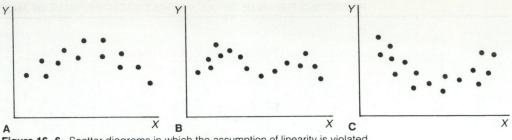

Figure 16–6. Scatter diagrams in which the assumption of linearity is violated.

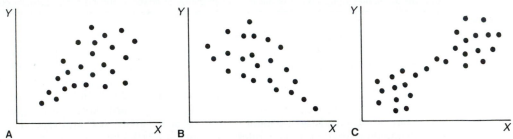

Figure 16–7. Scatter diagrams in which the assumption of homoscedasticity is violated.

patient. For example, a peak flow measurement of 82 (%) indicates that this expiratory rate is 82% of the expected value, given the individual's age, height, sex, and race.

Peak flow and FEV_1 measurements are plotted in a scatter diagram in Figure 16–8. The values of peak flow, the explanatory variable, appear on the X-axis; values of the outcome variable, FEV_1, are placed on the Y-axis. The pattern of the points provides information about the nature of the relationship, as well as obvious violations of linearity and homoscedasticity. The points appear to scatter around an invisible straight line that rises from left to right; as peak flow increases, FEV_1 values tend to increase. No obvious curvilinearity exists. The assumption of linearity appears reasonably well satisfied. Now visualize a straight line through these points, and the vertical dispersion about that line. The vertical scatter, for the most part, seems relatively equal throughout the range of X. No obvious departures, such as those depicted in Figure 16–7, are apparent. The assumption of homogeneity appears reasonably satisfied. Another approach to examining the assumption of homoscedasticity is presented in Chapter 19. Our "eyeball" test of linearity and homogeneity, however, suggests that it is appropriate to proceed with the analysis.

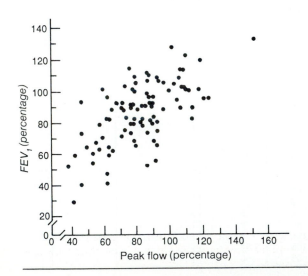

Figure 16–8. Scatter diagram of peak flow and FEV_1 measurements (n = 97).

Box 16–1. Developing the regression equation to predict FEV_1 from peak flow.

1. *Calculate and Organize the Sums, Sum-of-Squares, and Sum-of-the-Cross products*
Peak Flow (X, explanatory variable)
$\sum X = 74 + 84 + \ldots + 87 + 73 = 8032.00$
$\sum X^2 = 74^2 + 84^2 + \ldots + 87^2 + 73^2 = 707{,}182.00$

FEV_1 (Y, outcome variable)
$\sum Y = 83 + 78 + \ldots + 111 + 103 = 8345.00$
$\sum Y^2 = 83^2 + 78^2 + \ldots + 111^2 + 103^2 = 755{,}711.00$

Sum of the cross-products
$\sum XY = (74)(83) + (84)(78) + \ldots + (87)(111) + (73)(103) = 716{,}540.00$

Sample size
$n = 97$

2. *Calculate the Means and Standard Deviations*
Peak flow

$$\bar{X} = \frac{\sum X}{n} = \frac{8032}{97} = 82.8041$$

$$s_x^2 = \frac{\sum X^2 - \frac{(\sum X)^2}{n}}{n-1} = \frac{707{,}182 - \frac{8032^2}{97}}{96}$$

$$= \frac{42{,}099.2784}{96}$$

$$= 438.5341$$

$$s_x = \sqrt{438.5341} = 20.9412$$

FEV_1

$$\bar{Y} = \frac{8345}{97} = 86.0309$$

$$s_Y^2 = \frac{755{,}711 - \frac{8345^2}{97}}{96}$$

$$= \frac{37{,}782.9072}{96}$$

$$= 393.5720$$

$$s_Y = \sqrt{393.5720} = 19.8386$$

3. *Determine the Regression Line (Calculate the Slope and Intercept)*

$$b_{y.x} = \frac{\sum XY - \frac{(\sum x)(\sum y)}{n}}{\sum X^2 - \frac{(\sum x)^2}{n}}$$

$$= \frac{716{,}540 - \frac{8032(8345)}{97}}{707{,}182 - \frac{8082^2}{97}} = \frac{716{,}540 - \frac{8032(8345)}{97}}{42{,}099.2784} = 0.6067$$

$$a_{y.x} = \bar{Y} - b_{y.x}\bar{X} = 86.0309 - 0.6067(82.8041) = 35.7937$$

4. *Plot the Regression Line*
$\hat{Y}_i = 0.6067\,X_i + 35.7977$
$X_i = 46 \quad \hat{Y}_i = 0.6067(46) + 35.7977 = 63.71$
$X_i = 65 \quad \hat{Y}_i = 0.6067(65) + 35.7977 = 75.23$
$X_i = 88 \quad \hat{Y}_i = 0.6067(88) + 35.7977 = 89.19$
$X_i = 119 \quad \hat{Y}_i = 0.6067(119) + 35.7977 = 108.00$

STEP 2: DETERMINE THE REGRESSION LINE

Most statisticians and researchers utilize statistical software to perform a regression analysis. Hand calculations are presented below to demonstrate the procedures. Calculations are displayed in Box 16–1. Super- and subscripts are omitted in most formulae.

1. Calculate Sums, Sums-of-Squares, and Sum-of-Cross products

These quantities are used to calculate the means, standard deviations, slope, and intercept. The sum of the cross-products has not been calculated previously. It is the leftmost term in the numerator of the slope:

$$b_{y.x} = \frac{\sum X_i Y_i - \frac{(\sum X_i)(\sum Y_i)}{n}}{\sum X_i^2 - \frac{(\sum X_i)^2}{n}} .$$

We compute the sum-of-the-cross products by multiplying the peak flow and FEV_1 values for each patient and summing over all patients:

$$\sum X_i Y_i = X_1 Y_1 + X_2 Y_2 + \ldots + X_{96} Y_{96} + X_{97} Y_{97}$$
$$= (74)(83) + (84)(78) + \ldots + (87)(111) + (73)(103)$$
$$= 716{,}540.00$$

2. Calculate Means and Standard Deviations

The mean peak flow is 82.80, with a standard deviation of 20.94. The mean FEV_1 is 86.03, with a standard deviation of 19.84. These statistics help readers to assess how similar their patients are to individuals from whom data were collected. These statistics, plus demographic data like age, are important in evaluating external validity.

3. Determine the Regression Line

Calculate the Slope

Note that the denominator of the slope is the same as the numerator of the variance (standard deviation) of X (peak flow). Check the computations to verify that both are the same. Next, recall the nature of the pattern of the points in the scatter diagram (Figure 16–8)—as peak flow increases, FEV_1 tends to increase. This pattern suggests a positive relationship between these two variables. Thus, if our assessment is correct, the slope of the regression line should be positive. The slope is 0.6067; a one-unit increase in peak flow is associated with a 0.6067 increase in the predicted value of FEV_1.

Compute the Intercept

The regression line crosses the Y-axis at approximately 36 ($a_{y.x} = 35.7977$). The intercept will be reflected correctly on the scatter diagram only when the axes begin at (0,0) and no portion of the scale of measurement is omitted from either axis.

4. Plot the Regression Line

Select three or four peak flow values; use the regression equation to obtain the corresponding FEV_1 predicted values; plot the pairs of $(X_i, \hat{Y}_i)$; connect these pairs of points with a straight line; and check that the line passes through $(\bar{X}, \bar{Y})$. In Fig 16–9, the regression line has been plotted on the scatter diagram. Students often ask why we select more than two X values. If an error is made in calculating one of the $\hat{Y}_i$ values, the line drawn on the scatter diagram will be incorrect. Increasing the number of X values to three or four decreases the chance that the line will be plotted incorrectly. Check the line by hand to verify that it is correct if it is fitted by statistical software.

Which values of X should be selected? The selection of X values is somewhat arbitrary. Two guidelines exist. First, choose from *actual* values in the data set. The values should not be smaller or larger than those contained in the data, because the nature of the relationship between X and

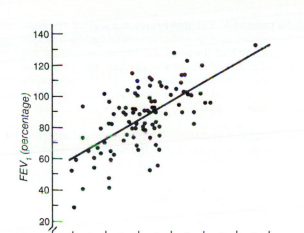

$$FEV_1 = 0.6067 \text{ (peak flow) } + 35.7977$$

Figure 16–9. Prediction of FEV_1 from peak flow (n = 97).

Y has not been established beyond the measurements contained in the data. Second, select values from the lower, middle, and upper range of X to increase plotting accuracy.

Why does a correctly drawn line pass through the intersection of the two means? If the value of X is set equal to its mean ($\overline{X} = 82.80$), the predicted value of Y equals its mean ($\overline{Y} = 86.03$):

$$\hat{Y}_i = 0.6067(82.80) + 35.7977 = 86.03$$

Verifying that the regression passes through $(\overline{X},\overline{Y})$ provides increased assurance that the line has been plotted correctly.

Visual inspection of Figure 16–9 confirms previous impressions. First, the pairs of peak flow and FEV_1 measurements appear to be described appropriately by a straight line (*linearity assumption*). Second, vertical dispersion about the line appears relatively equal throughout the range of peak flow values (*homoscedasticity assumption*). Contrast this scatter diagram with the diagrams in Figure 16–7, in which linearity exists but homoscedasticity does not.

Although the regression equation has been calculated and the line plotted, the question remains whether the regression line is useful statistically? Can peak flow be used effectively to predict FEV_1 measurements? We address these questions in the next chapter.

SUMMARY

We use regression analysis to predict an outcome (Y) from an explanatory variable (X). Linear regression is used with quantitative variables. The regression line satisfies the Least Squares Criterion; that is, the sum of the squared vertical deviations between values of Y and the regression line is as small as possible. The sum of these squared vertical deviations will be larger if determined from any other line. The regression line is characterized by its slope and intercept. The slope reflects the amount of change in the predicted value of Y, for each one unit change in X. The intercept indicates the point at which the line crosses the Y-axis. The five assumptions underlying the regression model are random sampling, independence, normality, linearity, and homoscedasticity. We assume that observations have been sampled randomly and independently, so that the values of Y for a specific value of X do not depend on the values of Y for any other value of X (independence). For each value of X, we assume the existence of a subpopulation of Y values distributed normally (normality). The means of the subpopulation of Y values for each X lie on the same straight line (linearity). Finally, we assume vertical deviations about the regression line are equal throughout the range of X (homoscedasticity). Consult a statistician if assumptions appear violated or questions exist about their tenability.

Begin the regression analysis by plotting the pairs of X, Y points to create a **scatter diagram,** which is a pattern of points that results from plotting two quantitative variables on a graph. Examine the scatter diagram for (1) obvious violations of linearity and homoscedasticity and (2) the basic nature of the relationship between X and Y. Next calculate the slope and intercept, if no obvious violations of linearity and homoscedasticity exist. Fit the regression line to the scatter diagram by choosing three or four X values; then calculate the corresponding predicted values of Y from the regression equation, plot the pairs of $(X_i, \hat{Y}_i)$, and connect these pairs of points with a straight line.

The assumptions underlying simple linear regression and formulae for slope and intercept are summarized in Table 16–2. We explore the statistical usefulness of the regression equation in the next chapter.

Table 16–2. Assumptions and formulas for developing a simple linear regression equation.

Assumptions	
Normality	
Linearity	
Homoscedasticity	
Independence	
Random sampling	
Formulae (sample)	
Regression of Y-on-X	$\hat{Y}_i = b_{y.x}X_i + a_{y.x}$
	$b_{y.x} = \dfrac{\sum X_i Y_i - \dfrac{(\sum X_i)(\sum Y_i)}{n}}{\sum X_i^2 - \dfrac{(\sum X_i)^2}{n}}$
Slope of Y-on-X (sample)	
Intercept of Y-on-X (sample)	$a_{y.x} = \bar{Y} - b_{y.x}\bar{X}$

REFERENCES

Altman DB: Statistics in medical journals: Developments in the 1980s. *Stat Med* 1991; **10**:1987.

Daniel D: *Biostatistics: A Foundation for Analysis in the Health Sciences,* 5th ed. Wiley, 1991.

Dawson-Saunders B, Trapp R: *Basic and Clinical Biostatistics,* 2nd ed. Appleton & Lange, 1994.

Emerson JD, Colditz BA: Use of statistical analysis in the *New England Journal of Medicine. N Engl J Med* 1983;**309**:709.

Minium E: *Statistical Reasoning in Psychology and Education,* 3rd ed. Wiley, 1993.

Moore JA, Essex-Sorlie D, Rolson A: Peak flow is a reliable asthma screen. *Proc Am Acad Pediatr* 1989.

Vogt WP: *Dictionary of Statistics and Methodology.* Sage, 1993.

Self-study Questions

Part I: Definitions

Define each of the following terms.

Correlation	Independence	Least Squares Line
Explanatory variable	Intercept	Linearity
Homoscedasticity	Least Squares Criterion	Line-of-best fit

Normality   Regression   Simple linear regression
Outcome variable   Regression equation   Slope
Random sampling   Scatter diagram

Part II: Thought Problems

Read each of the following hypothetical examples, examine the scatter diagram, determine if a *simple linear regression* analysis is appropriate, and briefly explain the basis for your assessment.

1. The effects of growth hormone (GH) replacement with recombinant human GH on bone and mineral metabolism were studied in 36 GH-deficient children. Several outcomes, including serum ionized calcium levels, were assessed at pretherapy (zero months) and 1, 3, 6, 9, and 12 months after the beginning of therapy. Simple linear regression was used to determine if changes in ionized calcium levels could be predicted from length of therapy. Each patient's ionized calcium level was employed in the analysis; mean calcium levels at each time period are displayed in Figure 16–10.

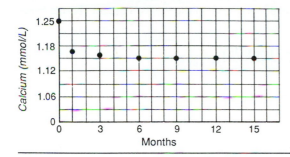

Figure 16–10. Mean levels of ionized calcium prior to (time = 0) and after therapy with growth hormone in children deficient in growth hormone (*n* = 36).

2. Because normal values for first-phase insulin release during an intravenous glucose tolerance test are not well defined for children and adolescents, investigators studied 100 healthy individuals, aged 7 to 18 years, with no family history of type I diabetes and a normal glycohemoglobin value. One objective was to determine if age is predictive of first-phase insulin release levels (eg, if levels are lower in younger children and higher in adolescents). The basic pattern evidenced by the data is displayed in Figure 16–11.

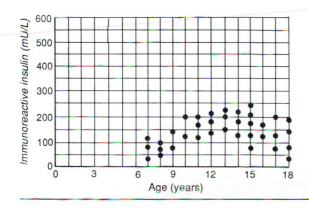

Figure 16–11. First-phase insulin release (expressed as 1-minute plus 3-minute IRI levels minus baseline level) by age (years).

3. Hypothermic circulatory arrest (HCA) is frequently used as a support technique during heart surgery in infants. HCA was studied in 150 infants who (1) were 3 months old or less, (2) weighed more than 2.5 kg at birth, and (3) were undergoing heart surgery to repair a ventricular septal defect. The investigators tried to assess whether length of the circulatory arrest could predicted time to recovery of first EEG activity. A representation of the data appears in Figure 16–12.

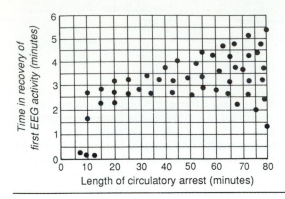

Figure 16–12. Time to recovery of first EEG activity and length of circulatory arrest.

4. Fifty volunteers with hyperlipidemia participated in a 4-month study in which they consumed diets high in soluable fiber, low in saturated fat, and high in carbohydrates. Low- and high-density lipoprotein levels (LDL and HDL, respectively) were monitored weekly. The data appear in Figure 16–13; time (weeks) is plotted on the x-axis and percent change from baseline in LDL levels is graphed on the y-axis. Percent change from baseline was calculated as

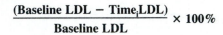

$$\frac{(\text{Baseline LDL} - \text{Time}_i\text{LDL})}{\text{Baseline LDL}} \times 100\%$$

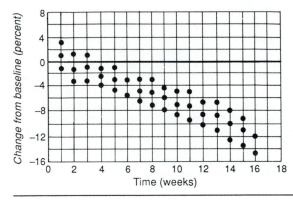

Figure 16–13. Change in LDL levels with respect to baseline for individuals on high soluble fiber diet.

5. The association between estimated gestational age (weeks) of the fetus and physical and neurologic examination score at birth (range, 0 to 70 points) was examined in 2500 newborns to determine the extent to which the score could be predicted from estimated age. The data appear in Figure 16–14.

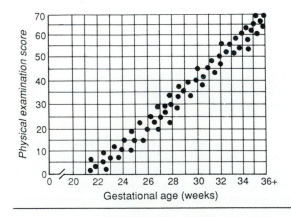

Figure 16–14. Gestational age and physical examination score of newborns.

Solutions

Part II: Thought Problems

1. A *repeated measures* design was used to study the effect of GH replacement therapy on 36 GH-deficient children. Serum ionized calcium levels were measured 6 times. Simple linear regression is not appropriate, because the assumption of independence is violated in this design. A comment is also in order about Figure 16–10. If a simple linear regression analysis were appropriate, the scatter diagram should contain the *observed* (X, Y) values, at a minimum. Although plotting mean values allows the investigator and reader to evaluate the assumption of linearity, it is impossible to assess homoscedasticity.

2. Examination of Figure 16–11 reveals clearly that the *assumption of linearity* is violated. The line-of-best fit for these data is curved, rather than straight. The curved line, when fitted to the data, will be similar to the one displayed in Figure 16–15.

3. Setting aside the three pairs of (X, Y) points near the bottom left-hand corner of the scatter diagram, it appears that linearity is reasonably satisfied. However, it is clear that the (X, Y) points are not homoscedastic. Vertical dispersion about an imaginary straight line fitted to the data is smaller for lower (X, Y) values and substantially greater in the upper range. Simple linear regression is not appropriate for these data, as plotted. The investigators should consult a statistician to determine if a suitable transformation will remedy the problem of heteroscedasticity (unequal vertical variation), or whether a different analysis should be used. Additionally, the three deviant (X, Y) points should be checked to ensure their validity. In Chapter 19, we discuss extremely deviant points and their effect on regression (and correlation).

4. This problem, like problem 1, involves taking repeated measurements over time; therefore, the assumption of independence is not met. Simple linear regression is *inappropriate*.

5. Linearity and homoscedasticity appear well satisfied, based on an examination of the scatter diagram (Figure 16–14). Independence has not been violated. Normality is assumed. Simple linear regression is appropriate in light of (1) the objective ("to determine the extent to which the [physical] examination score could be predicted from estimated age") and (2) the appearance of the scatter diagram.

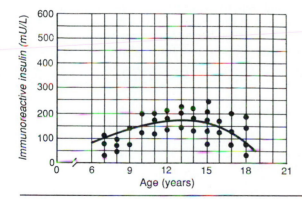

Figure 16–15. Line of best fit plotted for first-phase insulin release and age.

17 Evaluating the Equation for Predicting the Value of One Variable from the Value of Another

In the clinical example at the start of Chapter 16 we asked: "Is peak flow a useful predictor of FEV_1 in pediatric patients with asthma?" To answer this question, we follow four steps:

1. Construct a scatter diagram and examine it to determine if assumptions underlying the regression analysis are satisfied reasonably.

2. Determine the regression line from sample data.

3. Evaluate the regression line to determine its predictive utility.

4. Use the regression equation for prediction, if it has predictive utility.

Steps 1 and 2 were completed in Chapter 16. The scatter diagram appears in Figure 16–8. Examination of this figure reveals that FEV_1 values tend to increase as peak flow increases and decrease as peak flow decreases. No obvious curvilinearity or heteroscedasticity exists. We conclude from inspecting the scatter diagram that it is appropriate to determine the linear regression line (step 2); the slope and intercept are calculated as 0.6067 and 35.7977, respectively. Thus, the equation for the regression line is

$$\hat{Y}_i = 0.6067X_i + 35.7977$$

We use this equation to plot the regression line, which appears in Figure 16–9. Next, we assess its statistical utility by employing a conventional hypothesis test or by constructing a confidence interval. Both approaches are demonstrated in this chapter. A quantitative index that describes the amount of predictive error is developed first, because it figures into the hypothesis test and confidence interval. The regression equation is used for prediction at the end of the chapter.

OBJECTIVES

When you finish this chapter, you should be able to:

- Define and understand predictive error, standard error of estimate, and standard error of the slope.
- Explain the result of a test of the null hypothesis—that is, that the slope equals zero.
- Interpret a two-sided confidence interval about the slope with respect to the null hypothesis of zero slope.
- Describe why the confidence interval about a predicted mean value is narrower than the comparable interval about the predicted value for a single patient.
- Interpret a two-sided confidence interval about a predicted mean value.
- Interpret a two-sided confidence interval about the predicted value for a single patient.
- Work through a regression analysis and test the hypothesis of zero slope.

QUANTIFYING PREDICTIVE ERROR

Predictive error is the vertical dispersion about the regression line. As defined in Chapter 16, this error is the difference between the actual or observed value of Y and the corresponding predicted value:

$$e_i = Y_{obs} - \hat{Y}_i \qquad \qquad \textbf{17.1}$$

This difference is used to develop the **standard error of estimate.** The standard error of estimate is the standard deviation of the actual Y observations about the predicted Y values (Minium et al, 1993, p 183). It is symbolized as $\sigma_{y.x}$ for a *population* and $s_{y.x}$ in a *sample* in which Y is predicted from X. It is defined in a sample as

$$s_{y.x} = \sqrt{\frac{\sum(Y_i - \hat{Y}_i)^2}{n - 2}} \qquad \qquad \textbf{17.2}$$

Formula 17.2 is not convenient computationally because it involves subtracting every observed value of Y from the corresponding predicted value, squaring the difference, summing over all Y observations, and dividing by $n - 2$. A computational form is derived by first substituting $b_{y.x} X + a_{y.x}$ for $\hat{Y}_i$, replacing $b_{y.x}$ and $a_{y.x}$ by their computational equivalents, and simplifying the equation to produce the following:

$$s_{y.x} = \sqrt{\frac{1}{n - 2} \left(\sum(Y_i - \overline{Y})^2 - \frac{[\sum(X_i - \overline{X})(Y_i - \overline{Y})]^2}{\sum(X_i - \overline{X})^2} \right)} \qquad \qquad \textbf{17.3}$$

Although Formula 17.3 may appear formidable, keep in mind that we have already calculated all its components:

$\sum(X_i - \overline{X})^2$ **Numerator of the standard deviation of X**

$[\sum(X_i - \overline{X})(Y_i - \overline{X})]^2$ **Numerator of the slope, except for the squaring operation**

$\sum(Y_i - \overline{Y})^2$ **Numerator of the standard deviation of Y**

The standard error of estimate for the peak flow and FEV_1 data is calculated in Box 17–1.

Box 17–1. Calculating the standard error of estimate for the peak flow and FEV_1 data.

---

1. *Retrieve quantities used to calculate the standard deviations and slope*

$\sum(X_i - \overline{X})^2 = 42,099.2784$

$[\sum(X_i - \overline{X})(Y_i - \overline{Y})]^2 = 25,539.5876$

$\sum(Y_i - \overline{Y})^2 = 37,782.9072$

2. *Use these quantities to calculate the standard error of estimate*

$$s_{y.x} = \sqrt{\frac{1}{n - 2} \left(\sum(Y_i - \overline{Y})^2 - \frac{[\sum(X_i - \overline{X})(Y_i - \overline{Y})]^2}{\sum(X_i - \overline{X})^2} \right)}$$

$$s_{y.x} = \sqrt{\frac{1}{97 - 2} \left(37,782.9072 - \frac{25,539.5876^2}{42,099.2784} \right)}$$

$$= \sqrt{234.6240}$$

$$= 15.3174$$

Quantities used in its calculation were retrieved from Box 16–1 in Chapter 16. The standard error is 15.3174. The standard error of estimate is used to evaluate the regression line, as demonstrated in the remainder of this chapter. The standard error is revisited in Chapter 19.

What is the relationship between $s_{y.x}$ and the amount of vertical scatter about the regression line? If the actual Y observations equal the predicted values of Y, all points will fall directly on the regression line and no vertical dispersion will exist; thus, $(Y_i - \hat{Y}_i) = 0$ and $s_{y.x} = 0$. Therefore, the minimum value of the standard error of estimate is zero. As differences between the observed and predicted values of Y increase, vertical dispersion about the regression line increases and $s_{y.x}$ increases. Although it is not obvious, the standard error reaches its maximum value when the slope of the regression line equals zero. In this case, $s_{y.x} = s_y$. Demonstrating the connection between $s_{y.x}$ and s_y requires that the total variation in the linear model be partitioned into variation associated with regression and variation associated with error; however, doing so is beyond the scope of this chapter. Individuals who wish to pursue this topic should consult other sources, for example, Daniel (1991, pp 378–385).

TESTING THE HYPOTHESIS OF ZERO SLOPE

The slope of the regression line, fitted to a population of X, Y observations, will be either zero, positive, or negative. If β, the population slope, equals zero, samples selected from this population will yield, in the long run, regression equations that are not useful for prediction. In addition, the sample slope will tend to be compatiable, in the long run, with $\beta = 0$. Therefore, we evaluate the predictive utility of a regression equation against the null hypothesis that population slope equals zero.

The null and alternative hypothesis takes one of the following forms:

$$H_0: \beta = 0 \qquad H_0: \beta = 0 \qquad H_0: \beta = 0$$
$$H_A: \beta \neq 0 \qquad H_A: \beta > 0 \qquad H_A: \beta < 0$$

The null hypothesis states that the slope equals zero. The alternative hypothesis on the left postulates that the slope differs from zero; this results in a two-tailed test. The alternative hypothesis in the middle indicates that the slope is greater than zero; this produces a greater than one-tailed test. Therefore, the X, Y observations vary *directly* when the slope is greater than zero; that is, Y tends to increase as X increases, and Y tends to decrease as X decreases. The alternative hypothesis on the right posits that the X, Y observations vary *indirectly;* this yields a less than one-tailed test. When observations vary indirectly, the slope of the regression line is negative: Y tends to decrease as X increases and vice-versa.

The Student's t distribution and t statistic are used to evaluate the statistical hypotheses, if linearity, independence, and equal vertical dispersion (homoscedasticity) are satisfied. Often normality is assumed. These assumptions were discussed in Chapter 16 in the section "Assumptions Underlying the Simple Linear Regression Model." The t statistic is

$$t = \frac{b - \beta_0}{s_b}, \text{ with } df = n - 2 \qquad\qquad 17.4$$

where b is the sample slope, β_0 is the population slope given in the null hypothesis, and s_b is the **standard error of the slope.** Degrees of freedom are $n - 2$. The standard error of the slope is

$$s_b = \frac{s_{y.x}}{\sqrt{\sum X_i^2 - \dfrac{(\sum X_i)^2}{n}}}. \qquad\qquad 17.5$$

This standard error measures the spread of all possible values of the sample slope, b, about the population slope, β.

Box 17–2. Testing the null hypothesis of zero slope for the peak flow and FEV_1 data.

1. *Formulate the Scientific Hypothesis*
Peak flow is a viable predictor of FEV_1 measurements. The slope of the regression line for predicting FEV_1 values from peak flow measurements differs significantly from zero.

2. *Set up the Statistical Hypotheses*
H_0: $\beta = 0$
H_A: $\beta \neq 0$

3. *Determine the Test Criteria*
   a. Use the t distribution and t statistic.
   b. $\alpha = 0.05$.
   c. $df = n - 2$; $df = 97 - 2 = 95$; $t_{crit} = \pm 1.98$ (approximately) for a two-tailed test.

4. *Analyze the Data*
Calculate the standard error of the slope:

$$s_b = \frac{s_{y.x}}{\sqrt{\sum x_i^2 - \frac{(\sum x_i)^2}{n}}} = \frac{15.3174}{\sqrt{42,099.2784}} = 0.07465$$

Compute the t statistic:

$$t = \frac{b - \beta_0}{s_b} = \frac{0.6067 - 0}{0.07465} = 8.1273$$

5. *Evaluate the Statistics*
The null hypothesis of zero slope is rejected.

6. *Interpret the Statistics*
The slope of the regression equation for predicting FEV_1 from peak flow measurements differs significantly from zero (p-value < 0.001). Peak flow is a useful statistical predictor of FEV_1 measurements in pediatric patients with asthma.

A test of the null hypothesis that the population slope equals zero for the peak flow and FEV_1 data appears in Box 17–2. Note that the six-step process outlined in Chapter 10 is followed. The scientific hypothesis is formulated first, followed by the statistical hypotheses. A nondirectional alternative hypothesis is formulated because the investigators wish to detect a sample outcome in both directions, if possible. Test criteria are specified in step 3. In step 4, the investigators begin the analysis by computing the standard error of the slope. The t statistic is calculated next. This calculated value is compared in step 5 to the critical value and the null hypothesis of zero slope is rejected ($t_{calc} = 8.13$ versus $t_{crit} = \pm 1.98$). In step 6, the researchers conclude that the slope of the regression equation for predicting FEV_1 measurements from peak flow values differs significantly from zero (p-value < 0.001). Therefore, the researchers conclude that peak flow is a useful statistical predictor of FEV_1 measurements.

As discussed in previous chapters, we can construct a two-sided confidence interval to examine the null hypothesis and its nondirectional alternative. This approach is illustrated next.

CONSTRUCTING A TWO-SIDED CONFIDENCE INTERVAL ABOUT THE SLOPE

Like all other two-sided confidence intervals, the two-sided interval about the slope includes the sample statistic, its standard error, and the two-tailed critical value of the test statistic. The two-sided interval about the slope is:

$$100 (1 - \alpha)\% = (b - t_{\alpha/2}s_b \leq \beta \leq b + t_{\alpha/2}s_b) \text{ or} \qquad \text{17.6a}$$

$$100 (1 - \alpha)\% = b \pm t_{\alpha/2}s_b. \qquad \text{17.6b}$$

Recall that $t_{\alpha/2}$ is the two-tailed critical value of t for $df = n - 2$ and specified α.

Computation of the 95% two-sided confidence interval about the slope for the FEV_1 and

Box 17–3. Constructing the 95% two-sided interval about the slope.

1. *Assemble the Quantities Required to Calculate the Confidence Interval*
$b = 0.6067; t_{\alpha/2} = \pm1.98; s_b = 0.07465$

2. *Construct the 95% Confidence Interval*
$b \pm t_{\alpha/2}s_b = 0.6067 \pm 1.98 \, (0.07465) = 0.6067 \pm 0.1478 = 0.4589, 0.7545$

3. *Determine if β = 0 is Captured in the Interval*
Zero is not captured in the two-sided 95% confidence interval that extends from approximately 0.46 to 0.76.

4. *Make a decision about the null hypothesis that β = 0*
The null hypothesis of zero slope is rejected because the confidence interval does not capture zero.

peak flow data appears in Box 17–3. The quantities required to construct the interval are assembled in step 1. The interval is computed in the next step. The 95% two-sided interval extends from approximately 0.46 to 0.75. The *practical* interpretation of this interval is that we are 95% confident that the slope of the regression line for predicting FEV_1 measurements from peak flow is between approximately 0.46 and 0.75 in the population of pediatric patients with asthma (Daniel, 1991, p 134). The null hypothesis is rejected because β = 0 is not captured in the interval (steps 3 and 4). Thus, the decision about H_0: β = 0 is the same, regardless of whether we conduct a conventional significance test or construct a confidence interval.

We have established through the hypothesis test of H_0: β = 0, as well as through the 95% two-sided confidence interval about the slope, that the regression equation provides a statistically useful prediction of FEV_1 measurements. We can then use this equation to predict FEV_1 measurements, establish a confidence interval about the predicted mean FEV_1 measurement for a *group* of patients, and develop a confidence interval about the predicted value of FEV_1 for a *single* patient. These applications are demonstrated after the following word of caution.

A Word of Caution About Retaining The Null Hypothesis of Zero Slope

When retaining the null hypothesis of zero slope, beware of a common error in interpretation. Many individuals conclude when H_0: β = 0 is retained that no relationship exists between Y and X and, therefore, Y is of no value for predicting X. If we assume we did not commit a Type II error, however, we may retain the hypothesis of zero slope because: (1) the relationship between X and Y is not strong enough to be used for prediction, even though it may be linear; or (2) the relationship between X and Y is nonlinear, and therefore a linear equation has limited predictive value. Therefore, it is inappropriate to conclude that no relationship exists between X and Y when H_0: β = 0 is retained. If after examining a scatter diagram it is clear that X and Y are not related curvilinearly, we conclude that the strength of the linear relationship between X and Y is insufficient for prediction. Recall that we commit a type II error when we retain a false null hypothesis. Type II errors were discussed in Chapter 9 in the section "Hypothesis Testing: Correct Decisions and Errors."

USING THE REGRESSION EQUATION FOR PREDICTION

The regression equation can be used (1) to predict the mean Y value in a *group* of individuals, all of whom have the same X value; and (2) to construct a confidence interval about the predicted mean. Alternately, we can utilize the equation to predict a value for a *single* individual and develop a confidence interval about this value. The predicted mean for a group of individuals and the predicted value for an individual are numerically equivalent, but the confidence interval about the predicted value for an individual is wider than the interval about the predicted mean.

Predicting the Mean of Y for Given X

If we are interested in predicting the mean FEV_1 measurement for all patients who have a peak flow value of 74, we use the following regression equation:

$$\hat{Y}_i = 0.6067X_i + 35.7977$$

$$= 0.6067 \ (74) + 35.7977$$

$$= 80.69.$$

Thus, the predicted mean of all FEV_1 measurements is 80.69 for the group of patients who have a peak flow value of 74; this predicted mean is an estimate of $\mu_{Y|X}$ for the subpopulation of individuals for whom peak flow equals 74. We know, however, that if we repeat this $FEV_1/$ peak flow study in another group of patients sampled randomly from the same population as our current subjects, we will obtain a different regression equation and therefore a different estimate of the predicted mean FEV_1 value for patients whose peak flow value is 74. Consequently, we construct a confidence interval about the predicted mean; this provides a range of values in which we believe the population mean is captured. The formula for this confidence interval is:

$$\hat{Y} \pm t_{\alpha/2}s_{y.x} \sqrt{\frac{1}{n} + \frac{(X_i - \bar{X})^2}{\Sigma(X_i - \bar{X})^2}} \qquad 17.7$$

where $\hat{Y}$ is the predicted value of Y computed from the regression equation; $t_{\alpha/2}$ is the two-tailed critical value of t for $df = n - 2$ and specified α; $s_{y.x}$ is the standard error of estimate; X_i is the specific value of interest; $\bar{X}$ is the mean of X; and $\Sigma(X - \bar{X})^2$ is the numerator of the standard deviation of X. The 95% confidence interval for $\hat{Y} = 80.96$ given $X = 74$ is

$$80.69 \pm 1.98 \ (15.3174) \sqrt{\frac{1}{97} + \frac{(74 - 82.8041)^2}{42099.2784}}$$

$$80.69 \pm 3.3431$$

$$77.35, \ 84.03.$$

If we draw repeated random samples from the patient population, perform a regression analysis, and estimate $\mu_{Y|X}$ for $X = 74$ with a similarly constructed confidence interval, we find that 95% of all such intervals would capture the true mean FEV_1 measurement for the subpopulation of patients who have a peak flow of 74. The *practical interpretation* is that we are 95% confident that this confidence interval contains the mean FEV_1 value for the population of pediatric patients with asthma who have a peak flow measurement of 74 (Daniel, 1991, pp 394–395).

If we construct the 95% confidence interval for each subpopulation of patients with a given X measurement and plot the lower and upper boundaries on the scatter diagram with the regression line, we obtain a **confidence band** about the regression line by connecting all the lower boundaries with one curve and all the upper boundaries with another curve. The lower and upper boundaries of each interval about its corresponding predicted mean FEV_1 measurement appear in columns 5 and 6 of Table 17–1. For example, for the subpopulation of patients who have a peak flow of 87 (column 2), the predicted mean FEV_1 measurement is 88.58

Table 17–1. Peak flow and FEV₁ standardized for age, race, sex, and height and predicted value of FEV₁ (FEV₁ and predicted FEV₁ values expressed as a percentage).

Patient	Peak Flow	FEV$_1$	FEV$_1$ Predicted	95% Confidence Band About the Predicted Mean		95% Confidence Limit About Individual Values	
				Lower Limit	Upper Limit	Lower Limit	Upper Limit
1	74	83	80.69	77.35	84.03	50.18	111.20
2	84	78	86.76	83.65	89.84	56.27	117.24
3	91	68	91.00	87.70	94.31	60.49	121.51
4	84	82	86.76	83.68	89.84	56.27	117.24
5	72	92	79.48	76.01	82.94	48.95	110.00
6	151	132	127.40	116.88	137.93	95.29	159.51
7	78	79	83.12	79.96	86.28	52.62	113.61
8	76	114	81.90	78.83	84.98	51.40	112.40
9	88	96	89.18	86.01	92.36	58.69	119.68
10	87	106	88.58	85.44	91.72	58.09	119.07
11	121	95	109.20	102.78	115.62	78.20	140.21
12	97	88	94.64	90.92	98.36	64.09	125.20
13	63	64	74.02	69.77	78.27	43.39	104.64
14	79	100	83.72	80.59	86.85	53.23	114.21
15	68	92	77.05	73.28	80.82	46.49	107.61
16	90	90	90.40	87.14	93.65	59.89	120.90
17	78	101	83.12	79.96	86.28	52.62	113.61
18	38	52	58.85	51.56	66.14	27.65	90.05
19	78	91	83.12	79.96	86.28	52.62	113.61
20	94	106	92.82	89.33	96.31	62.29	123.35
21	90	92	90.39	87.14	93.65	59.89	120.90
22	89	92	89.79	86.58	93.00	59.29	120.29
23	110	122	102.53	97.47	107.59	71.78	133.28
24	53	54	67.95	62.58	73.33	37.15	98.75
25	63	59	74.02	69.77	78.27	43.39	104.64
26	79	68	83.72	80.59	86.85	53.23	114.21
27	106	108	100.10	95.49	104.71	69.43	130.78
28	107	113	100.71	95.99	105.43	70.02	131.40
29	46	40	63.70	57.45	69.95	32.74	94.67
30	65	62	75.23	71.18	79.28	44.63	105.83
31	46	73	63.70	57.45	69.95	32.74	94.67
32	77	79	82.51	79.31	85.71	52.01	113.01
33	62	82	73.41	69.06	77.76	42.77	104.05
34	80	65	84.33	81.22	87.44	53.84	114.82
35	71	89	78.87	75.33	82.41	48.34	109.40
36	77	89	82.51	79.31	84.03	52.01	113.01
37	72	88	79.48	76.01	89.84	48.95	110.00
38	90	79	90.40	87.14	94.31	59.89	120.90
39	53	60	67.95	62.58	89.84	37.15	98.75
40	108	102	101.32	96.48	106.15	70.61	132.03
41	109	102	101.92	96.98	106.87	71.19	132.65
42	103	104	98.28	93.99	102.57	67.65	128.91
43	87	98	88.58	85.44	91.72	58.09	119.07
44	41	29	60.67	53.77	67.57	29.57	91.77
45	57	63	70.38	65.47	75.28	39.65	101.10
46	83	80	86.15	83.07	89.23	55.67	116.63
47	87	73	88.58	85.44	91.72	58.09	119.07
48	93	74	92.22	88.79	95.64	61.69	122.74
49	57	79	70.38	65.47	75.28	39.65	101.10
50	119	119	107.99	101.82	114.16	77.04	138.94
51	65	88	75.23	71.18	79.28	44.63	105.83
52	84	90	86.76	83.67	89.84	56.27	117.24
53	97	105	94.64	90.92	98.37	64.09	125.20
54	77	73	82.51	79.31	85.71	52.01	113.01
55	108	113	82.51	79.31	85.71	52.01	113.01
56	42	59	101.32	96.48	106.15	70.61	132.03
57	42	59	61.28	54.51	68.05	30.20	92.35
58	114	89	104.96	99.41	110.50	74.12	135.79
59	62	47	73.41	69.06	77.76	42.77	104.05
60	102	127	97.68	93.49	101.86	67.06	128.29

(continued)

Table 17–1 (cont'd). Peak flow and FEV$_1$ standardized for age, race, sex, and height and predicted value of FEV$_1$ (FEV$_1$ and predicted FEV$_1$ values expressed as a percentage).

Patient	Peak Flow	FEV$_1$	FEV$_1$ Predicted	95% Confidence Band About the Predicted Mean		95% Confidence Limit About Individual Values	
				Lower Limit	Upper Limit	Lower Limit	Upper Limit
61	88	110	89.18	86.01	92.36	58.69	119.68
62	93	80	92.22	88.79	95.64	61.69	122.74
63	87	52	88.58	85.44	91.72	58.09	119.07
64	59	101	71.59	66.91	76.27	40.90	102.28
65	63	82	74.02	69.77	78.27	43.39	104.64
66	71	71	78.87	75.33	82.41	48.34	109.40
67	79	82	83.72	80.59	86.85	53.23	114.21
68	93	65	92.22	88.79	95.64	61.69	122.74
69	46	93	63.70	57.45	69.95	32.74	94.67
70	107	89	100.71	95.99	105.43	70.02	131.40
71	93	108	92.22	88.79	95.65	61.69	122.74
72	49	65	65.52	59.65	71.39	34.63	96.41
73	114	82	104.96	99.41	110.50	74.12	135.79
74	87	89	88.58	85.44	91.72	58.09	119.07
75	79	109	83.72	80.59	86.86	53.23	114.21
76	92	55	91.61	88.54	88.54	61.09	122.12
77	59	70	71.59	66.91	76.27	40.90	102.28
78	124	95	111.02	104.20	117.85	79.94	142.11
79	105	94	99.50	94.99	115.52	68.84	130.16
80	86	90	87.97	84.85	91.09	57.48	118.46
81	73	75	80.08	76.68	83.49	49.56	110.60
82	91	83	91.00	87.69	94.31	60.49	121.51
83	89	81	89.79	86.58	93.00	59.29	120.29
84	93	108	92.22	88.79	95.64	61.69	122.74
85	83	79	86.15	83.07	89.23	55.67	116.63
86	112	100	103.74	98.44	109.04	72.95	134.53
87	118	101	107.38	101.34	113.43	76.46	138.31
88	110	101	102.53	97.47	107.59	71.78	133.28
89	100	100	96.46	92.47	100.46	65.87	127.05
90	62	96	73.41	69.06	77.76	42.77	104.05
91	62	41	73.41	69.06	77.76	42.77	104.05
92	90	96	90.40	87.14	93.65	59.89	120.90
93	55	67	69.16	64.03	74.30	38.40	99.92
94	81	88	84.94	81.85	88.03	54.45	115.42
95	80	105	84.33	81.22	87.44	53.84	114.82
96	87	111	88.58	85.44	91.72	58.09	119.07
97	73	103	80.08	76.68	83.49	49.56	110.60

(column 4); the 95% interval about this mean extends from 85.44 to 91.72. The confidence band that results from plotting and connecting the upper and lower boundaries, respectively, appears in Figure 17–1.

Note that the confidence band is concave. It is narrowest when X_i equals $\overline{X}$ and widest at the ends. If we examine Formula 17.7, we see that the quantity under the square root is smallest when $X_i = \overline{X}$ because $(X - \overline{X})^2 = 0$; the right-hand fraction then divides to zero. As we move away from the mean of X, $(X - \overline{X})^2$ increases, the right-hand fraction increases, the quantity under the square root increases, and the interval width increases. The practical interpretation of this confidence band is: "We are 95% confident that the true regression line in the population is captured between the upper and lower boundaries of this confidence band."

We may also ask questions about confidence limits on our prediction for an *individual* patient, for example, one whose peak flow value is 74. Within what 95% confidence limits will the predicted FEV$_1$ measurement be captured? The development of these limits is highlighted in the next section.

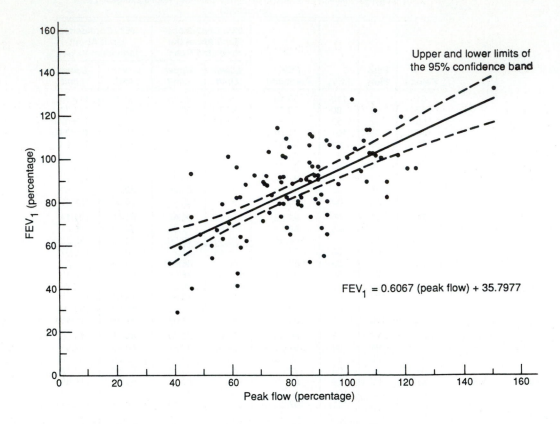

Figure 17–1. Ninety-five percent confidence band about the regression line.

Predicting Y for an Individual Patient

If we want to predict the FEV_1 measurement for a patient who has a peak flow value of 74, we use the regression equation as follows:

$$\hat{Y}_i = 0.6067X_i + 35.7977$$

$$= 0.6067\ (74) + 35.7977$$

$$= 80.69.$$

Thus, we employ the regression equation in the same way, regardless of whether we want to predict the (1) FEV_1 measurement for a single patient whose peak flow is 74 or (2) mean FEV_1 score for the subpopulation of patients who have a peak flow measurement of 74. However, the formula for confidence limits about the individual predicted value differs from that used to construct limits about the predicted mean value. The formula for computing the confidence limits about an individual's predicted Y measurement is

$$\hat{Y} \pm t_{\alpha/2} s_{y.x} \sqrt{1 + \frac{1}{n} + \frac{(X - \bar{X})^2}{\Sigma(X - \bar{X})^2}} \, . \qquad \qquad \text{17.8}$$

Examine Formulas 17.7 and 17.8 and note the inclusion of "1" under the square root sign in Formula 17.8. The confidence interval about a single observation is wider than the interval about the predicted mean for a subpopulation of individuals. We know from Chapters 10 and 11 that variation of individual observations is greater than variation of sample statistics. Thus, a confidence interval constructed about the individual patient will be wider than a comparably constructed interval about the mean of a subpopulation of individuals.

The 95% confidence interval about $\hat{Y} = 80.69$ for $X = 74$ is

$$80.69 \pm 1.98 \, (15.3174) \, \sqrt{1 + \frac{1}{97} + \frac{(74 - 82.8041)^2}{42099.2784}}$$

$$80.69 \pm 30.5121$$

$$50.18, \; 111.20$$

If we drew repeated random samples from our population of pediatric patients with asthma, performed the regression analysis, and constructed a 95% confidence interval for each patient whose peak flow equals 74, we would expect approximately 95% of these intervals to include the patient's FEV_1 measurement. The practical interpretation is that we are 95% confident that the single confidence interval captures the patient's FEV_1 measurement (Daniel, 1991, p 394).

The 95% confidence interval for each patient's FEV_1 measurement, corresponding to a given peak flow value, appears in the last two columns of Table 17–1. Compare the width of this interval to the interval about the predicted mean. For example, for Patient 50, peak flow equals 119 (column 2); the predicted FEV_1 measurement is 107.99 (column 4); the 95% confidence interval about this patient's FEV_1 measurement extends from approximately 77 to 139. The 95% confidence interval about the predicted mean FEV_1 value for the *subpopulation* of patients with a peak flow of 119 ranges from approximately 102 to 114.

If we plot the lower and upper limits of each interval on the scatter diagram with the regression line and connect all the lower limits with one line and upper limits with another line, we obtain a graphic representation of the confidence limits about the individual FEV_1 values for given peak flow measurements. Figure 17–2 contains the confidence limits depicted graphically. Observe that the upper and lower lines are slightly concave, indicating that the confidence intervals about the individual FEV_1 measurement are somewhat wider as we move in either direction away from the mean peak flow of 82.80.

SUMMARY

We compute the regression equation if the assumptions of linearity, independence, and homoscedasticity appear reasonably well satisfied from an examination of the scatter diagram. Normality typically is assumed. We test the null hypothesis of zero slope to determine if the regression equation is useful statistically. A conventional hypothesis test and two-sided confidence interval produce equivalent results, if a nondirectional alternative hypothesis is postulated. The Student's t statistic with $n - 2$ degrees of freedom is employed in the hypothesis test and the confidence interval. We conclude that the *linear* relationship between X and Y is not strong enough to use for prediction if the null hypothesis of zero slope is retained. We infer that the regression equation can be used for

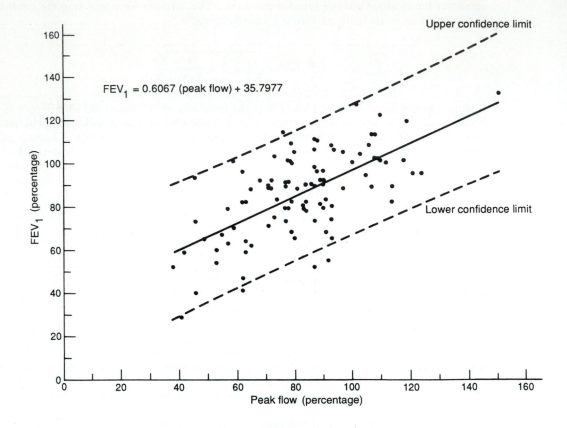

Figure 17–2. Ninety-five percent confidence limits about individual FEV_1 measurements.

prediction if the null hypothesis is rejected. The equation can be employed to predict the mean Y value for the subpopulation of individuals who have the same X value. In addition, the equation can be applied to obtain the predicted Y value for a single individual. Confidence intervals are then constructed about these predictions. The interval about the predicted mean value for a subpopulation of patients is narrower than the interval about an individual's predicted value, because variation among sample statistics is less than variation among individual observations. Procedures illustrated in this chapter are summarized in Table 17–2.

REFERENCES

Daniel W: *Biostatistics: A Foundation in the Health Sciences,* 5th ed. Wiley, 1991.
Minium E, King B, Bear G: *Statistical Reasoning in Psychology and Education,* 3rd ed. Wiley, 1993.

Table 17–2. Summary of procedures for testing the null hypothesis of zero slope and for constructing confidence intervals.

Assumptions

Linearity
Independence
Normality
Equal vertical dispersion (homoscedasticity)

Hypothesis	Formula	Probability Distribution and Tables
$H_0: \beta = 0$	$t = \dfrac{b - \beta_0}{s_b}$ with $df = n - 2$ $s_b = \dfrac{s_{y.x}}{\sqrt{\sum X_i - \dfrac{(\sum X_i)^2}{n}}}$ $s_{y.x} = \sqrt{\dfrac{1}{n-2}\left(\sum (Y_i - \overline{Y})^2 - \dfrac{[\sum(X_i - \overline{X})(Y_i - \overline{Y})]^2}{\sum (X_i - \overline{X})^2}\right)}$	Student's t distribution Student's t table
$H_0: \beta = 0$ $H_A: \beta \neq 0$	Confidence interval about the slope: $b \pm t_{\alpha/2}s_b$	Student's t distribution Student's t table

Confidence Intervals

About predicted mean Y values for given X	$\hat{Y}_i \pm t_{\alpha/2}s_{y.x}\sqrt{\dfrac{1}{n} + \dfrac{(X - \overline{X})^2}{\sum (X - \overline{X})^2}}$	Student's t distribution Student's t table
About individual Y values for given X	$\hat{Y}_i \pm t_{\alpha/2}s_{y.x}\sqrt{1 + \dfrac{1}{n} + \dfrac{(X - \overline{X})^2}{\sum (X - \overline{X})^2}}$	Student's t distribution Student's t table

Self-study Questions

Part I: Definitions

Define each of the following terms:

Confidence band
Predictive error
Standard error of estimate
Standard error of the slope

Part II: Application

Read each of the following descriptions and answer the questions, as indicated.

1. Investigators studied the relationship between body temperature and white blood cell count in patients with septic arthritis caused by clostridia. The goal was to determine if white blood cell count could be predicted from body temperature. The researchers hypothesized that the two variables would be related directly. *Write the statistical hypotheses.*
2. The relationship between anxiety (X) and scores on the Internal Medicine Subject Examination (Y) developed by the National Board of Medical Examiners was investigated in a midwestern college of medicine ($n = 179$). Subject examination scores and anxiety were measured continuously. The scatter diagram revealed that students who exhibited the

least anxiety tended to achieve low subject examination scores. Students who were moderately anxious earned the highest test scores. Students whose anxiety was highest tended to earn subject examinations scores comparable to students who demonstrated the least anxiety. A linear regression line was fitted to the X, Y observations to determine if subject examination scores could be predicted from anxiety level. The null hypothesis of zero slope versus a two-tailed alternative was tested. The null hypothesis was retained (p-value = 0.80). The investigators concluded that subject examination performance in internal medicine and anxiety are unrelated, and that anxiety is not a predictor of performance. *Comment on the appropriateness of the conclusion.*

3. The relationship between teenage drug and/or alcohol use (yes/no) and number of absences from high school classes was studied in 2076 freshman through senior high school students in an urban area on the West Coast. The objective was to determine if number of absences could be predicted from drug and/or alcohol use. *Comment on the appropriateness of performing a linear regression and testing the null hypothesis of zero slope.*

4. Investigators examined the effect of inhaled beclomethasone, a corticosteroid, on bone mineral density in 5-year-old children with asthma. All 48 children had been treated with inhaled beclomethasone, 300 to 800 µg/day, for a minimum of 9 months before the study began. Bone mineral density (Y) and cumulative beclomethasone dose (X) were examined to determine whether cumulative drug dose and bone mineral density varied indirectly. A regression analysis revealed a near zero slope for the prediction of bone mineral density from cumulative drug dose (p-value = 0.77). Assume the linear regression analysis is appropriate. *Interpret these findings.*

5. Cat scratch disease is diagnosed commonly in patients who have unexplained regional lymphadenopathy, after having been scratched or bitten by a cat or kitten. Serum from 67 patients diagnosed with the disease was tested weekly for antibodies to *Rochalimaea henselae* over a 25-week period after the onset of lymphadenopathy. The investigators found that time after onset of lymphadenopathy was highly predictive of antibody titer, with titer decreasing as time after onset increased ($b = -0.75$, p-value < 0.005). *Comment on the appropriateness of using the linear regression model to examine these data.*

6. A linear regression analysis was done to predict weight from height for 3059 females, ages 5 to 12 years. The scatter diagram revealed relatively small positive and negative differences between the actual and predicted weight for shorter females, and large positive and negative differences among taller females. The null hypothesis of zero slope versus the alternative of a greater than zero slope was tested; the null hypothesis was rejected ($b = 2.51$, p-value < 0.001). *Interpret the findings.*

Part III: Analysis

1. Clinicians studied cerebral blood flow in 42 patients who suffer acute panic attacks. The researchers hypothesized that increased blood flow would decrease the severity of the attack. Thirty-six patients who experience acute panic attacks received sodium lactate infusions at the onset of an acute attack. The investigators measured change in cerebral blood flow (X) and change in panic attack severity (Y) for each patient. Change in cerebral blood flow (X) was used to predict change in panic attack severity (Y). Follow the six-step process to test the null hypothesis of zero slope. Set $\alpha = 0.05$ and use the following information:

$$b_{y.x} = -0.8803$$

$$s_{y.x} = 8.5880$$

$$\sum X^2 - \frac{(\sum X)^2}{n} = 2939.1975$$

2. Easily determined from an x-ray, the distance from the upper pole calyx to the spine can be useful in diagnosing kidney disease in the pediatric patient, when gas and feces obscure the renal margins. Several observers have suggested that the upper pole calyces move closer to the spine when pyelonephritic scarring occurs. However, no definitive documen-

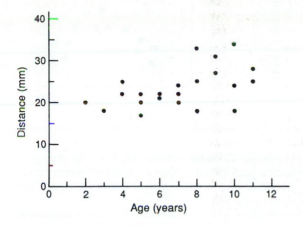

Figure 17–3. Scatter diagram of age and distance from the kidney to the spine in 24 healthy female patients, ages 2–11 years. (Adapted with permission from Friedland G, Filly R, Brown B. Distance of upper pole calyx to spine and lower pole calyx to ureter as indicators of parenchymal loss in children. *Pediatric Radiology* 1974;2:29–38.)

tation of these findings existed then the current investigation was designed. Three radiologists studied the x-rays of 177 females, ages birth to 11 years. The researchers measured the distance from the upper pole calyx of the kidney to the spine in healthy females and in those with parenchymal scarring. Among other things, the investigators hoped to determine if this distance could help differentiate healthy females from those with parenchmal scarring. A portion of the data for 24 healthy females, ages 2 to 11 years, appears in Figure 17–3.

a. Examine Fig 17–3 and comment on the appropriateness of a linear regression analysis. Note that 22 distinct pairs of points are plotted, because (5,20) and (5,20) overlie each other, as do (7,20) and (7,20).

b. Conduct a linear regression analysis.

c. Test the null hypothesis of zero slope using the Student's t test; set $\alpha = 0.05$. Use a two-tailed test.

d. Construct the 95% two-sided confidence interval about the slope and compare the result to the hypothesis test.

Summary data appear below:

X = age (years)
Y = distance (mm) from the inside wall of the kidney to the spine
$\Sigma X = 167$
$\Sigma X^2 = 1309$
$\Sigma Y = 556$
$\Sigma Y^2 = 13,384$
$\Sigma XY = 4010$

Solutions

Part II: Application

1. H_0: β = 0

   H_A: β > 0

2. As shown in Figure 17–4, Internal Medicine Subject Examination scores and anxiety are related curvilinearly, based on the description of the scatter diagram. The conclusion that the subject examination score and anxiety are unrelated is incorrect, as is the conclusion

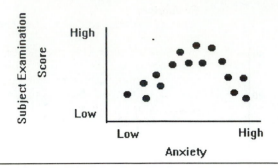

Figure 17–4. Prediction of internal medicine subject examination score from anxiety.

that anxiety is not a predictor of performance. Because a *linear* relationship does not occur, we cannot predict subject examination performance from a *linear* regression equation. We would find that anxiety is an excellent predictor of subject examination performance, if a *curvilinear* equation were fitted to the data.

3. The linear regression model requires that the criterion (Y) and predictor (X) be measured quantitatively. Teenage drug and/or alcohol use is a qualitative variable. The linear regression approach is not appropriate for these data.

4. The findings indicate that bone mineral density is not affected adversely by the cumulative dose of inhaled beclomethasone in 5-year-old children with asthma.

5. The linear regression model is not appropriate because the assumption of *independence* is violated in a repeated measures design. Serum from study participants was tested weekly for antibodies to *Rochalimaea henselae* over a 25-week period, after onset of lymphadenopathy.

6. The use of a linear regression analysis is troublesome because the errors of prediction are not homoscedastic. Vertical dispersion about the regression line is smaller for shorter females and larger for taller females, suggesting greater error in our predictions as age increases. Another analysis should be used because homoscedasticity is violated.

Part III: Analysis

1. *Acute Panic Attacks*
Scientific Hypothesis:
Increases in cerebral blood flow in patients receiving sodium lactate infusions at the onset of an acute panic attack are predictive of decreases in the severity of the attack.
Statistical Hypotheses:

$$H_0: \beta = 0$$

$$H_A: \beta < 0$$

Determine the Test Criteria:
a. Use the t distribution and t statistic.
b. $\alpha = 0.05$.
c. $df = n - 2 = 42 - 2 = 40$; $t_{crit} = -1.684$ (for a one-tailed test).
Analysis:
Calculate the standard error of the slope:

$$s_b = \frac{s_{y.x}}{\sqrt{\Sigma X^2 - \frac{(\Sigma X)^2}{n}}} = \frac{8.5880}{\sqrt{2939.1975}} = 0.1584$$

Compute the t statistic:

$$t = \frac{b - \beta_0}{s_b} = \frac{-0.8803}{0.1584} = -5.5574$$

Evaluation:
The null hypothesis of zero slope is rejected.
Interpretation:
The slope of the regression line for predicting changes in the severity of an acute panic attack from changes in cerebral blood flow following sodium lactate infusion is significantly less than zero ($b = -0.8803$, p-value < 0.0005). Increases in cerebral blood flow were associated significantly with decreases in panic attack severity.

2. *Kidney to Spine Distance*

   a. We see from Figure 17–3 that (X, Y) points vary directly; that is, as age increases, distance from the upper pole calyx to the spine tends to increase in these 24 healthy females. A straight, rather than curved, line appears to describe the relationship between age and distance. Vertical dispersion about an imaginary regression line appears somewhat greater for older children than younger children. However, the assumption of homoscedasticity appears to be reasonably satisfied in light of the relatively small number of observations.

   b. *Regression Analysis:*
      Assemble givens:

X = age (years)
Y = distance (mm) from the inside wall of the kidney to the spine
$\Sigma X = 167$
$\Sigma X^2 = 1309$
$\Sigma Y = 556$
$\Sigma Y^2 = 13,384$
$\Sigma XY = 4010$

Calculate means and standard deviations:
These are important because they help other clinicians judge the extent to which their patients resemble individuals from whom data were collected.

$$\bar{X} = \frac{167}{24} = 6.9583 \text{ years old}$$

$$s_x^2 = \frac{1309 - \dfrac{167^2}{24}}{24 - 1} = \frac{146.9583}{23} = 6.3895$$

$$s_X = 2.5277$$

$$\bar{Y} = \frac{556}{24} = 23.1667 \text{ mm}$$

$$s_Y^2 = \frac{13,384 - \dfrac{556^2}{24}}{24 - 1} = \frac{503.3333}{23} = 21.8841$$

$$s_Y = 4.6780$$

Compute the slope and intercept of the regression line:

$$b_{y.x} = \frac{4010 - \dfrac{167(556)}{24}}{1309 - \dfrac{167^2}{24}} = \frac{141.1667}{146.9583} = 0.9606$$

$$a_{y.x} = 23.1667 - 0.9606\,(6.9583) = 16.4826$$

The regression analysis reveals that a 1-year increase in age is associated with a 0.9606 mm increase in predicted distance from the kidney to the spine. The regression line appears in Figure 17–5. Does the slope differ significantly from zero? Is this regression equation useful statistically for predicting distance from age? These questions are answered by testing the null hypothesis of zero slope.

c. *Test the Null Hypothesis of Zero Slope:*
Scientific hypothesis:
The age of a healthy pediatric female patient, 2 to 11 years, is a useful statistical predictor of the distance from the upper pole calyx of the kidney to the spine (mm). The slope of the regression equation will differ significantly from zero.
Statistical hypotheses:

$$H_0: \beta = 0$$

$$H_A: \beta \neq 0$$

Determine the test criteria:

Use the Student's t distribution and t statistic
$\alpha = 0.05$
$df = 24 - 2 = 22;\ t_{crit} = \pm 2.074$

Analysis:
Calculate the standard error of estimate:

$$s_{y.x} = \sqrt{\frac{1}{22}\left(503.3333 - \frac{141.6667^2}{146.9583}\right)} = 4.0830$$

Compute the standard error of the slope:

$$s_b = \frac{4.0830}{\sqrt{146.9583}} = 0.3368$$

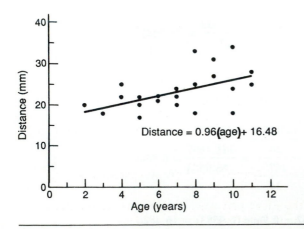

Distance = 0.96(age)+ 16.48

Figure 17–5. Regression analysis of kidney to spine distance and age in 24 healthy female patients, ages 2–11 years.

Obtain the t ratio:

$$t = \frac{0.9606 - 0}{0.3368} = 2.85$$

Evaluation:
The null hypothesis of zero slope is rejected ($t_{calc} = 2.85$, $t_{crit} = \pm 2.074$, $df = 22$, p-value < 0.01, $\alpha = 0.05$).
Interpretation:
The slope of the regression line for predicting the distance from the kidney to the spine from the age of healthy female pediatric patients, ages 2 to 11 years, differs significantly from zero (p-value < 0.01). Age in these patients is a useful statistical predictor of the kidney to spine distance.

  d. *Construct the two-sided 95% confidence interval about the slope:*

$$0.9606 \pm 2.074(0.3368) = 0.9606 \pm 0.6985$$

$$0.2621, 1.6591$$

$$(0.26 \leq \beta \leq 1.66)$$

Compare the results from the confidence interval and hypothesis test:
The confidence interval and hypothesis test provide equivalent findings with respect to the null hypothesis of zero slope. Based on the hypothesis test, the null hypothesis is rejected. It is rejected based on the 95% two-sided confidence interval because zero, the value given in the null hypothesis, is not captured in the interval that extends from approximately 0.26 to 1.66.

Describing the Relationship Between Two Quantitative Variables

18

Clinical Example: The Effect of Beclomethasone on Bone Mineral Content

Konig and associates (1993) investigated the effect of an inhaled corticosteroid, beclomethasone, on bone mineral content in two groups of chidren with asthma. Children in the experimental group were treated with inhaled beclomethasone; children in the control group did not receive corticosteroids. The Pearson correlation between bone mineral density measured radiographically and bone mineral content by single-photon densitometry in the combined group of beclomethasone-treated and control patients was 0.779.

Clinical Example: The Association Between FEV₁ and Peak Flow Measurements

The Pearson correlation between the FEV_1 and peak flow measurements presented in Chapters 16 and 17 is approximately 0.64.

What is a Pearson correlation coefficient? What does a Pearson correlation of approximately 0.64 or 0.78 indicate about the relationship between two variables? Are these coefficients statistically significant? For which clinical questions is correlation more appropriate than regression? These questions are addressed in this chapter.

OBJECTIVES

When you complete this chapter, you should be able to:

- Understand how to test a null hypothesis about a Pearson correlation coefficient.
- Understand how to construct a two-sided confidence interval about a Pearson correlation.
- Use a two-sided confidence interval to test a null hypothesis about a Pearson correlation.
- Translate the results from a test of a null hypothesis or confidence interval into nonstatistical terms.

CORRELATION VERSUS REGRESSION

We focused on simple linear regression in the last two chapters. Recall that regression is used when the goal is to *predict* values of a quantitative outcome (dependent variable) from values of a quantitative predictor (independent variable). The regression equation for predicting Y from X for a set of (X,Y) observations will differ from the equation for predicting X from Y for the same set of observations, unless our predictions are perfect, where $Y_i = \hat{Y}_i$ for every X_i. Thus, we must identify one variable as the outcome and the other as the predictor variable in regression. The goal of correlation, in contrast, is to describe *the strength of the relationship* between two quantitative variables. Daniel (1991) notes that "Correlation . . . implies a co-relationship between variables that puts them on an equal footing and does not distinguish between them by referring to one as the dependent and the other as the independent variable" (p 398). The correlation between X and Y for a set of (X,Y) observations is the same as the correlation between Y and X for the same set of observations.

Given their different goals, are regression and correlation incompatible? We do not perform a regression analysis unless we differentiate the outcome from the predictor, because the regression of X-on-Y and Y-on-X will differ unless the correlation is $\pm$ 1.00. However, we typically report the correlation coefficient as part of a regression analysis. The regression analysis addresses the question of predictability; the correlation focuses on the magnitude of the linear relationship. Correlation alone is employed, however, if the sole objective is to describe the strength of the relationship between two variables.

PEARSON CORRELATION COEFFICIENT

A common measure of association named after Karl Pearson, the **Pearson correlation** is also referred to as the "product-moment correlation," "Pearson's coefficient of correlation," or simply "correlation" (Minium et al, 1993, p 150). In this chapter, we use "correlation" as a synonym for "Pearson correlation." Because several correlation coefficients exist (eg, Spearman's rank correlation, eta, and phi), investigators should specify the type of correlation used in published studies. Other measures of association are listed in Table 18–1.

The Pearson correlation between X and Y is designated ρ_{XY} (rho$_{XY}$), when calculated from a *population* of X,Y observations, and r_{XY} when generated from a *sample of* (X,Y) observations; r_{XY} is an estimator of ρ_{XY}. The sample correlation is

$$r_{XY} = \frac{\sum(X_i - \overline{X})(Y_i - \overline{Y})}{\sqrt{\sum(X_i - \overline{X})^2 \, (Y_i - \overline{Y})^2}}$$

18.1

The super- and subscripts are omitted for convenience from the summation operator. Summation is over all (X,Y) pairs of points. A more convenient computational form is derived by performing the algebra, distributing the summation operator, replacing $\bar{X}$ and $\bar{Y}$ by their computational equivalents, and simplifying the equation to produce

$$r_{xy} = \frac{\sum X_i Y_i - \dfrac{(\sum X_i)(\sum Y_i)}{n}}{\sqrt{\left[\sum X_i^2 - \dfrac{(\sum X_i)^2}{n} \right]\left[\sum Y_i^2 - \dfrac{(\sum Y_i)^2}{n} \right]}} \qquad 18.2$$

All quantities have been defined in previous chapters:

$\sum X_i Y_i$ is the sum of the cross products.

$\sum X_i$ and $\sum Y_i$ are the sum of X and Y, respectively.

$\sum X_i^2$ and $\sum Y_i^2$ are the sum-of-squares of X and Y, respectively.

$(\sum X_i)^2$ and $(\sum Y_i)^2$ are the square-of-the-sum of X and Y, respectively.

$\sum X_i^2 - \dfrac{(\sum X_i)^2}{n}$ is the numerator of the standard deviation (or variance) of X.

$\sum Y_i^2 - \dfrac{(\sum Y_i)^2}{n}$ is the numerator of the standard deviation (or variance) of Y.

Properties of the Pearson Correlation

The following properties describe the Pearson correlation:

1. It is a measure of the strength of the *linear* relationship between two quantitative variables.

2. It is an index with no units of measurement.

Inspect either Formula 18.1 or 18.2; note that the units of measurement for X and Y cancel out when we divide the numerator by the denominator (Colton, 1974, p 206).

3. It varies between -1.00 and $+1.00$.

4. A zero correlation signals a lack of *linear* relationship.

5. A positive correlation indicates that X and Y are related directly, that is, as X tends to increase, Y tends to increase, and vice versa.

6. A negative correlation indicates that X and Y are related indirectly or inversely, that is, as X tends to increase, Y tends to decrease, and vice versa.

Because the Pearson correlation is a measure of linear association, we construct and examine scatter diagrams to detect departures from linearity, and to gain an understanding of the nature of the relationship between X and Y. Fig 18–1 contains plots of (X,Y) observations reflecting different degrees of association. A perfect positive correlation is depicted in diagram A. All points fall directly on a straight line that rises from left to right. A *direct* relationship exists among these points; that is, Y increases as X increases, and vice versa. A perfect negative correlation is graphed in diagram B. All points fall directly on a straight line that falls as we move from left to right. An inverse or indirect relationship exists; that is, Y decreases as X increases, and vice versa. The pattern of (X,Y) points resembles an oval when the correlation equals zero, as shown in C. The correlation also equals zero when the relationship between X and Y is markedly curvilinear, as shown in D. A transformation to achieve linearity or other coefficients, such as eta, may be appropriate if the relationship between X and Y is curvilinear. The plot of the (X,Y) pairs of points becomes more elongated and

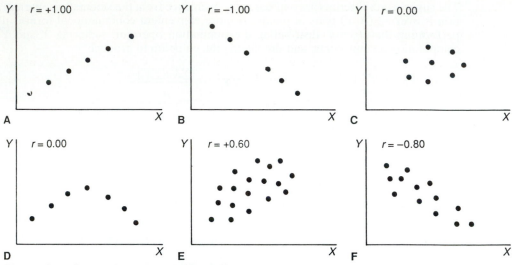

Figure 18–1. Scatter diagrams and different Pearson correlation coefficients.

narrower as the correlation approaches either +1.00 or −1.00, eg, diagrams E (r = +0.60) and F (r = −0.80).

Correlation coefficients are described frequently by adjectives such as indirect, direct, weak, moderate, or strong. Direct and indirect signal the *direction* or *sign* of the relationship. A positive correlation depicts a direct relationship; as noted above, values of X tend to increase as Y increases, and vice versa. An indirect relationship is described by a negative correlation; in this case, values of X tend to increase as Y decreases, and vice versa. Coefficients between ± 0.10 and ± 0.30 are typically considered weak; correlations between approximately ± 0.40 and ± 0.70 often are described as moderate; coefficients of ± 0.80 and above are considered strong.

Assumptions Underlying the Pearson Correlation

The (X,Y) points are assumed to vary together in what is known as a joint distribution. The joint distribution is referred to as a bivariate normal distribution if it is normal (ie, Gaussian). The following assumptions are required to test hypotheses about the Pearson correlation:

1. A normally distributed subpopulation of Y values exists for each value of X.

2. A normally distributed subpopulation of X values exists for each value of Y.

3. The joint distribution of X and Y is a bivariate normal distribution.

4. The subpopulations of Y values have the same variance.

5. The subpopulations of X values have the same variance.

If the above assumptions are not satisfied, at least reasonably, a test of the null hypothesis about a population correlation will produce invalid results, even though the Pearson correlation can still be computed as a descriptive statistic (Daniel, 1991, p 398). In such cases, consult a statistician to determine if a transformation would remedy a violation of assumptions or if another type of correlation coefficient may be computed.

Calculating the Pearson Correlation

The FEV_1/peak flow data are used to illustrate the calculation of the correlation. The following quantities were generated in Chapter 17:

Peak Flow	FEV$_1$
$\sum X_i = 8032.00$	$\sum Y_i = 8345.00$
$\sum X_i^2 = 707,182.00$	$\sum Y_i^2 = 755,711.00$

$$\sum X_i Y_i = 716,540.00$$

$$n = 97$$

$$\sum X_i^2 - \frac{(\sum X_i)^2}{n} = 42,099.2784 \quad \sum Y_i^2 - \frac{(\sum Y_i)^2}{n} = 37,782.9072$$

The correlation is

$$r_{xy} = \frac{716,540 - \frac{(8032)(8345)}{97}}{\sqrt{(42,099.27840)(37,782.9072)}} = 0.6404.$$

This coefficient indicates that a *moderate* direct relationship exists between FEV_1 and peak flow values. Is this coefficient of sufficient magnitude to indicate that these two variables are correlated in the population of pediatric patients with asthma? One of the most common approaches used to answer this question is to test the null hypothesis that the population correlation equals zero. This procedure is illustrated after a brief comment about the descriptive interpretation of the correlation.

COEFFICIENT OF DETERMINATION—r^2

The coefficient of determination, represented as r^2, is the proportion of variation in one variable associated with changes in the other variable. This coefficient is used descriptively to describe the strength of the linear relationship. For example, the Pearson correlation between FEV_1 and peak flow measurements is approximately 0.64; $r^2 \approx 0.41$. Thus, 41% (0.41 × 100%) of the variation in FEV_1 measurements is associated with changes in peak flow values. Recall the first clinical example at the beginning of the chapter. The correlation between bone mineral density measured radiographically and bone mineral content assessed by single-photon densitometry is 0.779. Thus, approximately 61% of variation in bone mineral density measured radiographically is associated with the values of bone mineral content as determined by single-photon densitometry. Although the coefficient of determination is a useful *descriptive* measure to depict the strength of the relationship between two quantitative variables, tests of significance and confidence intervals are used to determine the statistical significance of a Pearson correlation.

TESTING THE HYPOTHESIS THAT THE CORRELATION EQUALS ZERO

The Student's t statistic is used to test the null hypothesis of a zero correlation. The sampling distribution of the correlation is approximately normal, when the population correlation is zero. The t statistic is

$$t = r \sqrt{\frac{n-2}{1-r^2}}, \text{ with } df = n - 2 \qquad\qquad 18.3$$

where r is the Pearson correlation and n is the number of pairs of (X,Y) observations. The null hypothesis is $H_0 : \rho = 0$; the alternative hypothesis may be directional or nondirectional, depending on the question of interest. A test of the null hypothesis that $\rho = 0$ is presented in Box 18–1 for the FEV_1/peak flow data. A nondirectional scientific hypothesis is formulated because in this case a direct or indirect relationship would be clinically significant.

Box 18–1. Test of the null hypothesis that the population correlation equals zero for the FEV_1/peak flow data.

---

1. *State the Scientific Hypothesis*
   The correlation between FEV_1 and peak flow measurements differs from zero.

2. *Formulate the Statistical Hypotheses*
   $H_0 : = 0$
   $H_A : \neq 0$

3. *Determine the Test Criteria*
   a. Use the t distribution and t statistic.
   b. $\alpha = 0.05$.
   c. $df = n - 2$; $df = 97 - 2 = 95$; $t_{crit} = \pm 1.98$ (approximately for a two-tailed test).

4. *Analyze the Data*
   Compute the t statistic:
   $$t = \sqrt{0.6404 \frac{97-2}{1-0.6404^2}} = 0.6404 \sqrt{161.0476} = 0.6404 \, (12.6905) = 8.1270 \approx 8.13$$

5. *Evaluate the Statistics*
   The null hypothesis of a zero population correlation is rejected.

6. *Interpret the Statistics*
   The correlation between FEV_1 and peak flow measurements ($r = 0.64$) differs significantly from zero ($t_{calc} \cong 8.13$, $t_{crit} = \pm 1.98$, p-value < 0.001, $\alpha = 0.05$).

The scientific hypothesis is stated in step 1. The null and alternative hypothesis appear in step 2. The test criteria are formulated in the third step, including the critical value of the test statistic. We approximate the critical value by utilizing the one that corresponds to $df = 120$ for a two-tailed test with $\alpha = 0.05$. The computed t statistic equals approximately 8.13. The calculated value is compared to the critical value of t in step 5 and the null hypothesis is rejected ($t_{calc} \approx 8.13$ versus $t_{crit} \approx \pm 1.98$). The statistical result is interpreted in the last step. We note that the correlation between FEV_1 and peak flow measurements differs significantly from zero (p-value < 0.001, $\alpha = 0.05$). We obtain the p-value by (1) consulting Table A–2 in the appendix of statistical tables and (2) observing that the calculated value of 8.13 exceeds the critical value of ± 3.373 for $df = 120$ and $\alpha = 0.001$; therefore, the p-value is less than 0.001.

In summary, the Student's t distribution and t statistic with $df = n - 2$ are appropriate to test a null hypothesis about a Pearson correlation only when H_0: $\rho = 0$. The approach employed to test a null hypothesis when ρ is some value other than zero is demonstrated next.

TESTING THE HYPOTHESIS THAT THE CORRELATION EQUALS A NONZERO VALUE

Because the sampling distribution of the correlation is skewed when ρ is nonzero, the t test is inappropriate. For example, consider that $\rho = 0.70$. Samples of the same size drawn randomly from this population will produce sample coefficients that can exceed 0.70, up to a maximum of +1.00. Thus, +1.00 acts as a "positive ceiling." Keep in mind, however, that coefficients may vary in the opposite direction, between 0.70 and −1.00. Therefore, the distribution of the sample correlations is skewed. Consequently, we address this problem by transforming the sample correlations to produce a distribution of values that is approximately normal. We can then rely on a variant of the z statistic to determine the tenability of the null hypothesis.

The first step is to use **Fisher's transformation** to transform the sample correlation:

$$Z_r = \frac{1}{2} \ln \frac{1 + r}{1 - r} \qquad \qquad \textbf{18.4}$$

where Z_r is Fisher's transformed value, ln is the natural logarithm, and r is the sample correlation. It can be shown that Z_r is distributed approximately normally with a mean of $\frac{1}{2} \ln \frac{1 + \rho}{1 - \rho}$ and standard deviation of $\frac{1}{\sqrt{n - 3}}$ (Daniel, 1991, p 404).

The second step is to use Fisher's transformation to transform the value of ρ given in the null hypothesis. The third step is to use the two transformed values to compute the z statistic (Marascuilo & Serlin, 1988, pp 330–332):

$$z = \frac{Z_r - Z_\rho}{1/\sqrt{n - 3}} \qquad \qquad \textbf{18.5}$$

Fisher's Z values, calculated for values of the correlation between 0.00 and 0.99, appear in Table A–4 in the appendix of statistical tables. The values of r appear in one column and corresponding values of Z_r appear in the next column. For example, if $r = 0.20$, then $Z_r = 0.2027$. We can use these tabled values or Formula 18.4 to transform the Pearson correlations. Testing a null hypothesis about a nonzero correlation is demonstrated in the next example.

Clinical Example: Testing Human Sera for Tuberculin Antibody

Consider that it is well established that two commonly used methods to test human sera for tuberculin antibody produce results that correlate at 0.93. As director of your hospital's clinical laboratory, you conduct studies regularly to determine if laboratory results meet established norms. You are particularly concerned when correlations between different methods are less than well-established values. You randomly select 25 specimens of human sera tested for tuberculin antibody and correlate the logarithms of the titers obtained by both methods. The Pearson correlation is 0.80. Is this correlation compatible with a population correlation of 0.93, or is it significantly less—requiring further study of laboratory procedures?

The question is addressed in Box 18–2. As in previous examples, we begin by formulating the scientific and statistical hypotheses (steps 1 and 2). In step 3 we specify the test criteria; the critical value of z is −1.645 for a one-tailed, less than, test with $\alpha = 0.05$. The sample and population correlations are transformed to Fisher's Z values in the next step. Table A–4 is consulted. For example, the Fisher's Z value is 1.0990 for $r = 0.80$. The transformed values are used to compute the z statistic; the calculated value is approximately −2.62. The null hypothesis that $\rho = 0.93$ is rejected in step 5, because the calculated value falls in the region of rejection ($z_{crit} = -1.645$). Thus, the correlation between results from the two methods to test tuberculin antibody in human sera is significantly less in this laboratory than the well accepted norm ($r = 0.80$, $\rho = 0.93$, p-value < 0.004, $\alpha = 0.05$).

In addition to employing Fisher's transformation and the z statistic to test a null hypothesis about a nonzero population correlation, we can use the transformed values to construct a confidence interval about the observed correlation. Two-sided confidence intervals are demonstrated next with the FEV_1/peak flow data.

Box 18–2. Testing the null hypothesis that the correlation between two methods for testing tuberculin antibody equals 0.93.

1. *State the Scientific Hypothesis*
The correlation between two commonly used methods to test human sera for tuberculin antibody is less than 0.93.
2. *Formulate the Statistical Hypotheses*
H_0: $\rho = 0.93$
H_A: $\rho < 0.93$
3. *Determine the Test Criteria*
   a. Use the z distribution and z statistic.
   b. $\alpha = 0.05$.
   c. $z_{crit} = -1.645$ (for a one-tailed, less than, test).
4. *Analyze the Data*
Consult Table A–4 to transform the sample correlation to a Fisher's Z value:
$r = 0.80$ $Z_r = 1.0990$
Consult Table A–4 to transform the population correlation to a Fisher's Z value:
$\rho = 0.93$ $Z_\rho = 1.6580$
Compute z:

$$z = \sqrt{\frac{1.0990 - 1.6580}{1/\sqrt{25 - 3}}} = \frac{-0.5590}{0.2132} = -2.6219$$

5. *Evaluate the Statistics*
The null hypothesis that the population correlation is 0.93 is rejected.
6. *Interpret the Statistics*
The correlation between results from the two methods to test tuberculin antibody in human sera ($r = 0.80$) is significantly less in this clinical laboratory than the well established norm of 0.93 ($z_{calc} \approx -2.62$, $z_{crit} = -1.645$, p-value < 0.004, $\alpha = 0.05$).

CONSTRUCTING TWO-SIDED CONFIDENCE INTERVALS

Because Fisher's transformation, which is more flexible than the t statistic, can be used to test zero and nonzero null hypotheses, the transformation is employed to form confidence intervals. The two-sided confidence interval is

$$(Z_r - z_{\alpha/2}\frac{1}{\sqrt{n-3}} \leq \rho \leq Z_r + z_{\alpha/2}\frac{1}{\sqrt{n-3}}) \text{ or} \qquad \textbf{18.6a}$$

$$Z_r \pm z_{\alpha/2}\frac{1}{\sqrt{n-3}} \qquad \textbf{18.6b}$$

where Z_r is the Fisher's transformed value of r and $z_{\alpha/2}$ is the two-tailed critical value of z. Note that the limits of the confidence interval, identified as Fisher's transformed values, must be transformed back to values that correspond to the Pearson correlation. The 95% confidence interval for the FEV_1/peak flow data appears in Box 18–3.

As calculated earlier, the Pearson correlation between FEV_1 and peak flow measurements equals 0.6404 (step 1). The value of r is transformed into a Fisher's value in the second step. Formula 18.4 is used to calculate Z_r: $Z_r = 0.7589$. We identify the critical value of z in step 3 ($z_{\alpha/2} = \pm1.96$). The upper and lower limit of the interval are calculated in step 4; the upper limit equals 0.9611 and the lower limit is 0.5567. Next we must change Fisher's transformed values into values that correspond to the Pearson correlation. We approximate these values from Table A–4; the lower and upper limit are approximately 0.51 and 0.75, respectively. We are 95% confident that the correlation between FEV_1 and peak flow measurements is between approximately 0.51 and 0.75 in the population of pediatric patients with asthma. Note that the confidence interval is not symmetric about the sample correlation ($r = 0.6404$) because the sampling distribution of the correlation is skewed.

Recall that we could have used the 95% two-sided confidence interval to test the null hypothesis of zero correlation with $\alpha = 0.05$, versus the alternative that the correlation differs

Box 18–3. Constructing a 95% two-sided confidence interval for FEV_1 and peak flow measurements.

---

1. *Calculate the Pearson Correlation Coefficient*
The Pearson correlation, as calculated earlier in this chapter, equals 0.6404.

2. *Transform r Into a Fisher's Transformed Value*
$r = 0.6404$ $Z_{r= 0.6404} = 0.7589$ (calculated from Formula 18.4)

3. *Identify the Critical Value of z for a 95% Two-sided Interval*
$z_{crit} = \pm 1.96$

4. *Calculate the Upper and Lower Limit of the Confidence Interval*

$$Z_r \pm z_{\alpha/2} \frac{1}{\sqrt{n-3}} = 0.7589 \pm 1.96 \frac{1}{\sqrt{97-3}} = 0.7589 \pm 0.2022 = (0.5567, 0.9611)$$

5. *Transform the Fisher's Value Back to Values Corresponding to the Pearson Correlation*
$Z = 0.5567$ $r \approx 0.51$ (from Table A–4)
$Z = 0.9611$ $r \approx 0.75$ (from Table A–4)

6. *Interpret the Confidence Interval*
We are 95% confident that the correlation between FEV_1 and peak flow measurements in the population of pediatric patients with asthma is between approximately 0.51 and 0.75.

---

from zero. We would reject the null hypothesis if we relied on the confidence interval, because the hypothesized value of ρ (= 0) is not captured in the interval.

OTHER TYPES OF CORRELATION COEFFICIENTS

A brief summary of other types of correlation coefficients is presented in Table 18–1. Individuals who wish to pursue this topic further should consult other sources (eg, Minium et al, 1993; Hays, 1981; or Marascuilo & Serlin, 1988).

Table 18–1. Other measures of association.

Measure of Association	Brief Description
Spearman's rank correlation; also called Spearman's rho or rank order correlation	Correlation between two sets of measurements that have been assigned ranks, such as a rank of 1 for the largest value, a rank of 2 for the second largest value, and so forth. Ranking is done separately for each variable
Phi (ϕ) coefficient	Measure of association between two qualitative variables that are dichotomous (ie, have only two categories)
Contingency coefficient (ϕ')	Measure of association in $r \times c$ contingency tables in which both variables have no underlying numerical continuum; typically used when one variable has 3 or more categories
Point-biserial correlation	Measure of association for which one variable is quantitative and the other is qualitative and dichotomous, with no underlying numerical continuum
Biserial correlation	Measure of association for which one variable is quantitative and the other, which is also quantitative, has been reduced to two categories (eg, below the median and above the median)
Tetrachoric correlation	Measure of association between two quantitative variables; *each* has been reduced to two categories (eg, above the median and below the median)
Correlation ratio; also called eta (η)	Measure of *curvilinear* association between two quantitative variables
Multiple correlation (R)	Correlation between a quantitative outcome variable and best-weighted combination of two or more predictor variables
Partial correlation	Correlation between two quantitative variables, X_1 and X_2, where the linear relationship with a third quantitative variable has been removed statistically from both X_1 and X_2
Part correlation, also called semipartial correlation	Correlation between two quantitative variables, X_1 and X_2, where the linear relationship with a third quantitative variable has been removed statistically from either X_1 or X_2, but not both

SUMMARY

Although they share many similarities, correlation and regression have different objectives. *Predicting* the value of an outcome or dependent variable from the value of an independent or predictor variable is the goal of regression. Determining the *strength of the linear association* between two quantitative variables, neither of which is identified as the independent or dependent variable, is the goal of correlation. The Pearson correlation is a measure of strength of this linear relationship. The Pearson correlation is an index that varies between -1.00 and $+1.00$. A positive coefficient indicates that X and Y are related directly: X tends to increase as Y tends to increase, and vice versa. In contrast, a negative coefficient signals that X and Y are related indirectly; as X tends to increase, Y tends to decrease, and vice versa. Although we assume linearity when we compute and use a correlation as a descriptive measure, we make 5 additional assumptions to test hypotheses about the Pearson correlation, including the following: the subpopulations of Y values have the same variance; the subpopulations of X values have the same variance; and X and Y are distributed as a bivariate normal distribution. If these assumptions are not reasonably satisfied, a test of the null hypothesis about the population correlation will produce invalid results.

The Student's t distribution and t statistic with $df = n - 2$ are used to test the null hypotheses that the population correlation equals zero. The t distribution and t statistic cannot be employed to test a null hypothesis that the population correlation equals a nonzero value, because the distribution of sample correlations is skewed. In this situation, Fisher's transformation is used to transform the sample and population coefficient. Because the distribution of the transformed sample correlations is approximately normal, we can utilize a variant of the z statistic to test the null hypothesis of a nonzero population correlation. Because the z statistic is more flexible than the Student's t, we also use the z statistic to construct confidence intervals.

Assumptions underlying the Pearson correlation and tests about a population correlation are summarized in Table 18–2.

Table 18–2. Summary of Assumptions and Formulae for Calculating and Testing a Pearson Correlation.

Assumptions	Formula	
A normally distributed subpopulation of Y values exists for each value of X. A normally distributed subpopulation of X values exists for each value of Y. The joint distribution of X and Y is a bivariate normal distribution. The subpopulation of Y values have the same variance. The subpopulation of X values have the same variance.		
Pearson Correlation	$r_{xy} = \dfrac{\sum X_i Y_i - \dfrac{(\sum X_i)(\sum Y_i)}{n}}{\sqrt{\left[\sum X_i^2 - \dfrac{(\sum X_i)^2}{n}\right]\left[\sum Y_i^2 - \dfrac{(\sum Y_i)^2}{n}\right]}}$	

Hypothesis	Formula	Probability Distribution and Tables
$H_0 : \rho = 0$	$t = r\sqrt{\dfrac{n-2}{1-r^2}}$ with $df = n-2$	Student's t distribution and t table
$H_0 : \rho = Nonzero$	$Z_r = \dfrac{1}{2}\ln\dfrac{1+r}{1-r}$ $z = \dfrac{Z_r - Z_\rho}{1/\sqrt{n-3}}$	Standard normal curve Table of the standard normal curve
Two-Sided Confidence Interval	$Z_r = \dfrac{1}{2}\ln\dfrac{1+r}{1-r}$ $Z_r \pm z_{\alpha/2}\dfrac{1}{\sqrt{n-3}}$	Standard normal curve Table of the standard normal curve

REFERENCES

Colton T: *Statistics in Medicine.* Little, Brown, 1974.

Daniel W: *Biostatistics: A Foundation for Analysis in the Health Sciences,* 5th ed. Wiley, 1991.

Hays W: *Statistics,* 3rd ed. Holt, Rinehart and Winston, 1981.

Konig P et al: Bone metabolism in children with asthma treated with inhaled beclomethasone dipropionate. *J Pediatr* 1993;**122**:219.

Marascuilo L, Serlin R: *Statistical Methods for the Social and Behavioral Sciences.* Freeman, 1988.

Minium E, King B, Bear G: *Statistical Reasoning in Psychology and Education,* 3rd ed. Wiley, 1993.

Self-study Questions

Part I: Definitions

Define the following terms:

Coefficient of determination   Fisher's transformation   Pearson correlation

Part II: Explanation

Describe briefly when and why Fisher's transformation is used to examine hypotheses about a correlation coefficient.

Part III: Correlation Versus Regression—Which Analysis Should Be Used?

Read each of the following descriptions and indicate whether correlation or regression is the most appropriate analysis.

1. Investigators evaluated the association between a woman's exposure to cigarette smoke and traces of that exposure in newborns within 3 days of birth. The level of cotinine (nanograms), a form of broken-down nicotine, was measured in 194 women and their newborns.
2. A radiologist investigated the utility of noninvasive ultrasound to predict the size of the lumen of the aorta. Data were collected from 28 patients; observations consisted of measurements on an aortogram and ultrasound measurements above the renal arteries.
3. Investigators studied 253 adults with aggressive non-Hodgkin's lymphoma to identify indicators of relapse-free survival. In one analysis, serum concentrations of lactate dehydrogenase (U/mL) were used to estimate relapse-free survival (months) following therapy. In a second analysis, investigators sought to predict relapse-free survival, from tumor size (cm).
4. The relationship between cigarette smoking and shoulder muscle injury was investigated in 67 men with rotator cuff injuries. In the first analysis, the extent of the rotator cuff tear (cm) and number of cigarettes smoked per day were examined. In the second analysis, the extent of the rotator cuff tear (cm) and pack years of smoking were scrutinized.
5. Height, weight, fat-free mass, and age of 139 obese and nonobese prepubertal children, ages 5 to 10 years, were assessed to identify the single best predictor of resting metabolic rate (RMR). Data for boys and girls were analyzed separately.

Part IV: Is the Pearson Correlation Appropriate?

Read each of the following descriptions and determine if the Pearson correlation is the appropriate analysis. If the Pearson correlation coefficient seems appropriate, conclude that assumptions required for its use are reasonably satisfied.

1. At the National Institutes of Health, 480 HIV-positive, pregnant women participated in a clinical trial to determine if taking AZT (yes/no) during pregnancy correlates with the HIV status of newborns (positive/negative). The Pearson correlation was used to examine maternal AZT status (1 = AZT yes/0 = AZT no) and newborn HIV status (1 = positive/0 = negative).
2. The association between symptom-free survival (months) and the use of balloon angioplasty or a new class of drugs (lazaroids) to clear blocked arteries to the brain was investigated in 36 stroke patients. Investigators computed the Pearson correlation between treatment type (1 = angioplasty/0 = drugs) and symptom-free survival (months).
3. The relationship between niacin intake (mg/day) and liver function—defined as serum bilirubin (mg/dL), albumin (g/dL), and alkaline phosphatase (IU/L)—was studied in 76 patients who were taking niacin to lower cholesterol levels. Pearson correlations were calculated between niacin intake (mg/day) and serum bilirubin levels, niacin intake and serum albumin levels, and niacin intake and alkaline phosphatase.
4. The incidence of complications in central vein nutritional support was studied in 22 medical centers over a 12-month period. The Pearson correlation was calculated between the number of patients who had catheter-related complications after receiving central vein nutritional support, and the number of central vein catheters inserted by physicians during this period.
5. Data from 22 countries were used to quantify the relationship during a 12-month period between estimated, average red meat consumption per person (pounds per year) and deaths due to coronary heart disease (per 100,000 population) in patients aged 35 to 64 years. For example, the following data were recorded for one country: an estimated average of 25 pounds of red meat per person per year; 10 deaths due to coronary heart disease per 100,000 persons, ages 35 to 64 years.

Part V: Interpretation

Read the following description and comment on the appropriateness of the conclusions, in light of the information presented.

In 1984, investigators studied the relationship between number of cigarettes smoked per day and number of absences from work over a 12-month period; the study involved 1531 adults, ages 21 to 55 years, who worked on automotive assembly lines in two plants. The Pearson correlation was 0.83 (p-value < 0.001, two-tailed). The investigators concluded that a significant relationship exists between number of cigarettes smoked per day and absences from work in a 1-year period.

The study was repeated in 1994 in the same automotive plants. Seven hundred thirty-six adults, ages 21 to 55 years, were sampled. Cigarettes smoked per day was coded as 0 (0 cigarettes per day) or 1 (1 or more cigarettes per day). The Pearson correlation between number of absences from work in a 12-month period and cigarettes smoked per day was 0.05 (p-value ≈ 0.34, two-tailed).

The researchers stated that the strong relationship that existed 10 years earlier between the number of cigarettes smoked per day and absences from work no longer exists in workers who are employed on automotive assembly lines. The investigators attributed the change to increased public awareness of health risks associated with cigarette smoking and the availability of a "stop smoking" program in the two automotive plants where study participants worked.

Part VI: Extended Analysis

Use the kidney-to-spine distance and the age data in the self-study questions at the end of Chapter 17 to do the following.

1. Calculate the Pearson correlation between distance and age.
2. Test the null hypothesis that the population correlation equals zero against the alternative that the population correlation differs from zero; set $\alpha = 0.05$.
3. Construct the 95% two-sided interval about the sample coefficient.
4. Use the 95% interval to test the statistical hypotheses just described.
5. Compare the results of the conventional significance test to results from the confidence interval.

Summary information appears below for the 24 children included in this portion of the investigation:

X = age (years)
Y = distance (mm) from the inside wall of the kidney to the spine
$\sum X = 167$
$\sum X^2 = 1309$
$\sum Y = 556$
$\sum Y^2 = 13,384$
$\sum XY = 4010$

Solutions

Part II: Explanation

Fisher's transformation is used when the null hypothesis indicates that the population correlations (ρ) is nonzero. The distribution of sample correlation is skewed when ρ is nonzero; consequently, the Student's t distribution and t statistic cannot be used. Because the distribution of Fisher's transformed values is approximately normal, we can use a variation of the z statistic.

Part III: Correlation Versus Regression

1. *Correlation* is more appropriate because the objective is to quantify the strength of the relationship between two quantitative variables.
2. *Regression* analysis is warranted because the radiologist wants to predict the size of the lumen of the aorta from ultrasound measurements.
3. *Regression* is justified for both analyses because the goal is to predict months of relapse-free survival from serum concentrations of lactate dehydrogenase (U/mL) and tumor size (cm).
4. *Correlation* is the appropriate analysis in the investigation of smoking and shoulder muscle injury.
5. *Regression* analyses are indicated in the study of resting metabolic rate. The goal is to identify the single best predictor of resting metabolic rate from among four independent variables: height, weight, fat-free mass, and age.

Part IV: Is the Pearson Correlation Appropriate?

1. The Pearson correlation is *inappropriate* for these data because the two variables are dichotomous, rather than quantitative.
2. Although symptom-free survival was measured quantitatively, treatment type (angioplasty versus drug therapy) is a qualitative variable with two categories. The assignment of numbers to treatment type (1 = angioplasty/0 = drugs) does not render the variable quantitative. Therefore, the Pearson correlation is *inappropriate*.
3. The Pearson correlation is *appropriate* in the niacin study. Niacin intake and all three indicators of liver function were measured quantitatively.

4. Both variables were measured quantitatively in the study of catheter-related complications. Thus, the Pearson correlation is *appropriate*.
5. If we accept that the average estimates of red meat consumption and the data on cause of death are reliable, the Pearson correlation is appropriate because both variables (red meat consumption and deaths) are measured quantitatively. Observe that deaths due to coronary heart disease are reported per 100,000 individuals, because population size differs from country to country.

Part V: Interpretation

The conclusion is unfounded given the results of analyses from which it was developed. A critical error was made in the 1994 study when cigarettes smoked per day was treated as a dichotomous variable. Thus, the Pearson correlation should not have been calculated.

Part VI: Extended Analysis

1. *Obtain the Pearson correlation*

$$r = \frac{4010 - \dfrac{(167)(556)}{24}}{\sqrt{\left[1309 - \dfrac{167^2}{24}\right]\left[13{,}384 - \dfrac{556^2}{24}\right]}} = \frac{141.1667}{\sqrt{146.9853\,(503.333)}} = 0.5190 \approx 0.52$$

2. *Test the Null Hypothesis* (The six-step process is used)
Formulate the scientific hypothesis:
The age of healthy pediatric female patients, 2 to 11 years, is correlated with the distance (mm) from the upper pole calyx of the kidney to the spine.
State the statistical hypotheses:
$H_0: \rho = 0$
$H_A: \rho \neq 0$
Determine the test criteria:
a. Use the Student's t distribution and t statistic.
b. $\alpha = 0.05$.
c. $df = n - 2 = 24 - 2 = 22$; $t_{crit} = \pm 2.074$.

Analyze the Data
Compute the t *statistic:*

$$t = 0.5190 \sqrt{\frac{24 - 2}{1 - 0.5190^2}} = 0.5190\,(5.4873) = 2.8479$$

Evaluate the Statistics
The null hypothesis of a zero population correlation is rejected ($t_{calc} = 2.85$; $t_{crit} = \pm 2.074$, $df = 22$, p-value < 0.01, $\alpha = 0.05$).
Interpret the Statistics
The Pearson correlation ($r = 0.52$) between the distance (mm) from the upper pole calyx to the spine and age in healthy pediatric female patients, 2 to 11 years, differs significantly from zero (p-value < 0.01).
3. *Construct the 95% Two-sided Interval*
Calculate the Fisher's transformed value for r = 0.5190:

$$Z_r = \frac{1}{2}\ln\frac{1+r}{1-r} = \frac{1}{2}\ln\frac{1 + 0.5190}{1 - 0.5190} = 0.5750$$

Construct the interval using the transformed value:

$$Z_r \pm z_{\alpha/2} \frac{1}{\sqrt{n-3}} = 0.5750 \pm 1.96 \frac{1}{\sqrt{24-3}}$$

$$= 0.5750 \pm 1.96 \,(0.2182) = 0.5750 \pm 0.4277$$

$$= 0.1473, \, 1.0027$$

Translate the Fisher's transformed values back to sample correlations:
Use Table A–4 to approximate the sample correlations:

$$Z_r \approx 0.15 \qquad r \approx 0.15$$
$$Z_r \approx 1.02 \qquad r \approx 0.77$$

4. We are 95% confident that the population correlation between the distance (mm) from the upper pole calyx to the spine and age in healthy pediatric female patients, 2 to 11 years, is between approximately 0.15 and 0.77.
5. *Compare the Results from the Confidence Interval and Hypothesis Test*
   The significance test led to the rejection of the null hypothesis that the population correlation equals zero. Based on the 95% two-sided confidence interval, the null hypothesis is also rejected because $\rho = 0$ is not contained in the interval. Both approaches lead to the same conclusion, that is, the null hypothesis is not tenable.

19 Identifying Regression and Correlation Problems in Research

Clinical Example: Hypercholesterolemia and Soy Protein and Soy Fiber

Investigators studied the effects of soy protein and fiber consumption on plasma lipids in 32 hypercholesterolemic men. The researchers hypothesized that the consumption of soy protein and fiber would contribute to (1) a decrease in total serum cholesterol, triglycerides, and low-density lipoprotein levels; and (2) an increase in high-density lipoprotein levels. Study participants followed an 8-week dietary regimen that included 50 g of isolated soy protein and 20 g of soy cotyledon fiber per day. Among their findings the researchers noted that posttreatment total cholesterol was significantly less than the pretreatment level ($\overline{X}_{PRE} = 440 \text{ mg/dL}, \overline{X}_{POST} = 400 \text{ mg/dL}, s_{\overline{d}} = 9.37, t = 4.27, t_{crit} = 1.697, p\text{-value} < 0.0005, \alpha = 0.05$).

What aspect of regression or correlation affects our interpretation of these findings? The answer is a phenomenon known as regression toward the mean. This topic and others, including linearity, causation, sample size, range restriction, and combining samples, are addressed briefly in this chapter.

We noted in Chapter 16 that regression and correlation appear frequently in the medical literature. Altman (1991) estimated that these methods were employed in approximately 35% of the articles published in the past several years in *The New England Journal of Medicine*. Unfortunately, regression and correlation are often abused and misinterpreted. Individuals who read the literature or employ these methods must be aware of the problems associated with the use of these valuable procedures. Because regression and correlation share many features, the problems that affect them are also similar.

OBJECTIVES

When you complete this chapter, you should be able to:

- Describe the three conditions necessary to claim causation.
- Explain why results based on correlation and regression alone should not be used to infer a causal relationship.
- Define and recognize regression toward the mean and range restriction.
- Explain how the absence of linearity affects the magnitude of the Pearson correlation and the slope of the regression line.
- Describe the effect(s) of combining different samples on the magnitude of the Pearson correlation and the usefulness of the regression equation.
- Define outliers and indicate how they affect a correlation and regression analysis.
- Identify problems that affect regression and correlation studies from a description of a study, to its findings, and its conclusions.

CAUSATION

Cause: "An event, such as a change in one variable, that produces another event, such as a change in a second variable" (Vogt, 1993, p 31). Results from regression and correlation studies are insufficient by themselves for establishing a causal relationship.

Although a high Pearson correlation suggests that two quantitative variables are related linearly, it is *never* appropriate to infer a causal relationship solely on the basis of a correlation coefficient. Similarly, if X is a predictor of Y, it is *never* appropriate to assert that X causes Y based only on a regression analysis. Colton (1974, p 214) notes that "correlation indicates that two variables tend to be related. One may directly influence or 'cause' the other to vary, but it is also possible that some other variable, or a whole host of other variables, may influence the two that are correlated."

Vogt (1993, p 31) comments that highly respected researchers and philosophers disagree about what constitutes a cause, and about conditions that must prevail before claiming cause. He suggests, however, that many investigators would agree that three conditions are necessary, but not sufficient, to attribute cause, that is, for X to cause Y: (1) X must precede Y; (2) X and Y must vary together (covary); and (3) no rival explanations exist to account for the covariation of X and Y.

LINEARITY

Linearity: Two quantitative variables are related linearly if their relationship can be described appropriately by a straight line. The discrepancy between the observed and predicted values in a linear regression model will generally increase as the departure from linearity increases. The Pearson correlation will underestimate the strength of the relationship, if it is curvilinear.

A method of describing the relationship between two quantitative variables, simple linear regression requires fitting the best *straight line* to the data; values of the independent variables are used to predict values of the outcome (dependent) variable. Pearson correlation is a method of characterizing the strength of the linear relationship between two quantitative variables.

In general, the more closely the (X,Y) observations follow a straight line when plotted, the higher the Pearson correlation. However, a "high" correlation does not necessarily imply that the line of best fit is a straight one; the relationship between X and Y may depart slightly from linearity and may produce a curved line. Additionally, a "low" correlation does not indicate with certainty that X and Y are unrelated. For example, if we assume we did not commit a Type II error, a test of the null hypothesis of $\beta = 0$ or $\rho = 0$ may be *retained* because (1) the relationship between X and Y is not strong enough to be used for prediction, even though it may be linear; or (2) the association is nonlinear and methods that characterize a linear relationship are inappropriate.

Before calculations begin, a scatter diagram should *always* be constructed and examined for linearity (and homoscedasticity). If a straight line is fitted to a curvilinear relationship, the discrepancy between the observed and predicted values will generally increase as the departure from linearity increases. Further, the Pearson correlation will underestimate the strength of the relationship if it is curvilinear—the more marked the departure from linearity, the greater the underestimation. Although it may be possible to achieve linearity by transforming the data, a statistician should be consulted to determine if a transformation is warranted or if another measure of association is more suitable.

SAMPLE SIZE

Regression and correlation results based on small samples may be misleading; such results must be generalized cautiously.

Like all other statistics, regression coefficients (eg, the slope) and the correlation coefficient are subject to sampling fluctuation; that is, respective values can vary from sample to sample. Moreover, sampling fluctuation typically increases when sample sizes are smaller. Consider the following illustration of the effect of sampling fluctuation and sample size on the Pearson correlation.

Suppose that the population correlation between two quantitative variables is zero. Assume that we obtain repeated random samples of size 5 from this population. Ninety-five percent of these samples will have a sample correlation between -0.88 and $+0.88$ (Edwards, 1976, p 56). Thus, a moderately high sample correlation of 0.80 would not be highly unusual in a sample of 5 observations, even though the population correlation equals zero. If the sample size is increased to 15, 95% of the samples will yield a correlation between -0.51 and $+0.51$ (Minium et al, 1993, p 163). Further, 95% of the samples will yield a correlation between -0.28 and $+0.28$ if the size of each sample is increased to 50, even though $\rho = 0$. Consequently, regression and correlation results derived from small samples must be generalized cautiously; because statistics derived from these samples are relatively unstable, they may not be representative of the population from which the sample was obtained.

COMBINING DIFFERENT SAMPLES

The effect of combining different samples on regression and correlation statistics depends on where the sample values lie relative to one another in both the X and Y dimensions.

The utility of a regression equation and magnitude of the Pearson correlation may be influenced when a sample of observations actually consists of two more subsamples, in which either $\overline{X}$ or $\overline{Y}$ or both differ from sample to sample. A situation like this may occur when, for example, men and women or diseased and nondiseased patients are pooled or combined and treated as if they represent one population. Figure 19–1 contains three diagrams depicting different ways in which samples may be combined. Diagram A contains three samples that have different Y means, but the same X mean. Each sample is represented by an oval drawn

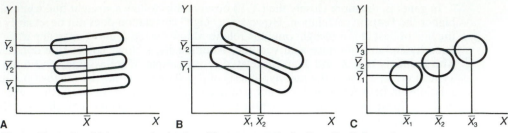

Figure 19–1. Combining samples having different means in the X and/or Y dimension.

to depict the outline of a plot of (X,Y) points. Suppose that these samples represent three populations in which patients have the same approximate mean total cholesterol level (X), but different mean potassium levels due to different diseases. Imagine a regression line drawn through each sample of (X,Y) points. Note the relatively small amount of vertical dispersion about each imaginary regression line. Based on an visual assessment, we would suggest that total cholesterol is a predictor of potassium level in each sample. In addition, a moderate positive correlation exists between cholesterol and potassium levels in each sample.

When the samples are combined as if they represent one population, however, the regression line falls in the middle of the second oval. Vertical dispersion about this line is considerably greater than the vertical dispersion about the imaginary regression line for each sample. Further, the correlation in the combined samples approaches zero. A similar situation exists in diagram B, with the exception that the slope of the regression line and Pearson correlation are negative in each sample. The Pearson correlation decreases substantially when the samples are combined; also, the usefulness of the regression equation diminishes markedly in the combined samples. A rather different scenario is depicted in diagram C. The slope and Pearson correlation are approximately zero in each sample. The Pearson correlation in the combined samples is positive and moderate and X is a relatively good predictor of Y.

In summary, the effect of pooling samples on regression and correlation coefficients is situation-specific. The magnitude of the slope of the regression equation and the Pearson correlation may be inflated spuriously (as in diagram C) or decreased substantially (as in A), depending on the relative positions of the sample values in both the X and Y dimensions (Minium et al, 1993, p 197).

RANGE RESTRICTION

Range restriction occurs when a portion of a distribution formed by the (X,Y) pairs, usually the extreme upper or lower segment, is studied. The greater the restriction in range in X and/or Y, the lower the Pearson correlation.

The extent to which a variable can predict another variable, as well as the magnitude of the Pearson correlation, depends upon (1) the degree of variation describing each variable and (2) the nature of the relationship between the two variables (Edwards, 1976, p 60; Minium et al, 1993, p 194). We illustrate this with a hypothetical case. Suppose an obstetrician/gynecologist wishes to investigate the relationship between estriol level (ng/mL) in 450 pregnant women near term, and subsequent infant birth weight (g). A Pearson correlation of approximately 0.60 is obtained. The outline of the scatter diagram appears in Fig 19–2, diagram A. Consider now that only women whose estriol levels fall to the right of the vertical line are studied (diagram B). In this select group of patients, the Pearson correlation between estriol level and infant birth weight approaches zero, suggesting that no linear relationship exists between these two variables.

In general, the greater the restriction in variation in X and/or Y, the lower the Pearson correlation; in this setting, the regression equation becomes less useful. In situations like this,

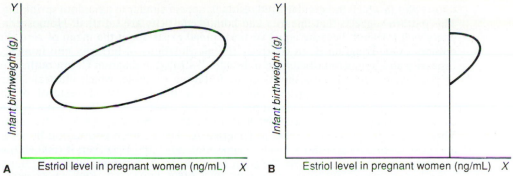

Figure 19–2. Illustration of range restriction when variation in estriol level and infant birthweight are restricted.

the error results *not* from studying a select group of patients, but from generalizing findings from a "restricted group" to an "unrestricted group," and vice versa.

OUTLIERS

Outliers are extremely deviant data points. Their presence typically inflates the Pearson correlation and the slope of the regression line.

An outlier is an observation that has an extreme value on X or Y. A simple and effective method for detecting outliers, as well as violations of linearity and homoscedasticity, is to compute and examine a graph of standardized residuals plotted against X. A **standardized residual,** designated e_{is}, is the difference between the observed and predicted value, divided by the standard error of estimate:

$$e_{is} = \frac{(Y_i - Y_i^3)}{s_{y.x}}$$

19.1

With a mean of zero and a standard deviation of one, standardized residuals are distributed approximately as independent, standard, normal deviates in moderately sized samples. When sample sizes are moderate, approximately 95% of the (X,Y) points will have standardized residuals between +2.00 and −2.00; approximately 99% of the (X,Y) points will have standardized residuals between +3.00 and −3.00. Thus, some statisticians define an extreme data point as one that has a standardized residual of ±3.00 or greater.

Fig 19–3 contains three diagrams of standardized residuals plotted against X. Diagram A con-

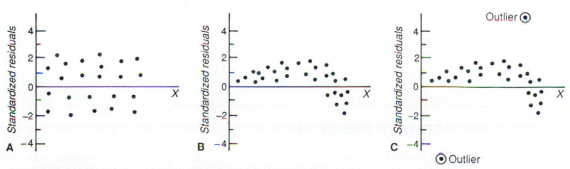

Figure 19–3. Graphs of standardized residuals plotted against X.

tains a plot in which the standardized residuals appear similar to a random sprinkling of points. This pattern suggests that linearity and homoscedasticity are satisfied. Homoscedasticity appears well satisfied, because equal vertical spread exists about the mean of zero. Further, no outliers exist. Diagram B, in contrast, reveals violations of linearity and homoscedasticity. Linearity and homoscedasticity are reasonably satisfied in diagram C, but outliers exist.

The impact of outliers is shown in the following example, which illustrates the effect of dietary inclusion of soy protein and soy fiber on the total cholesterol of five hyper-cholesterolemic men (Fig 19–4). Suppose that the baseline and 10-week posttreatment total cholesterol (mg/dL) values are (400,400); (450, 440); (460, 400); (465, 450); and (600, 600). These five pairs of points appear in Diagram A. The Pearson correlation between baseline and posttreatment cholesterol levels is approximately 0.95. However, if (600,600) is omitted, the Pearson correlation is 0.56. Diagram B also contains five pairs of points, but the outlier occurs at the lower end of the plot: (400,400); (450, 440); (460, 400); (465, 450); and (400, 200). The Pearson correlation is approximately 0.69 with all five points included in the calculation, and approximately 0.56 when the deviant pair is excluded.

Controversy exists about the proper handling of outliers. Should they be omitted? Do they suggest a highly important clinical finding? All extreme data points should be verified to determine if they are erroneous (eg, due to an error in transcribing or coding data). Researchers are advised to correct outliers due to recording, coding, or transcription errors, and to reanalyze the affected data. The researcher may want to consider the following strategy when legitimate outliers occur:

Analyze the data with and without outliers, and report both sets of findings.
Describe the differences and similarities between both sets of findings, so that others can gauge the impact of the extreme data points.
Develop a case study report for each outlier or group of similar outliers, so their clinical significance may be assessed.

In summary, outliers are extreme data points whose presence inflates the Pearson correlation. Because they can distort summary statistics, outliers can contribute to misleading conclusions.

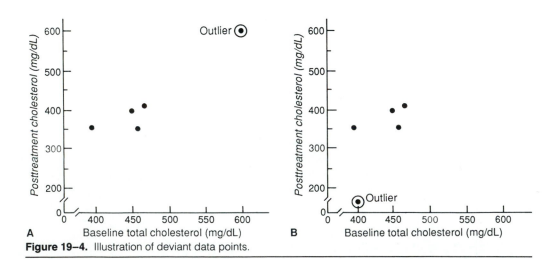

A Baseline total cholesterol (mg/dL) **B** Baseline total cholesterol (mg/dL)
Figure 19–4. Illustration of deviant data points.

REGRESSION TOWARD THE MEAN

Regression toward the mean is the tendency for extreme values of a variable to move closer to the center of a distribution, when the variable is measured a second time. Regression toward the mean can make a treatment appear useful, when in fact it is not.

Regression toward the mean, known also as regression on the mean, is illustrated in the hypothetical clinical problem at the beginning of the chapter. It is the tendency for extreme values of a variable to move closer to the center of a distribution, when the variable is measured a second time (Michael et al, 1984, p 75). In one-group, pre-posttest studies, regression toward the mean is particularly problematic because it prevents us from separating out treatment effectiveness from regression effects (Campbell & Stanley, 1963, pp 6–12). Regression toward the mean occurs because the relationship between two measurements is affected by random variation (Ingelfinger et al, 1987, p 192). Consequently, the correlation between two measurements is not perfect; extreme values at pretreatment rarely correspond perfectly to extreme values at posttreatment.

Suppose a moderate-sized group of men participate in a study to examine the effects of diet on total cholesterol. Consider that the total cholesterol of all men is measured at baseline and again several weeks later. Because an individual's total cholesterol is subject to considerable random variation, we would expect about half those initially screened to have higher and about half to have lower total cholesterol levels, when cholesterol is measured a second time. Thus, the increases and decreases balance out in the total group, and minimal change is observed in a summary statistic, eg, the overall group mean. Suppose, however, that only men whose cholesterol level is elevated, perhaps equal to or greater than 400, are measured a second time. Their total cholesterol level will appear to have dropped, even though the "true" level has not changed; the apparent decrease is due solely to random variation between the first and second measurements. Researchers can guard against regression toward the mean by including a control (reference) group in their experimental design (Dawson-Saunders and Trapp, 1994, p 180).

SUMMARY

Causal relationships, linearity, sample size, combining different samples, range restriction, outliers, and regression toward the mean are discussed in this chapter. It is *never* appropriate to use the results from regression and correlation studies to infer a causal relationship. Although disagreement exists about the conditions necessary to establish a causal relationship, many researchers agree that if X is the cause of Y, then X must precede Y, X and Y must covary, and no rival explanations exist to account for the covariation of X and Y.

Linearity is a basic assumption of simple linear regression and Pearson correlation. Although relatively simple to discern from a scatter diagram, linearity often is overlooked. The greater the departure from linearity, the greater the inadequacy of the linear regression model and the more the Pearson correlation will underestimate the strength of the true relationship between two quantitative variables. Consult a statistician to determine if a transformation to achieve linearity is appropriate or if another measure of association is indicated.

Regression coefficients and the Pearson correlation are subject to sampling fluctuation, like all other statistics. These values tend to vary more from sample to sample, when sample sizes are small. Results from small samples should be applied cautiously, because statistics derived from them may not characterize the population from which the sample was obtained.

The effect of combining different samples depends on where the sample values lie in relation to one another in both the X and Y dimensions. The slope of the regression line and the Pearson correlation may be inflated markedly by pooling samples, or they may be decreased considerably and approach zero. In contrast, range restriction occurs when a subset of a distribution, typically the extreme upper or lower portion, is studied. The greater the restriction in range, the lower the Pearson correlation; when this occurs, it is more difficult to utilize one variable to predict another variable. In each situation, error can occur if findings are generalized inappropriately from one group of patients (eg, patients who are diseased) to another group with different characteristics (eg, individuals in the general population).

Extreme data points, known as outliers, often go undetected because investigators do not examine plots of their data. Outliers may inflate the slope of the regression line and the magnitude of the Pearson correlation. Researchers disagree on how to treat outliers. If the outlier is a genuine observation, consider reporting results with and without it, so that others can understand directly the outlier's impact on the results. If it represents a significant clinical finding, describe the outlier in a case study.

Regression toward the mean occurs when patients are selected because of extreme values on characteristics that are subject to random variation when measured over time. Extreme values of these characteristics tend to regress toward, or move closer to, the center of the population when measured a second time (Ingelfinger et al, 1987, p 193). In one-group, pre-post designs, treatment effectiveness is often confounded because it cannot be separated from regression effects. Researchers can often sort out regression and treatment effects by including a control group and by comparing outcomes in the treatment and control group.

REFERENCES

Altman DB: Statistics in medical journals: Developments in the 1980s. *Stat Med* 1991;**10**: 1987.

Campbell D, Stanley J: *Experimental and Quasi-experimental Designs for Research.* Rand McNally, 1966.

Colton T: *Statistics in Medicine.* Little, Brown, 1974.

Daniel D: *Biostatistics: A Foundation for Analysis in the Health Sciences,* 5th ed. Wiley, 1991.

Dawson-Saunders B, Trapp R: *Basic and Clinical Biostatistics,* 2nd ed. Appleton & Lange, 1994.

Edwards A: *An Introduction to Linear Regression and Correlation.* Freeman, 1976.

Ingelfinger J et al: *Biostatistics in Clinical Medicine,* 2nd ed. Macmillan 1987.

Michael M, Boyce W, Wilcox A: *Biomedical Bestiary: An Epidemiologic Guide to Flaws and Fallacies in the Medical Literature.* Little, Brown, 1984.

Minium E, King B, Bear G: *Statistical Reasoning in Psychology and Education,* 3rd ed. Wiley, 1993.

Vogt WP: *Dictionary of Statistics and Methodology.* Sage, 1993.

Self-study Questions

Part I: Definitions

Define each of the following terms:

Cause	Outlier	Regression toward the mean
Linearity	Range restriction	Standardized residual

Part II: Explanation

1. Explain briefly why correlation or regression results should be interpreted cautiously when the study involves a small sample.
2. Describe briefly a study in which regression toward the mean may confound the interpretation of findings; recommend a modification in design to address the problem.
3. Describe range restriction and discuss how it affects the application of results from an investigation which involves a highly select group of patients.
4. Identify the effect of outliers on the slope of the regression line and Pearson correlation.

Part III. Problems in Regression/Correlation Research

Read each of the following descriptions and comment on the appropriateness of the generalizations. Pay particular attention to problems that may affect regression and correlation studies.

1. The effectiveness of sustained-release nicardipine, a calcium channel antagonist, was evaluated in 42 men with severe hypertension. The investigators hypothesized that a

significant decrease in diastolic blood pressure would occur after a 10-week treatment regimen with nicardipine. Pretreatment, mean diastolic blood pressure was 130 mm Hg. Posttreatment, mean diastolic blood pressure was 123 mm Hg. The clinicians concluded that a significant decrease in diastolic blood pressure occurred in men with severe hypertension after 10 weeks of treatment with nicardipine ($\bar{d} = \bar{X}_{PRE} - \bar{X}_{POST} = -7$, $s_{\bar{d}} = 2.06$, $t_{calc} \approx -3.40$, $t_{crit} = -1.684$, p-value < 0.0005, $\alpha = 0.05$).

2. The relationship between a patient's rating of fatigue and external locus of control on Levenson's scale was studied in 79 women with a clinical diagnosis of chronic fatigue syndrome (CFS). The clinicians hypothesized that an indirect relationship exists between the two variables. The Pearson correlation was -0.79 (p-value < 0.005). The investigators suggested that a low sense of ability to control external factors (low score on Levenson's scale) was the fundamental source of CFS. They also suggested that successful psychiatric intervention with women who have a low sense of control of external factors may eliminate the development of CFS in these women.

3. Researchers have shown that perinatal mortality and morbidity are higher in pregnant women with gestational diabetes than other healthy pregnant women who do not have gestational diabetes. Consequently, standardized management protocols recommend that pregnant women with a 2-hour postprandial glucose level of 120 mg/dL or greater be considered for insulin therapy. A clinician who questions the wisdom of this practice screened a large sample of pregnant women with the 2-hour postprandial glucose test, and selected patients for further study if their glucose level was 140 mg/dL or greater. Approximately 3% of those screened qualified. The Pearson correlation between infant birthweight and 2-hour postprandial glucose level in these women was 0.05 [$t_{calc} = 0.18$, $t_{crit} = 1.771$ (one-tailed), $df = 13$, $\alpha = 0.05$]. The clinician concluded that no relationship exists between 2-hour postprandial glucose levels and infant birthweight. Further, he found that these pregnant women with gestational diabetes were not at risk for delivering low-birthweight infants. Therefore, the clinician recommended against using the 2-hour postprandial glucose test to screen pregnant women suspected of having gestational diabetes or to monitor pregnant women with gestational diabetes.

4. A neurologist hypothesized that an indirect relationship exists between antemortem volumetric measurements of the hippocampus (made using magnetic resonance imaging) and severity of memory loss in 5 patients with Alzheimer's disease. Memory loss was graded by a skilled clinician who used a reliable scale; ratings ranged from zero (no memory loss) to 100 (complete memory loss). A Pearson correlation of -0.87 was obtained, indicating that greater memory loss was associated with smaller volumetric measurements of the hippocampus (p-value < 0.005, one-tail). The neurologist concluded that antemortem volumetric measurements of the hippocampus should be used to differentiate Alzheimer's from non-Alzheimer's patients and to characterize objectively the degree of memory loss.

5. Attitude toward smoking and self-image was examined in healthy adolescents, adolescents with active asthma, and adolescents with a past history of asthma who had no asthmatic episodes in the past 9 months. An indirect relationship was postulated. Attitude and self-image were measured quantitatively on reliable, standardized instruments. Higher attitude scores signaled more positive attitudes toward smoking; higher self-image scores indicated a more positive opinion about one's self. The graph of attitude and self-image scores appears in Fig 19–5. The Pearson correlation was -0.12 (p-value ≈ 0.21,

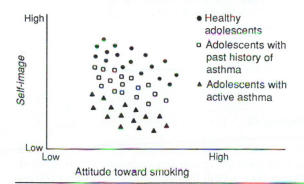

Figure 19–5. Self-image and attitude toward smoking in adolescents.

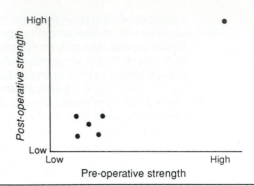

Figure 19–6. Pre- and postoperative strength in 6 elderly patients.

one-tailed). The investigators concluded that attitude toward smoking was not related to self-image in healthy adolescents and adolescents with a past or current history of asthma.

6. Two geriatricians studied the relationship between pre- and postoperative strength in 6 elderly patients to determine if preoperative strength predicted postoperative strength 6 days after surgery. Their data appear in Fig 19–6. The slope of the regression line fitted to these data was positive and significantly greater than zero ($\alpha = 0.05$, one-tailed). The Pearson correlation was positive and significantly greater than zero ($r = 0.85$, p-value < 0.025, one-tailed). The clinicians concluded that pre-operative strength was a strong, positive predictor of postoperative strength 6 days after surgery.

7. The association between red wine consumption (ounces per week) and total cholesterol (mg/dL) was investigated in a large sample of adults. A moderate positive correlation was obtained. The investigators concluded that a moderate direct association exists between total cholesterol and red wine consumption ($r = 0.59$, p-value < 0.001). The researchers suggested that increased red wine consumption may contribute to decreases in total cholesterol, particularly in persons whose total cholesterol level is elevated. A representation of the scatter diagram appears in Fig 19–7.

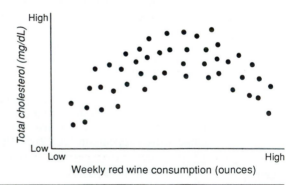

Figure 19–7. Pre- and post-operative strength in six elderly patients.

Solutions

Part III: Problems in Regression/Correlation Research

1. A one-group, pre-post experimental design was used to evaluate the effectiveness of sustained release nicardipine for the treatment of severe hypertension (pretreatment mean diastolic blood pressure was 115 mm Hg). Recall that extreme values of a variable tend to move closer to the center of a distribution when measured a second time. This

phenomenon is referred to as *regression toward the mean*. It is not possible to separate treatment effectiveness from regression toward the mean in one-group, pre-post studies involving a highly select group of patients. Therefore, the findings in this study are confounded by regression toward the mean.

2. The clinicians who examined the relationship between fatigue and external locus of control in women with chronic fatigue syndrome have drawn a *causal conclusion* based on the Pearson correlation. Causal conclusions cannot be supported solely based on regression and/or correlation studies. In this study, there is no evidence that low sense of control of external factors causes chronic fatigue syndrome (CFS), and that increasing a woman's ability to control external factors in her environment will eliminate CFS.

3. The principal problem in this study is *range restriction*. Only 3% of the pregnant women screened met the criterion for participating in the study. It is not surprising that the Pearson correlation between 2-hour postprandial glucose levels and infant birthweight approached zero in this sample. However, the results in this highly selected group of women were generalized to pregnant women suspected of having gestational diabetes and to pregnant women with gestational diabetes. Keep in mind that it is appropriate to study patients with particularly high or low values on a variable of interest; the error occurs when results from a restricted group are applied broadly to patients with different clinical characteristics.

4. *Small sample size* is a major problem in extending the results from five patients with Alzheimer's disease to all diseased patients. Recall that approximately 95% of sample correlation coefficients will vary between -0.88 and $+0.88$ in samples of size 5, if sampling has been from a population in which the correlation equals zero. Regression and correlation statistics, like other statistics, vary from sample to sample, with less stability in small samples. Although these results in Alzheimer's patients may be promising, they should not be applied broadly. Note also that results were extended to non-Alzheimer's patients, even though none was included in the investigation.

5. *Combining different samples* takes its toll in this problem. Note that the three groups of adolescents in Figure 19–5 constitute three clearly differentiated samples. Observe also that a moderate to strong negative relationship appears to exist in each sample between attitude toward smoking and self-image. The pattern of points in the combined sample, however, is similar to what we expect to see when the Pearson correlation approaches zero. Combining the samples into one group obscures the relationship in each sample.

6. An *outlier* inflates the slope and Pearson correlation in this investigation of pre- and postoperative strength in 6 elderly patients. Five of the six points cluster at the lower end of the scatter diagram in a rectangular-like pattern. The sixth point in the far upper right of the diagram is clearly different from the other five. The magnitude of the slope and Pearson correlation can be attributed clearly to the presence of this extremely deviant data point.

7. The relationship between weekly red wine consumption and total cholesterol is *curvilinear*, as shown in Figure 19–7. The Pearson correlation underestimates the strength of a curvilinear association. A measure of association appropriate for nonlinear data should be used.

Reading and Evaluating the Medical Literature

20

Mud Wrestling?

Michael and associates note that "most medical students regard epidemiology as somewhere between mud-wrestling and mah-jongg in its relevance to medicine" (1984, p ix). For various reasons, many medical students feel the same way about statistics. Some students contend that practicing clinicians never do research. Others believe that "real doctors" (usually defined as those who care for patients) seldom read journal articles. Still others believe that clinicians do not have to understand statistics and epidemiology because journals only publish articles that have been carefully reviewed before publication.

Why Read Published Articles Critically?

Although manuscripts are reviewed by reviewers and editors, many articles, including ones published in highly respected journals, contain serious errors in design and analysis. Thorough reviews of published medical literature have found consistently that, in approximately 50% of the papers examined, incorrect statistical methods were used (Glantz, 1981, p 7). Williamson and co-workers (1986) found that approximately 80% of the medical papers they reviewed were scientifically flawed.

Who Reads the Literature and Why?

Most clinicians and other health care professionals read published papers. The reasons for reading a paper vary. Individuals may want to keep informed of advances in particular areas; find out if clinical observations about a particular phenomenon are documented in the literature; plan a research project; or evaluate a treatment, drug, procedure, or diagnostic test to determine whether to modify patient care. Clinicians who want to decide whether to use a new drug, for example, must be able to identify well-done studies and interpret the results in order to make informed decisions. Thus, clinicians, students, and other health care professionals must be able to judge whether investigations are properly designed, data are correctly analyzed, and conclusions are justified and appropriately generalized. Doing so requires knowledge of statistics and epidemiology.

In this chapter, we outline the sections of a published paper, note common study biases and flaws, and provide a checklist, in question format, for evaluating published papers.

Common Types of Studies

In Chapter 1, we discussed common types of studies and indicated that investigations can be divided into experiments and observational studies, based on whether patients are merely observed or whether some kind of intervention is performed. Knowledge of common study types is important because different kinds of questions require different study designs. Common study types are summarized in Table 20–1, along with the advantages and disadvantages of each study type.

OBJECTIVES

When you complete this chapter, you should be able to:

- Identify common biases often found in published reports.
- Discuss the types of errors that can result from respective biases.
- List the main ways to evaluate whether the statistical assumptions, methods and conclusions of a study are sound.

Table 20–1. Common types of studies.

Type	Description	Advantages	Disadvantages
Experiments Clinical trials	A study in which the investigator manipulates or controls an intervention.	• Design of choice when the goal is to evaluate the effectiveness of a treatment or procedure. • May provide the strongest evidence of causal linkages.	• Expensive. • Some important questions cannot be studied in experiments. • Not well suited to rare diseases. • May require more time to complete than other types of studies.
Observational Studies	A study in which participants are merely observed and their experiences recorded; they are not assigned to an intervention; investigator does not manipulate or control an intervention.		
Case report	Interesting characteristics in a single patient are described in detail.	• May lead to formalized research to identify causes of disease, diagnose disease, or treat disease. • May lead to the detection of unusual patterns of disease.	• Interesting findings may be due to chance. • Cannot generalize findings.
Case series	Interesting characteristics in a series of patients are described in detail.	• May lead to formalized research to identify causes of disease, diagnose disease, or treat disease. • May lead to the detection of unusual patterns of disease.	• Interesting findings may be due to chance. • Cannot generalize findings.
Ecologic	Data collected routinely are used to study disease occurrence and possible causes in groups of individuals.	• Relatively inexpensive because they rely on extant data. • Appropriate for preliminary or exploratory studies.	• Findings from may not be generalizable to individuals. • Depend on the quality of extant data. • Findings require confirmation by other types of studies.
Case control	Cases (diseased) and controls (disease-free) are compared to tease out differences in their backgrounds that are thought to be associated with disease.	• Efficient design, particularly to study rare diseases. • May be appropriate to study preliminary hypotheses. • Among the least expensive to conduct.	• Depend on the quality of extant records. • Difficult to identify appropriate control groups.
Cross-sectional	Characteristics of participants are studied at a point in time to look for associations between disease and possible causes.	• Appropriate for preliminary investigations. • Relatively inexpensive and easy to conduct. • Useful for estimating the prevalence of disease at a point in time. • Useful for evaluating a new diagnostic procedure.	• May lead to erroneous conclusions because we may not be able to determine sequence of events.
Prospective cohort	Exposed and unexposed individuals are followed prospectively; occurrence of new disease is studied to determine it disease is linked to different exposures.	• Best observational study for investigating possible causes of disease, course of disease, and risk factors.	• Expensive. • Patient attrition. • Require a long time to complete. • Not suited to the study of rare diseases or diseases with long latency periods. • Does not establish cause, because there is no active intervention.
Retrospective cohort	Exposed and unexposed individuals are followed retrospectively; occurrence of new disease during retrospective period is studied to determine if disease is linked to different exposures.	• Best observational study for investigating possible causes of disease, course of disease, and risk factors.	• Depend on the quality of historical records. • Expensive. • Patient attrition. • Not suited to the study of rare diseases or diseases with long latency periods. • Does not establish cause, because there is no active intervention.

SECTIONS OF A PUBLISHED PAPER

Most published papers contain (1) an abstract, (2) an introduction, (3) a methods section, (4) the results, and (5) a discussion and conclusions.

Abstract

The abstract is a brief, comprehensive summary of an article. The major purpose of the abstract is to highlight the study's objectives, hypotheses, methods, major findings, and important conclusions.

Introduction

The introduction usually includes (1) a succinct review of the relevant literature, (2) a statement of purpose, (3) the research hypotheses, and (4) a statement about the significance of the problem being investigated.

Typically brief, the *review of literature* describes current knowledge by citing and summarizing relevant research. The review establishes the context of the study and describes the *purpose* of the current investigation. The investigation may have been done to:

Clarify conflicting findings in recent studies.
Build on previous investigations by refining experimental methods, observational procedures, operational definition of outcomes, or measurement of outcomes.
Investigate a previously unstudied phenomenon or one that has received little attention.
Test a new theory or examine one that is thought to be wrong or archaic.
Evaluate new therapies, diagnostic procedures, or suspected causes of disease or other health outcomes.
Study therapies that have shown promise in small-scale human or animal trials.

The review of literature builds to the *problem statement*. This statement is clear and concise. It includes the objectives of the research, variables studied, and the relationship of these variables to theory or clinical observation. The problem statement, in turn, leads to clearly formulated and understandable *hypotheses*. Hypotheses are "clear, concise, operational definition[s] of a study's purpose" (Bausell, 1994, p 41). In addition, hypotheses indicate the expected findings.

Many introductions conclude with two or three sentences that highlight the potential *significance* of the study. Greenberg (1993, p 121) points out that significance may be clinical, biologic, or statistical. Findings that are clinically significant lead to changes in clinical practice. Biologically significant discoveries clarify causal mechanisms, for example, by identifying genetic markers of susceptibility or risk factors associated with disease development. Statistically significant results exclude chance as an explanation for the findings.

Methods

The methods section includes a description of (1) study participants, (2) study design, (3) procedures, and (4) statistical analyses.

Many methods sections begin with a *description of study participants*. This description includes the total number of participants, how they were chosen and, if applicable, how they were assigned to study groups. We must know the characteristics of participants if we are to identify the target population and generalize findings. If random sampling and random assignment are used, they should be described in enough detail to assure readers that they fulfill the definition of randomization and that they actually occurred. Random selection and assignment minimize extraneous variation, minimize initial differences between study groups, maximize the likelihood that differences between study groups are due to the independent variable (eg, treatment or exposure), and increase generalizability.

In addition, methods of obtaining informed consent from study participants are detailed. Inducements offered to study participants are indicated (eg, money, theater tickets, complimentary dinner for two).

Inclusion and exclusion criteria are described as well. These may include age, race, sex, family income, current disease or health status, family history, medical history of participants, education, geography, work history, smoking history, and so forth. After reviewing these criteria, the reader should be able to determine whether any hypothetical individual would be included or excluded from the study.

The next component of the methods section is *study design*. The description of the design may highlight key elements of the design; greater detail may be provided in the procedures portion of the methods section. The type of design is identified (eg, prospective cohort or controlled randomized clinical trial). Data sources are noted, such as medical records, death certificates, or questionnaires. Assumptions are indicated. For example, researchers assume that clinicians participating in a multicenter investigation adhere to the experimental protocol, use identical diagnostic criteria to identify disease, and accurately report all information. In addition, limitations of the study and potential biases are reported (eg, patient attrition may limit generalizability). The study design may also incorporate the operational definition of independent, dependent, and confounding variables, or these definitions may be included in the procedures component of the methods section.

The *procedures* used in the study are also described in the methods section. The procedures include a description of the treatments or other interventions, experimental protocol, operational definition of variables, diagnostic criteria, unusual instruments, instructions to patients, and source of equipment and supplies. Indications for discontinuing treatment or switching a study participant from one group to another are summarized. In addition, procedures used to mask or blind patients, caregivers, radiologists, technicians, and so forth, are specified. The absence of blinding may introduce biases that affect study outcomes. For example, a radiologist who knows patient group assignments may look more critically for evidence of disease progression in the x-rays of control group participants and brush over many similar indications in the radiographs of individuals in the treatment group. In this case, treatment effects will be exaggerated. In short, the procedures component of the methods section details what was done and how it was done.

The methods section typically concludes with the *statistical analyses*. The analyses used to examine the data are specified. If not widely known, the techniques are referenced. Statistical significance is noted (eg, $\alpha = 0.05$) in all analyses. The number of study participants included in each analysis is reported. Methods for handling missing data, such as those due to patient attrition, are presented. Criteria for excluding observations (eg, outliers) are detailed. The reader should be able to determine if the data are analyzed appropriately after reading the description of analyses.

Results

The results section is a straightforward reporting of findings as they relate to the hypotheses stated in the introduction. Authors summarize results in tables and graphs, as well as in the text. Descriptive and inferential findings are presented. For example, descriptive statistics include the mean, standard deviation, minimum and maximum values, and range for quantitative outcomes. Frequencies and proportions may be presented for qualitative data. Inferential findings include calculated values of test statistics, degrees of freedom, and *p*-values.

Discussion and Conclusions

In this final section of a published paper, conclusions are presented, discussed, and related to the hypotheses. Results are generalized and alternative explanations for findings are offered. Statistical significance is differentiated from clinical and biologic significance. Limitations of the investigation are summarized and recommendations for further study are made.

COMMON BIASES IN PUBLISHED STUDIES

Bias is "anything that produces systematic error in a research finding" (Vogt, 1993, p 21) and thus threatens internal or external validity. Bias may occur in the selection of study participants, definition of variables, analysis of data, results, or conclusions. No study is immune to bias; some study designs are more susceptible to it than others. For example, case-control studies are threatened by bias in the selection of study participants; in such studies, for example, spurious associations can be demonstrated between disease and exposure if controls differ from cases with respect to important clinical and demographic characteristics.

In the following presentation, potential biases are grouped according to the section of a paper in which they are usually found. The biases are also summarized in Table 20–2. Individuals interested in reading more about potential flaws in published research may want to consult Sackett (1979) and Michael and associates (1984).

Selecting Study Participants

Because investigators cannot study all individuals with a particular disease, risk factor, or exposure, they select samples and examine only a portion of the population of interest. Selection of study participants depends on the purpose of the study, the study's design, the problem under investigation, the study's setting, and the disease or exposure of interest. The process used to select study participants may *increase* or *decrease* the chance of detecting a significant relationship between the independent and dependent variables, for example, between exposure and disease (Greenberg, 1993, p 112).

HEALTHY WORKER BIAS

The healthy worker bias may occur when findings from an epidemiologic study of workplace exposures are extended to the general population. Investigators may find that workers have more favorable outcomes, compared to individuals in the general population. For example, researchers may observe that workers in a hazardous environment survive longer than individuals in the general population. Findings like these can occur because good health is a prerequisite for employment, but not for being a member of the general population.

MEMBERSHIP BIAS

Membership bias can occur when study participants are selected from preexisting groups (eg, joggers, smokers, or unemployed individuals). This bias occurs when factors associated with group membership affect the outcome of interest. For example, some factors may imply a degree of health that differs significantly between individuals in a sampled group and those in other groups or the general population. According to Dawson-Saunders and Trapp, some researchers believe that smoking does not cause cancer; rather, these researchers may suggest that another factor more common in smokers than nonsmokers contributes to cancer development (1994, p 268). We cannot easily disprove this contention, because no clinical trial with humans has been conducted to examine the relationship between smoking and cancer development. Nor is one likely to occur, given the weight of current epidemiologic evidence, plus the ethical considerations and potential cost of such a trial. Because it cannot be prevented, membership bias makes the investigation of disease and risk factors difficult, given that many risk factors are related to lifestyle. Membership bias affects cohort and case-control studies (Sackett, 1979, p 55).

VOLUNTEER EFFECT

This effect occurs when exposures or outcomes in a study differ systematically between volunteers and nonvolunteers. The opposite effect is **nonresponse bias,** which occurs when characteristics of persons who refuse to respond differ systematically from characteristics of respondents; these characteristics may include exposures, education, income, health, or lifestyle. Initial differences between volunteers and nonvolunteers, or respondents and nonrespondents, prevent investigators from untangling effects of treatment from differences between the groups. Further, the volunteer effect and nonresponse bias may lead to under- or overestimates of the association between risk factors and disease or other outcomes.

In a controlled clinical trial, investigators can minimize the volunteer effect by randomly choosing participants and randomly assigning them to study groups. In observational studies, researchers can reduce this effect by carefully identifying the characteristics of eligible participants before enrolling them in the study. Nonresponse bias can be minimized through the use of questionnaires and follow-up surveys designed to increase the number of respondents. To minimize nonresponse bias, Sackett (1979, p 54) suggests that investigators achieve response rates of at least 80%.

PROCEDURE SELECTION BIAS

This bias occurs when study group assignment is not randomized, but rather is based on particular characteristics of participants (eg, prognosis). When this happens, certain clinical procedures may be offered to those who are poor risks. For example, suppose investigators want to compare medical and surgical management of a disease. Rather than randomly assigning patients to a therapy, they choose participants from (1) individuals who are receiving or will soon receive medical therapy and (2) those who have recently had or will soon have surgery. If surgery is the treatment of last resort, that is, if surgery is used only after medical intervention fails, the prognosis of patients who have surgery may be much less favorable than the prognosis of participants who receive and benefit from medical therapy. In this case, medical intervention may prove more effective than surgery.

ADMISSION BIAS OR BERKSON'S PARADOX

Named after the individual who first identified it in 1946, Berkson's paradox occurs in hospital- or clinic-based studies when hospital admission rates differ among exposed cases, unexposed cases, and controls. Compared to population-based trials, clinic-based studies tend to have a higher frequency of adverse outcomes (Greenberg, 1993, p 113). Therefore, findings from clinic-based studies may overestimate disease frequency and other outcomes (eg, mortality). Hospital-based studies may include patients who have two or more diseases, because these individuals tend to be hospitalized more frequently. Clinicians may detect an association that does not exist in the general population—perhaps an association between the diseases or between disease and another factor in hospitalized patients. Such an association may occur, for example, in a hospital-based study in which cigarette smoking, which is frequently linked with respiratory disease, seems to correlate with bone disease, because bone and respiratory disease are related in certain hospitalized patients (Greenberg, 1993, p 113). Although smoking and bone disease may be correlated in hospitalized patients, they are not associated in the general population. Admission bias may lead to over- as well as underestimates of the association between disease and other factors, such as exposure.

Admission bias is a serious threat to case-control studies, because cases are often identified from clinic or hospital records. We have already noted that findings from clinic- and hospital-based studies may not apply to the general population. In addition, cases selected from clinic or hospital records may not represent the population of patients with disease, because some clinics and hospitals are more likely to treat certain patients. This can occur because of the location of the institution, the expertise of the staff, physician referral patterns, or other factors.

PREVALENCE-INCIDENCE (NEYMAN) BIAS

Prevalence bias occurs when a condition is characterized by early fatalities, that is, individuals die *before they are diagnosed;* the fatalities are often missed because of the time interval between exposure and an investigation of its consequences. This type of bias can also occur if mild cases or cases of occult (undiscovered) disease are missed. In addition, prevalence bias affects a study when evidence of exposure disappears after the event or onset of disease (Sackett, 1979, p 52). Because disease status is the starting point in case-control investigations, prevalence bias may distort findings from these studies by increasing or decreasing estimates of risk. If cases die early, the association between exposure and disease may be underestimated. If exposure leads to selective survival rather than selective mortality, the estimate of risk may be spuriously high. Prevalence bias can be minimized in case-control studies by limiting eligibility to incident cases, that is, to individuals with newly diagnosed disease (Greenberg, 1993, p 113). Prevalence bias does not occur in cohort studies, because the correct time sequence between exposure and disease development is preserved. Recall that cohort studies begin with exposed and unexposed individuals; the occurrence of new disease is then charted over a specified follow-up period.

Procedural Biases

IDENTIFYING AND MEASURING VARIABLES

The following biases may occur when identifying or measuring patient characteristics, disease, or risk factors; these distortions are sometimes referred to as *measurement biases, information biases,* or *misclassification biases* (Greenberg, 1993, p 124).

Recall Bias

Recall bias may occur when patients are asked to recall events (eg, exposures or medical history) and the individuals in one study group are more likely than those in another group to remember the event. For example, Klemetti and Saxen (1967) studied women whose pregnancy ended in fetal death (cases) and women whose pregnancies ended normally (controls). They found that 28% of cases and 20% of controls reported exposures to drugs that could not be substantiated in prospective interviews or through medical records.

Family Information Bias

Family information bias occurs when information about exposures and disease is stimulated by, or directed to, a new case in the family. Family history may vary markedly, depending on whether the individual providing it is diseased or disease-free. For example, patients with rheumatoid arthritis are more likely than their unaffected siblings to report that their parents have arthritis (Schull & Cobb, 1969). Likewise, when asked about family history, women with breast cancer may be more likely than disease-free women to mistake benign forms of breast disease for breast cancer. Family history bias can be minimized by relying on medical records.

Diagnostic Suspicion Bias

This bias occurs when knowledge of an individual's *exposure* to a suspected risk factor influences the intensity and outcome of the diagnostic process. For example, investigators conducting a cohort study to examine the link between asbestos exposure and lung disease may use more sensitive imaging methods to detect disease in exposed workers. As a result, they may underestimate disease occurrence in the unexposed group. Although usually associated with cohort investigations, diagnostic suspicion bias can affect the selection of cases and controls in case-control studies, if the suspected risk factor has received widespread publicity.

Exposure Suspicion Bias

Exposure suspicion bias may occur when knowledge of *disease status* influences the intensity and outcome of the search for exposure to a suspected risk factor. Sackett (1979, p 56) points out that this bias "may operate whenever patients appear with disorders whose 'causes' are 'known.'" For example, if researchers believe an association exists between thyroid cancer and prior irradiation, they may search more vigorously to identify prior irradiation. In an actual study that involved routine questioning and medical record searches, investigators found that none of 22 children with thyroid cancer had prior irradiation. More intensive questioning and additional review of medical records revealed, however, that 50% of the affected children had indeed been exposed to radiation (Raventos et al, 1962).

Insensitive Measure Bias

Insensitive measure bias occurs when outcome measures are incapable of detecting disease or significant clinical changes. For example, although urine dipstick tests are a useful way to screen for protein, albumin, and intact globulin, the dipstick tests miss the light chains of immunoglobulin present in the urine of patients with multiple myeloma (Freeman, 1993, p 708). If the urine dipstick test were used to screen for multiple myeloma, insensitive measure bias would occur. Consider another example. Conventional x-ray examinations miss many cases of osteoporosis, because approximately 30% of bone loss occurs before osteoporosis can be detected by x-ray (Dawson-Saunders & Trapp, 1994, p 270). If conventional x-rays are used to screen for osteoporosis, disease frequency may be underestimated.

Detection Bias

Detection bias may occur with the introduction of new, more sensitive diagnostic technologies that allow disease to be identified at an earlier stage. Because disease is detected earlier, duration of survival of affected patients may appear to increase. For example, before advances in diagnostic radiology, conventional x-rays of the abdomen were used in some cases to evaluate kidney disease. Because this imaging modality is not sensitive to many changes associated with this disease, it misses a large proportion of diseased patients. Today, with widespread availability of magnetic resonance imaging (MRI), kidney disease is detected much earlier. Even if treatment advances have not occurred, patient outcomes, such as survival, may appear more favorable because improved diagnostic technology leads to earlier detection of disease.

Detection bias may play a major role in investigations that compare changes in outcomes in different time periods (eg, length of survival of patients with a particular brain cancer diagnosed in 1950 versus patients diagnosed in 1990), or changes in the incidence of disease in different groups separated by time (eg, incidence of regional enteritis in 1940 versus 1990). Detection bias may also affect case-control investigations, when cases and controls are not contemporaneous.

Measurement Biases Versus Sampling Biases

Measurement biases are often easier to prevent than sampling biases. Effective strategies for minimizing or preventing measurement biases include "blinding" study participants and investigators to the participants' diagnoses and prior exposures. Investigations in which only the participants are unaware of the treatment they receive are *single-blind* studies. In a *double-blind* study, the investigators and the participants do not know which treatment is being received by the respective patients. Measurement bias may also be minimized by (1) establishing explicit, objective criteria for exposures and outcomes and (2) obtaining information about exposure, medical history, and family history from independent sources (eg, medical records that are unaffected by memory or the flow of information in the family) (Sackett, 1979, p 58).

Although blinding minimizes the effects of *a priori* beliefs and expectations, blinding patients and researchers is not always possible. It is obvious, for example, to patients and investigators when the experimental intervention is a surgical procedure and the control condition consists of medical therapy. Blinding is less critical when outcomes can be measured objectively (eg, mortality or number of hospitalizations). Blinding is more important when subjective outcomes are assessed, such as quality-of-life measures that may include a patient's assessment of pain, ability to enjoy life, or sense of well-being. Although patients and investigators who deliver the treatments may not be blinded, blinding can be introduced if outcomes are assessed by an individual who is unaware of the study's purpose and patient group assignments.

Sampling biases are more problematic than measurement biases, because many sampling biases cannot be addressed without altering the nature of the study. For example, admission bias can be prevented if case-control studies are replaced by investigations in the general population. Time-and-cost advantages of case-control studies are lost, however, in population-based investigations. Membership bias can be prevented if investigators match on, or statistically adjust for, all important confounding variables—clearly an unrealistic expectation because we do not currently understand enough about determinants of group membership to identify and control all of them! Prevalence bias can be minimized in case-control studies if eligibility is limited to incident cases, that is, individuals with newly diagnosed disease who undergo similar diagnostic examinations. This restriction, however, may result in overmatching of cases and controls. Overmatching occurs when controls and cases are excessively similar (Michael et al, 1984, p 121). Case-control studies in which cases and controls are excessively similar may fail to detect real associations between disease and exposure.

In summary, measurement biases are usually easier to prevent than sampling biases. Measurement biases can be minimized or prevented by blinding; by establishing explicit, objective criteria for exposures and outcomes; and by obtaining information about exposure, medical history, and family history from independent sources. Methods used to minimize or eliminate many sampling biases may alter the fundamental nature of case-control investigations; this may require that investigators conduct other types of studies that cost more and take longer to complete.

MANIPULATING THE EXPERIMENTAL TREATMENT OR EXPOSURE

Errors in experimental design or treatment procedures may lead to the following biases, which may be difficult or impossible to detect, especially because many investigators do not report them.

Compliance Bias

Compliance bias occurs when study participants find it easier or more pleasant to comply with one treatment than another (Dawson-Saunders & Trapp, 1994, p 270). For example, in the treatment of glaucoma, patients receiving an experimental eyedrop that blurs vision and causes the eyes to tear and sting may use the eyedrop less frequently or discontinue use altogether. The standard eyedrop causes none of these side effects. Comparisons between the standard and the experimental eyedrop may show that the standard medication is more effective than the experimental preparation; yet the experimental eyedrop may be more effective in compliant patients.

Contamination Bias

This bias occurs when members of the control group inadvertently receive the experimental intervention. For example, in a controlled clinical trial of the effectiveness of aspirin in patients at risk for a heart attack, differences in outcomes between the aspirin and control group may be systematically reduced if control patients mistakenly receive aspirin.

Hawthorne Effect or Attention Bias

The Hawthorne effect, or attention bias, occurs when study participants change their behavior simply because they are observed. Thus, some participants may improve as a result of being studied. For example, individuals taking an experimental drug may receive more attention than individuals taking a placebo. Even if the experimental drug is ineffective, patients in the experimental group may improve simply because investigators spend more time asking them questions and monitoring outcomes of interest. The Hawthorne effect can be minimized by treating all study participants identically, except for the experimental intervention.

Therapeutic Personality Bias

When investigators conducting an experiment are not "blinded" to the treatment or purpose of the study, their convictions about efficacy may systematically influence the measurement of outcomes. For example, researchers who believe high doses of vitamins and minerals will alleviate symptoms of premenstrual syndrome (PMS) may communicate a positive attitude to treatment-group patients and a negative attitude to patients receiving a placebo. This positive attitude toward the treatment group may contribute to apparent improvements, if it leads these women to minimize or underreport their symptoms. Similarly, the investigators' predisposition may cause them to evaluate similar changes in both groups as being more favorable when they are experienced by women in the treatment group.

ANALYZING THE DATA

Statements like the following are often heard: "Health statistics may be hazardous to our mental health" (Paulos, 1994, p 30). "If you torture your data long enough, they will tell you whatever you want to hear" (Mills, 1993, p 1196). Many individuals harbor these and similar sentiments, in part because they do not know how to detect biases that may affect statistical analyses.

Opportunitist Data Torturing—the Fishing expedition

Opportunistic data torturing occurs when "the perpetrator simply pores over data until a 'significant' association is found between variables and then devises a biologically plausible hypothesis to fit the association" (Mills, 1993, p 1197).

To determine whether opportunistic data torturing has occurred in a study, ask the following questions (Mills, 1993, pp 1197–1198):

1. Is the finding a chance result with an *a posteriori* hypothesis to give it credibility?

2. Are the results biologically and clinically plausible?

3. Is the finding supported by data from other human or animal studies?

4. How many comparisons are significant, given the number of tests that were performed?

Readers should suspect data torturing if they can answer "yes" to the first question and "no" to the second and third. Regarding question number four, which involves *multiple statistical comparisons,* readers should be alert to data torturing if a large number of tests are performed but the number of "significant" results is relatively small. Multiple independent comparisons increase the probability of a Type I error, that is, the conclusion that significant differences exist when they do not. The opportunistic data torturer can obtain erroneous "significant" findings by simply increasing the number of independent comparisons.

Procrustean Data Torturing

Procrustean data torturing occurs when the investigator manipulates the data so that they support the desired hypothesis (Mills, 1993, p 1197). When done skillfully, Procrustean data torturing is more difficult to detect than opportunistic data torturing, because the former involves selective suppression of data that contradict the desired hypothesis. Procrustean data torturing can take several forms:

1. Exposure may be redefined to strengthen the association between outcomes and exposure.

2. Disease outcomes may be lumped together, split, or omitted to produce desired results.

3. Normal ranges for laboratory results may be altered.

4. Study participants may be dropped or withdrawn from the study (withdrawal bias); or participants may be reallocated to the control group (bogus control bias).

Withdrawal bias and bogus control bias are described below. To try to detect Procrustean data torturing, ask the following questions (Mills, 1993, p 1198):

1. Why were study participants dropped or excluded from analyses?

2. Does the classification of exposure and disease make sense?

3. Are cutoff points for laboratory tests reasonable and customary?

4. Is a convincing rationale presented for examining patient subgroups?

5. Is there a meaningful and clear biologic explanation for significant effects that occur in one subgroup but not in other subgroups?

The reader should suspect data torturing when study participants are dropped without clear reasons, or when a large proportion of participants are excluded for any reason. Suspect data torturing when clear reasons are not provided for evaluating certain exposure groups only (eg, men who worked for 5 years or more) or individuals who have certain characteristics (eg, diastolic blood pressure above 100 mm Hg). Were individuals with fewer than 5 years of exposure omitted because their data did not fit the hypothesis? Sackett (1979, p 62) refers to the exclusion of participants whose data do not fit the hypothesis as "tidying-up bias." Suspect data manipulation, too, when significant findings are noted in only one of several patient groups (eg, men over 65 years of age). Is there a clear biologic explanation that could account for an effect in only one group? If not, the significant finding may be due to chance or it may result from multiple comparisons.

Withdrawal Bias

Withdrawal bias occurs when the investigator withdraws participants because they experience undesirable outcomes and omits them from all analyses. Patients who are withdrawn from the study may differ systematically from individuals who remain *Sackett, 1979, p 62). For example, suppose that carotid thromboendarterectomy (a surgical procedure) is compared to medical intervention in patients experiencing carotid ischemic attacks; patients who die or have a stroke following surgery are withdrawn by the investigators, or identified as "unavailable for follow-up," and excluded from analyses. In this scenario, thromboendarterectomy may appear more favorable than it actually is, because patients with undesirable outcomes are excluded from analyses.

Bogus Control Bias

This bias, which is similar to withdrawal bias, occurs when patients in the *experimental* group sicken or die before or during the administration of the experimental procedure and are subsequently omitted from the study or reallocated to the control group. In this case, positive benefits associated with the experimental maneuver will be exaggerated and the procedure will appear spuriously superior. Consider a clinical trial to compare vitamin and conventional therapy to treat a particular cancer. If patients in the vitamin group who experience cancer recurrence during follow-up are omitted from this group, the effectiveness of vitamin therapy will be exaggerated. As a result, it may appear more effective than conventional treatment.

Migration Bias

Migration bias occurs when participants in one group cross over to another group. For example, suppose that clinicians compare medical treatment with balloon angioplasty in patients with coronary artery disease. During the study, the condition of a patient receiving medical therapy worsens and she undergoes angioplasty. Migration bias has occurred because the patient crossed over from the medical to the surgical treatment group. In such cases, the patient's data should be analyzed with the group to which he or she was assigned initially (Dawson-Saunders & Trapp, 1994, p 272).

Biases Affecting Results and Conclusions

The results and conclusions of a study are not immune to biases. The biases described below may be less subtle and, therefore, easier to detect than some procedural biases (eg, therapeutic personality bias or bogus control bias).

SIGNIFICANCE BIAS

Significance bias occurs when statistical significance is confused with biological or clinical significance. Sackett (1979, p 63) points out that statistically significant results that are viewed without regard to biologic and clinical significance can lead to fruitless conclusions and useless studies.

To increase the value of statistical findings, many journal require that investigators provide confidence intervals and *p*-values. Confidence intervals indicate a range of values within which the population parameter is likely to occur. *Narrow intervals provide a more precise estimate of this range than wide intervals.* For example, a 95% confidence interval of 4.2 to 7.9 for a relative risk clearly defines an increased risk. Although an investigator might argue that an interval that extends from 1.1 to 12.7 indicates an increased risk, the interval is too wide to be useful clinically. In addition, *p*-values also help us gauge statistical significance. They reflect the probability that a finding is due to chance (Michael et al, 1984, p 155). However, even *p*-values can be abused by investigators who conduct multiple comparisons and fail to adjust for the number of tests performed. Always keep in mind *the role that sample size plays in statistical significance:* Even trivial differences can appear "significant" if the sample size is large enough, because large samples can lead to "narrow" confidence intervals and small *p*-values.

Table 20–2. Common biases that affect medical studies.

Bias	Brief Definition
Selecting Study Participants	
Healthy worker effect	Comparisons of health outcomes between workers and the general population often show that workers have more favorable outcomes, simply because they are healthy enough to be employed.
Membership bias	Characteristics associated with group membership (eg, employed, joggers, smokers) may imply a degree of health that differs systematically from other groups, as well as from the general population.
Volunteer effect	Volunteers from a sample may exhibit exposures or outcomes that differ systematically from nonvolunteers.
Nonresponse bias	Nonrespondents from a sample may exhibit exposures or outcomes that differ systematically from respondents.
Procedure selection bias	Characteristics of individuals, rather than random assignment, are used to determine if a patient receives a particular clinical procedure (eg, only patients whose prognosis is poor are offered an experimental therapy).
Admission bias (Berkson's paradox)	This can occur in hospital- and clinic-based studies when hospitalization rates differ among different exposure or disease groups.
Prevalence-incidence (Neyman) bias	This bias can exist when (1) a condition under investigation includes early fatalities that were missed because of a time lag between exposure and a study of its consequences; (2) silent (undiscovered) cases exist; or (3) evidence of exposure disappears after the event or disease onset.
Procedural Biases	
Measuring Variables	
Recall bias	When asked to recall events (eg, exposures), individuals in one group are more likely than those in another group to remember the event.
Family information bias	Family history varies markedly depending on whether it is provided by an individual with disease or a person who is disease free.
Diagnostic suspicion bias	Knowledge of a patient's *exposure* to a suspected risk factor influences the intensity and outcome of the diagnostic process.
Exposure suspicion bias	Knowledge of a patient's *disease status* affects the intensity and outcome of the search for exposures.
Insensitive measure bias	Outcome measures are incapable of detecting disease or clinically significant changes (eg, conventional x-ray to detect osteoporosis).
Detection bias	Health outcomes appear more favorable simply because new, more sensitive diagnostic technologies detect disease sooner than older technologies.
Delivering the Treatment	
Compliance bias	Compliance with treatment varies between groups, because participants in one group find it easier or more pleasant to comply than individuals in other study groups.
Contamination bias	Members of the control group inadvertently receive the experimental intervention.
Hawthorne effect (attention bias)	Study participants change their behavior simply because they are observed.
Therapeutic personality bias	Outcomes and their measurement are influenced by the researcher's convictions about the effectiveness of the intervention.
Analyzing Data	
Opportunistic data torturing	Data are analyzed in several different ways to detect statistical significance and to devise biologically plausible hypotheses to fit the association.
Procrustean data torturing	Data that contradict desired hypotheses are selectively suppressed.
Withdrawal bias	Participants who experience undesirable outcomes or who are lost to follow-up are "withdrawn" from the study and omitted from analyses.
Bogus control bias	Patients (in the treatment or experimental group) who sicken or die before or during the administration of the experimental maneuver are omitted from the study or reallocated to the control group.
Migration bias	Participants in one group cross over to another group.
Results and Conclusions	
Significance bias	Statistical significance is confused with biologic or clinical significance.
Correlation bias	Correlation (association) is equated with causation.
Ecological fallacy	Inferences about outcomes in groups are generalized inappropriately to individuals.

CORRELATION BIAS

This error occurs when correlation is equated with causation. We stressed in Chapter 19 that it is *never* appropriate to use correlation coefficients to infer causation. Many investigators agree that three conditions are necessary, but not sufficient, to establish that X causes Y: (1) X must precede Y; (2) X and Y must vary together (ie, covary); and (3) no rival explanations can exist to account for the covariation of X and Y (Vogt, 1993, p 31). Thus, correlation results used to assert causation should always be questioned.

ECOLOGIC FALLACY

The ecologic fallacy is a "mistaken conclusion that . . . [is] reached when one infers the behavior or experience of individuals from the behavior or experience of groups" (Michael et al, 1984, p 105). For example, investigators have consistently found a strong, direct relationship between dietary fat consumption per capita and breast cancer occurrence in different countries (Greenberg, 1993, pp 126–127). Researchers then conclude that an association exists between dietary fat intake and breast cancer. Because investigators classify countries by estimates of the general level of fat intake per capita, however, these studies do not demonstrate that increased fat intake in *individuals* is associated with cancer occurrence in these same *individuals*.

USING A CHECKLIST TO EVALUATE PUBLISHED ARTICLES

The following guide is designed to help individuals evaluate published articles. The guide is organized by sections of a published paper and presented in question form. Depending on the study design, some questions may not apply. Keep in mind that researchers do not operate in an ideal world and they cannot control all potential sources of contamination, confounding, or bias. Maintain a clear and realistic view of the constraints that may impact the researchers' ability to plan and conduct an investigation. At the same time, read critically and be alert to biases that may affect a study.

I. *Abstract*
    A. Assuming the study is well done, are the findings worth knowing about?
    B. Do statistically significant results have biologic or clinical significance?

II. *Introduction*
    A. Does the literature review establish a clear need for the study?
    B. How does this study differ from previous investigations?
    C. Is the problem stated clearly?
    D. Is the purpose clearly articulated?
    E. Are the hypotheses stated clearly and concisely? Are the hypotheses developed from previous literature or from sound clinical observation?
    F. Are the hypotheses plausible?
    G. Is the potential significance of the study described? (This may be found in the Discussion and Conclusions section.)

III. *Methods*
    A. *Study participants*
       1. Are the sampling methods clearly described? How were study participants recruited? How were they sampled? What is the total number of participants?
       2. Did patients participate voluntarily? If inducements were offered, are these described? Did study participants give informed consent?
       3. Are eligibility criteria detailed? What limitations may occur because of these criteria?
       4. How were study participants assigned to groups? Were patients matched or

paired? Was group assignment random? Was a control (reference) group included? If control subjects were included, were they appropriate controls?

    5. Are all relevant characteristics of participants described (eg, age, gender, education, disease or health status, and race)?

    6. Do the samples represent the target population?

    7. Are the samples large enough to support generalizations?

    8. Did investigators control for biases that can affect selection of participants? If so, how?

B. *Study design*

    1. Is the study design described thoroughly?

    2. Is the design appropriate, given the objectives of the study?

    3. Are the data sources appropriate (eg, death certificates, medical records, self-report data, surveys, questionnaires, occupational histories)?

    4. Are the independent and dependent variables operationally defined? How were these variables measured? Is the reliability of measurements established? (These issues may be described in the Procedures section.)

    5. How was patient compliance monitored? How were patients followed? How was patient attrition handled (eg, Were subjects labeled as "lost to follow-up" and excluded from all analyses?)

    6. Were study participants treated identically, except for the experimental maneuver?

    7. How were measurement biases controlled?

C. *Procedures*

    1. Are references or explanations given for unusual study methods?

    2. Do the investigators describe the sources for (and type of) equipment and supplies?

    3. Was blinding used when feasible? Are descriptions of blinding clear and realistic? If blinding was not used, what biases may threaten the study?

    4. Are experimental maneuvers thoroughly defined? Are procedures standardized and consistent?

    5. What quality assurance procedures were used in a multicenter study, if more than one individual executed the experimental maneuver, or if more than one individual measured and evaluated outcomes?

    6. Are definitions of terms, measurement procedures, and diagnostic criteria appropriate, given the study design and objectives?

    7. Do the investigators describe contraindications that may have led to the modification or discontinuation of treatment for certain participants?

    8. Are instructions that were given to patients summarized or quoted?

    9. Do the procedures comply with federal guidelines for the use of human subjects?

    10. How were procedural biases minimized?

D. *Statistical analyses*

    1. Are the analyses described fully? Are they understandable? Are analyses referenced if they are not widely used? Which descriptive procedures are used? Which inferential procedures are used?

    2. Are the analyses appropriate given the study design, objectives, and hypotheses?

    3. Is statistical significance defined (eg, $\alpha = 0.05$)?

    4. Do all comparisons involve the same number of individuals? If not, are discrepancies explained and appropriate?

    5. Were multiple independent comparisons done? If so, are appropriate adjustments made to the level of significance to take into account the total number of comparisons?

    6. Are confounding variables identified and handled appropriately?

IV. *Results*

A. Do the results relate to the objectives and hypotheses?

B. Are summary data presented (eg, means, standard deviations, frequencies, range) and not just statistical test results?

C. Do the findings derive from the analyses? (When obtained results are not consistent with hypothesized outcomes, some investigators ignore obtained results and describe findings that are not actually observed.)

   D. Are appropriate, clearly labeled tables and charts used to present important findings?
   E. Are calculated values of test statistics reported?
   F. Are *p*-values presented? Are confidence intervals constructed, when appropriate?
   G. Can significant differences between study groups be attributed to initial lack of comparability between these groups?
   H. Are results consistent internally, that is, from analysis to analysis?
   I. What precautions were taken to minimize analysis biases?
V. *Discussion and Conclusions*
   A. Are conclusions supported by data and statistical analysis?
   B. Do the investigators distinguish between statistical and clinical or biologic significance?
   C. Are results extrapolated appropriately? Are the findings extended to the appropriate target population? Do the investigators overgeneralize?
   D. Are conclusions biologically or clinically plausible?
   E. Is our understanding of the problem enhanced by this study? Are conflicting findings in recent studies clarified?
   F. Are competing or alternative explanations for the findings discussed?
   G. Do the investigators address shortcomings and limitations of their study? Do the investigators provide constructive suggestions for future research?

REFERENCES

Bausell R: *Conducting Meaningful Experiments: 40 Steps to Becoming a Scientist.* Sage, 1994.

Dawson-Saunders B, Trapp R: *Basic and Clinical Biostatistics,* 2nd ed. Appleton & Lange, 1994.

Fitzgerald P: Endocrine disorders. In: *Current Medical Diagnosis and Treatment.* Tierney L Jr et al (editors). Appleton & Lange, 1993.

Freeman R: Evaluation of the kidney. In: *Current Medical Diagnosis and Treatment.* Tierney L Jr et al (editors). Appleton & Lange, 1993.

Glantz S: *Primer of Biostatistics,* 3rd ed. McGraw-Hill, 1981.

Greenberg R: *Medical Epidemiology.* Appleton & Lange, 1993.

Klemetti A, Saxen L: Prospective versus retrospective approach in the search for environmental causes of malformations. *Am J Pub Health* 1967;**57:**2071.

Michael M, Boyce W, Wilcox A: *Biomedical Bestiary: An Epidemiologic Guide to Flaws and Fallacies in the Medical Literature.* Little, Brown, 1984.

Mills J: Data torturing. *N Engl J Med* 1993;**329:**1196.

Paulos J: Counting on dyscalculia. *Discover,* March 1994:30.

Raventos A, Horn R Jr, Ravdin I: Carcinoma of the thyroid gland in youth: A second look ten years later. *J Clin Endocrin Metab* 1962;**22:**886.

Sackett D: Bias in analytic research. *J Chron Dis* 1979;**32:**51.

Schull W, Cobb S: The intrafamilial transmission of rheumatoid arthritis. *J Chron Dis* 1969;**22:**217.

Vogt W: *Dictionary of Statistics and Methodology: A Nontechnical Guide for the Social Sciences.* Sage, 1993.

Williamson J, Goldschmidt P, Colton T: The quality of medical literature. An analysis of validation assessments. In: *Medical Uses of Statistics.* Bailar J, Mosteller F (editors). Massachusetts Medical Society, 1986.

Practice Examination

Directions: For questions 1 to 92, select the one best lettered answer for each question.

Data for Questions 1 through 8

A surgical oncologist studied three groups of women whose disease status is known to determine if p65, a protein in the blood, is a useful indicator of breast cancer. Data appear in the following table.

Breast disease status and p65 test results in three groups of women.

Test Result[a]	Breast Disease Status			Total
	Cancer	Benign	Disease-Free	
p65 positive	212	13	21	246
p65 negative	23	62	179	264
TOTAL	235	75	200	510

[a]Positive = test result above normal; negative = test result within normal range.

1. This study is an example of a _____ investigation.
   a. retrospective cohort
   b. prospective cohort
   c. clinical trial
   d. case-control
   e. cross-sectional
2. If the investigator wishes to determine whether p65 levels (positive/negative) are associated with disease status in women with benign diseases and women with cancer, she should calculate the
   a. relative risk.
   b. odds.
   c. risk difference.
   d. odds-ratio.
3. What is the cumulative incidence of breast cancer in this study?
   a. 212/510 = 0.42.
   b. 235/510 = 0.46.
   c. 212/246 = 0.86.
   d. 212/235 = 0.90.
   e. Cumulative incidence of disease cannot be calculated from an investigation with this type of study design.
4. What is the probability that a woman selected at random has benign breast disease?
   a. 13/510 = 0.03.
   b. 62/510 = 0.12.
   c. 75/510 = 0.15.
   d. 62/264 = 0.23.
5. What is the probability that a woman has breast cancer given a positive p65 test result?
   a. 212/510 = 0.42.
   b. 212/246 = 0.86.
   c. 212/235 = 0.90.
   d. 235/246 = 0.96.

6. What is the probability that a woman is disease-free and has a negative p65 test result?
   a. $179/510 = 0.35$.
   b. $179/264 = 0.68$.
   c. $179/246 = 0.73$.
   d. $179/200 = 0.90$.

7. The fraction $13/246$ is the probability that a woman has
   a. benign disease and a positive p65 test result.
   b. a positive p65 test result, given that she has benign disease.
   c. benign disease, given that she has a positive p65 test.
   d. benign disease.

8. The investigator compared women with breast cancer and women who are disease-free and found that women with breast cancer are approximately 79 times more likely to have a positive p65 test result than disease-free women. The correct interpretation of this finding is
   a. there are approximately 79 women who have breast cancer and a positive p65 test for every one woman who has cancer and a negative p65 test.
   b. the association between p65 and breast cancer disease status is so strong that we may conclude that p65 causes breast cancer.
   c. women who test positive for p65 are approximately 79 times more likely to develop disease than women who test negative.
   d. the odds of a positive p65 test result in breast cancer patients are approximately 79 times greater than the odds of a positive test result in disease-free women.

9. An epidemiologist studied the relationship between body weight and longevity in men and found that very thin and very heavy men have the shortest life spans. Perplexed by these findings, she reexamined her data and found that cigarette smoking is associated with longevity. She reanalyzed the data, while controlling for cigarette smoking, and found that lean men live the longest. In this study, cigarette smoking is a (an) _____ variable.
   a. dependent
   b. independent
   c. predictor
   d. confounding

Data for Questions 10 and 11

Patients with a rare and often fatal eye cancer known as ocular melanoma were assigned randomly to undergo conventional treatment, which involves removing the affected eyeball, or an experimental therapy, in which a small plastic disc containing radioactive iodine is attached surgically to the back of the eyeball, which is left in place. Patients are followed for 10 years to determine the proportion of participants alive at the end of the follow-up period and mean survival time (months).

10. This study is an example of a (an) _____.
    a. prospective cohort investigation.
    b. case-control investigation.
    c. uncontrolled clinical trial.
    d. controlled clinical trial.
    e. cross-sectional investigation.

11. In reviewing all patient records and data, auditors from the National Cancer Institute discover that several patients receiving the experimental treatment died within 5 to 7 months of the beginning of the study. After death, these patients were then reallocated to the conventional therapy group by the principal investigator and their results were analyzed with this group. Reallocating these patients to the conventional treatment group is an example of _____ bias.
    a. withdrawal
    b. bogus control
    c. migration
    d. tidying-up

12. Stimulated by case series reports that men with prostate cancer appear to have a family history of prostate cancer, two urologists asked newly diagnosed cases and controls, ages 50 to 80 years, whether men in their family have ever been diagnosed with prostate cancer. They found that men with prostate cancer are three times more likely than disease-free men to have a family history of this disease. Their results may be affected by _____ bias.
    a. exposure suspicion
    b. diagnostic suspicion
    c. family information
    d. disease significance

13. Because three cases of a very rare brain cancer have been detected in children living in a small community located near a hazardous waste disposal site, local clinicians want to determine if they can identify risk factors associated with cancer development. They should conduct a _____ to address this question.
    a. case-control investigation
    b. controlled clinical trial
    c. prospective cohort study
    d. cross-sectional study

Data for Questions 14 through 18

The use of inhaled corticosteroids is studied in 35 outpatients, ages 2 to 7 years. Study participants have severe perennial asthma, defined as asthma that has not been controlled for at least 3 months by treatment. Children self-administer a nebulized solution of budesonide twice daily. They are then examined monthly during the first year of treatment and every 3 months thereafter for 4 years. Height, weight, height velocity, bone age, and pulmonary function measurements are considered in separate analyses. Pre- and posttrial values are compared for each variable.

14. The independent variable(s) is (are)
    a. asthma status: severe perennial asthma (yes/no).
    b. age (2 to 7 years).
    c. budesonide therapy.
    d. height, weight, height velocity, bone age, and pulmonary function measurements.

15. Which statistical test is appropriate to examine the questions of interest?
    a. Student's t test for means, matched/paired data.
    b. Student's t test for means, independent groups.
    c. z test for means, independent groups.
    d. Pearson correlation.

16. In one analysis, the investigators compared mean bone age pre- and posttrial to determine if the posttrial mean is significantly greater than the pretrial mean. The p-value is 0.002 ($\alpha = 0.05$). The correct interpretation of this finding is
    a. the null hypothesis of no mean difference is retained.
    b. normal biologic variation is a probable explanation for this result.
    c. pre- and posttrial differences are due to chance variation.
    d. the posttrial mean is significantly greater than the pretrial mean.
    e. the pretrial mean is significantly greater than the posttrial mean.

17. To maximize the external validity of their findings, the investigators should extend their conclusions about budesonide treatment to
    a. children with asthma.
    b. children, ages 2 to 7 years, with asthma.
    c. children who have asthma, who are outpatients, and who are between the ages of 2 and 7 years.
    d. children who have severe perennial asthma, who are outpatients, and who are between the ages of 2 and 7 years.

18. A colleague suggests that it may be worthwhile to plot bone age and time (months), beginning at time zero (pretherapy) and including each follow-up examination (eg, 1 month, 2 months, and so forth). He suggests using linear regression with bone age as the dependent variable and time as the predictor, if the data are linear and homoscedastic. His recommendation is
    a. a sound one, if these two important assumptions are satisfied.
    b. inappropriate, because chi-square is better suited than regression to determine if bone age and time are associated.
    c. inappropriate, because *time* is a repeated measure and values of bone age at each time are not independent.
    d. inappropriate, because estimates of the slope and intercept are subject to too much sampling fluctuation with a sample size as small as 35.

19. In an investigation of the role of agricultural exposures to pesticides in the development of neurologic disorders, one important difference between an observational and experimental study is that
    a. the treatment and control groups are the same size in an experimental study.
    b. the researchers determine who is and is not exposed to pesticides in an experimental study.
    c. the experimental study is prospective.
    d. study participants are selected based on their hisotry of agricultural exposure to pesticides in an experimental investigation.

20. Random assignment of individuals to treatment and control groups in experimental investigations
    a. ensures that assignment to the treatment and control condition occurs by chance.
    b. ensures that the treatment and control groups are as similar as possible, except for the experimental maneuver.
    c. minimizes or eliminates admission bias.
    d. minimizes or eliminates the Hawthorne effect as a possible explanation for post-treatment differences between groups.

21. In cohort studies
    a. clinicians compare factors present in the history of participants with and without disease to identify risk factors.
    b. participants with known exposures are followed over time to chart the development of new disease.
    c. researchers are able to determine the prevalence of disease by recording the number of new cases and dividing that value by the number of persons observed.
    d. investigators determine who will and will not be exposed to suspected risk factors, and then record the number of new cases of disease in exposed and unexposed groups.

Data for Question 22

Oncologists studied 30,000 patient charts to examine the relationship between adolescent mononucleosis (M+) and adult onset of non-Hodgkin's lymphoma (L+). They obtained the following results: $pr(M+) = 0.15$; $pr(L+) = 0.01$; and $pr(L+|M+) = 0.15$.

22. The appropriate interpretation of these findings is that
    a. 15% of individuals in this sample had mononucleosis and adult onset non-Hodgkin's lymphoma.
    b. 15% of individuals in this sample who had mononucleosis as an adolescent subsequently developed non-Hodgkin's lymphoma as an adult.
    c. the occurrence of adolescent mononucleosis and adult onset non-Hodgkin's lymphoma appear to be independent because $pr(M+)$ and $pr(L+|M+) = 0.15$ are equal.
    d. the percentage of individuals who developed adult onset non-Hodgkin's lymphoma is so small (1%) that reliable statements cannot be made about the relationship between this disease and adolescent mononucleosis.

23. A pharmaceutical company claims that an experimental influenza vaccine produces immunity (elevated antibody titer) in 95% of adults. If the company's claims are true, the distribution of the number of vaccinated adults who will obtain *inadequate* immunity in a sample of 20 is
    a. binomial with $p = 0.05$ and $n = 20$.
    b. binomial with $p = 0.95$ and $n = 20$.
    c. binomial with $p = 0.50$ and $n = 20$.
    d. continuous with values ranging from 0 to 20 adults.

Data for Question 24

Clinicians examine total cholesterol levels for each of 2000 elementary school children, grades 1 to 8, with a hypercholesterolemic mother. Total cholesterol is measured quantitatively. Values range from 140 to 300 mg/dL. Approximately 10% of these values fall between 140 and 160 mg/dL; 60% occur between 220 and 260 mg/dL; and 15% are greater than 261 mg/dL.

24. Which measure of central tendency should the clinicians use to describe the "average" total cholesterol of these children?
    a. Mode.
    b. Median.
    c. Mean.
    d. Weighted mean, with weights proportional to the number of children in each grade.

Data for Question 25

Two cardiologists investigated the relationship between heart attack in 1500 men, ages 55 to 75 years, and activity level 24 hours preceding the attack. Activity level was classified as heavy exertion, moderate exertion, or mild to very light exertion. Fifty percent of heart attacks occurred when the patient had been involved in activities demanding heavy exertion within 24 hours of the attack; 35% in activities requiring moderate exertion; and 15% in activities demanding mild to very light exertion.

25. Which graph is appropriate to display the heart attack by activity level data?
    a. Bar diagram.
    b. Histogram.
    c. Frequency polygon with raw frequency on the y-axis.
    d. Frequency polygon with percentage frequency on the y-axis.

Data for Question 26

The number of children with central nervous system (CNS) tumors who were admitted to a large metropolitan hospital for tumor-related treatment is displayed in the following table.

Hospital admissions for tumor-related treatment in children with CNS tumors.

Age (years)	Number of Children Admitted in Interval			
	1975–1979	1980–1984	1985–1990	Total
0–4	24	34	66	124
5–9	16	28	70	114
10–14	24	18	14	56
TOTAL	64	80	150	294

26. These data support which of the following conclusions?
   a. The prevalence of CNS tumors increased between 1975 and 1990.
   b. The prevalence of CNS tumors is higher in children who are 0 to 4 years old than in children who are 10 to 14 years old.
   c. Between 1975 and 1990, the cumulative incidence of CNS tumors increased in children who are 5 to 9 years old.
   d. Between 1975 and 1990, the cumulative incidence of CNS tumors decreased in children who are 10 to 14 years old.
   e. Between 1975 and 1990, the number of hospital admissions for tumor-related treatment increased in children with CNS tumors.

27. Investigators studied three groups of men, ages 30 to 50 years, to examine the relationship between smoking and high-density lipoprotein (HDL) levels (mg/dL): group 1 never smoked cigarettes, $n = 332$; group 2 was made up of ex-cigarette smokers who had quit for at least 1 year, $n = 221$; and group 3 consisted of current smokers, $n = 493$. To plot the distribution of HDL data for each study group on the same set of axes, the researchers should construct a _____ for each group.
   a. bar diagram with percentage frequency on the y-axis and HDL values on the x-axis
   b. histogram with raw frequency on the y-axis and HDL values on the x-axis
   c. frequency polygon with percentage frequency on the y-axis and HDL values on the x-axis
   d. frequency polygon with raw frequency on the y-axis and HDL values on the x-axis

Data for Question 28

Epidemiologists examined deaths in 1990 by sex and race for malignant neoplasms, cardiovascular disease, accidents, and homicides. Data are displayed in the figure.

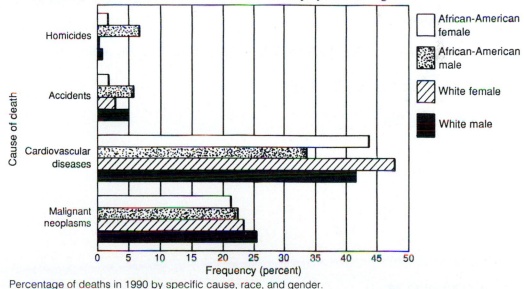

Percentage of deaths in 1990 by specific cause, race, and gender.

Source: Table 9, Advance Report on Final Mortality Statistics, Monthly Vital Statistics Report, Centers for Disease Control and Prevention, 1993, 41 (Supplement): 24–25.)

28. The appropriate interpretation of these findings is that
   a. the percentage of deaths due to accidents is lower in white females than African-American females.
   b. the incidence density of deaths due to homicides is lower in white females than white males.
   c. the percentage of deaths due to malignant neoplasms is between 20 and 25% in all four groups.
   d. in African-American men the prevalence of death due to cardiovascular diseases is approximately 5.5 times higher than the risk of death due to accidents.

29. An important difference between cumulative incidence and incidence density is
    a. the type of study design from which each is determined.
    b. the definition of the denominator.
    c. the definition of the numerator.
    d. that only incidence density describes the occurrence of new disease; cumulative incidence reflects already existing disease.

Data for Questions 30 through 33

At the beginning of a randomized controlled clinical trial, a gynecologist asked women with clinically diagnosed premenstrual syndrome (PMS) to rate the quality of their life, with zero indicating very poor and 10 being very good. The ratings of 5 participants are 2, 2, 3, 5, and 6.

30. The mean quality-of-life rating is
    a. $(2 + 2 + 3 + 5)/4 = 12/4 = 3.0$.
    b. $(2 + 2 + 3 + 5 + 6)/5 = 18/5 = 3.6$.
    c. $(2 + 3 + 3 + 5 + 6)/5 = 19/5 = 3.8$.
    d. $(2 + 3 + 5 + 6)/4 = 16/4 = 4.0$.
31. The median rating is
    a. 2.
    b. 3.
    c. $(3 + 5)/2 = 4.0$.
32. The modal rating is
    a. 2.
    b. 3.
    c. 5.
    d. 6.
33. Given that $(\Sigma X)^2 = 324$ and $\Sigma X^2 = 78$, the variance of the quality-of-life ratings is

    a. $\sqrt{\dfrac{78 - \dfrac{324}{5}}{4}} = \sqrt{3.3} = 1.82$

    b. $\sqrt{\dfrac{78 - \dfrac{324}{5}}{5}} = \sqrt{2.64} = 1.62$

    c. $\dfrac{78 - \dfrac{324}{5}}{4} = 3.3$

    d. $\dfrac{78 - \dfrac{324}{5}}{5} = 2.64$

Data for Question 34

In response to a complaint from a patient about the cost of a common over-the-counter antihistamine, a family practitioner surveyed the pharmacies in the community in which he practices. The cost of 16 brand-name tablets, available in only one strength, are $1.46, $1.79, $1.99, $2.29, $2.99, and $8.99.

34. The most appropriate measure of central tendency for these data is the
    a. mode.
    b. median.
    c. mean.
    d. weighted mean.

Data for Questions 35 and 36

Women participating in a 6-month, supervised weight-loss program were measured before the program began and after it ended. Included in the measurements are diastolic blood pressure, weight, and total cholesterol. End-of-program data appear in the table below.

End-of-weight-loss program measurements for 25 female participants.

	Diastolic Blood Pressure (mm Hg)	Mean Weight Loss (kg)	Cholesterol (mg/dL)
Mean	85.0	7.0	270.0
SD	13.0	2.0	26.0
Number	25	25	25

35. Which of the following statements is true regarding the variation in these end-of-program measurements?
    a. The weight-loss data exhibit the least variation.
    b. The cholesterol values show the greatest variation.
    c. The variation in blood pressure readings is greater than weight lost, but less than the variation in cholesterol values.
    d. The total cholesterol readings are less variable than the blood pressure and weight lost.
    e. Descriptive comparisons about variation cannot be made because each variable has a different measurement metric (kilograms versus mg/dL versus mm Hg).
36. Based on the means and standard deviations presented in the table, what can be inferred about the shape of these three distributions?
    a. The distribution of total cholesterol values is probably skewed, because its standard deviation is so much larger than the standard deviation of the other two variables.
    b. The weight loss distribution is probably bell-shaped, because the standard deviation is small in relation to the standard deviation of the other two variables.
    c. The distribution of total cholesterol values is probably bell-shaped, because its standard deviation is not particularly large in relation to its mean.
    d. No inferences about the shape of a distribution can be made from the information given in the table.

Data for Questions 37 through 39

Diastolic blood pressure is distributed normally in a group of female automotive assembly line workers, with a mean of 80 mm Hg and standard deviation of 10 ($n = 75$).

37. What is the probability that a worker selected at random from this group has a diastolic blood pressure of 90 mm Hg or greater?
    a. $1/75 = 0.0133$.
    b. Approximately 0.16.
    c. Approximately 0.34.
    d. Approximately 0.66.
    e. Approximately 0.84.
38. Approximately what percentage of workers have a diastolic blood pressure of 70 mm Hg or greater?
    a. 16%.
    b. 34%.
    c. 48%.
    d. 84%.
39. Approximately what percentage of workers have a diastolic blood pressure between 60 and 90 mm Hg?
    a. 32%.
    b. 48%.
    c. 64%.
    d. 82%.

Data for Questions 40 through 41

After extensive study, gastroenterologists note that the mean age at onset for a particular intestinal disorder is 25 years. The median age at onset is 17.6 years; the modal age is 15.1 years. The disease typically attacks patients between the ages of 8 and 45 years.

40. The distribution of age at onset for this particular intestinal disorder is
   a. approximately bell-shaped.
   b. positively skewed.
   c. negatively skewed.
   d. asymmetrical, but the type of skewness (positive or negative) can be determined only from a graph of these data.
41. Although all measures of central tendency have been calculated for the age at onset data, the preferred measure of central tendency is the
   a. mean.
   b. mode.
   c. median.

Data for Questions 42 through 45

Within a community of 1000 adults, an initial clinical examination reveals that 250 have hypertension, defined as a diastolic blood pressure greater than 90 mm Hg and a systolic blood pressure greater than 140 mm Hg. All adults are followed for 5 years. During this follow-up period, 50 additional adults develop hypertension; 5 of these individuals die within 2 years of diagnosis of coronary heart disease or a cerebrovascular accident.

42. The initial prevalence of hypertension is
   a. 50/250.
   b. 50/750.
   c. 50/1000.
   d. 250/750.
   e. 250/1000.
43. The cumulative incidence of hypertension is
   a. 50/250.
   b. 50/750.
   c. 50/1000.
   d. 250/1000.
44. The cumulative incidence of hypertension is the _____ of developing hypertension within 5 years.
   a. risk
   b. relative risk
   c. odds
   d. odds ratio
45. The 2-year case fatality of incident cases is
   a. 5/50.
   b. 5/(50 + 250).
   c. 5/750.
   d. 5/1000.

Data for Questions 46 through 54

Polymerase chain reaction (PCR) DNA amplification, an experimental method, and Southern blot hybridization are used to screen for human papillomavirus (HPV) in 467 undergraduate women who are seen by a physician for a routine gynecologic examination at a university health service. Because the Southern blot technique is currently considered the "gold standard," this technique is used to define true infection status. Results appear in the table.

Test characteristics of PCR in screening for human
papillomavirus in undergraduate college women.

Test Result	True Infection Status		Total
	Diseased	Disease-free	
PCR positive	190	23	213
PCR negative	10	244	254
TOTAL	200	267	467

46. The true prevalence of HPV in the study group is
    a. 190/467 = 0.41.
    b. 200/467 = 0.43.
    c. 213/467 = 0.46.
    d. 190/213 = 0.89.
    e. 190/200 = 0.95.
47. The prevalence of HPV as estimated by the PCR test is
    a. 190/467 = 0.41.
    b. 200/467 = 0.43.
    c. 213/467 = 0.46.
    d. 190/213 = 0.89.
    e. 190/200 = 0.95.
48. The sensitivity of PCR is
    a. 190/467 = 0.41.
    b. 200/467 = 0.43.
    c. 213/467 = 0.46.
    d. 190/213 = 0.89.
    e. 190/200 = 0.95.
49. If a woman who is disease-free has a positive PCR test, her test result is referred to as a
    a. false negative.
    b. false positive.
    c. true negative.
    d. true positive.
50. What is the probability that a woman who is disease-free will have a negative test result?
    a. 244/467 = 0.52.
    b. 254/467 = 0.54.
    c. 254/467 = 0.57.
    d. 244/267 = 0.91.
    e. 244/254 = 0.96.
51. What is the probability that a woman is diseased, given that her PCR test is positive?
    a. 190/467 = 0.41.
    b. 200/467 = 0.43.
    c. 213/467 = 0.46.
    d. 190/213 = 0.89.
    e. 190/200 = 0.96.
52. The probability that a woman has HPV given a positive PCR test is the _____ of the test.
    a. sensitivity
    b. specificity
    c. positive predictive value
    d. true positive value
    e. negative predictive value
53. What proportion of test results are false negatives?
    a. 10/254 = 0.04.
    b. 10/200 = 0.05.
    c. 23/267 = 0.09.
    d. 244/267 = 0.91.
    e. 244/254 = 0.96.

54. Suppose that with increased screening and highly effective treatment, the prevalence of HPV in the target population decreases from 42 cases per 100 women to 5 cases per 100 women. Which of the following statements is true about the effect of this decrease in prevalence on the performance characteristics of the PCR test?
    a. The sensitivity of the PCR test will decrease.
    b. The specificity of the PCR test will decrease.
    c. The specificity of the PCR test will increase and sensitivity will decrease.
    d. The positive predictive value will decrease.
    e. The negative predictive value will decrease.

55. A couple seeks genetic counseling because both are carriers of a particular disease. They would like to have 4 children. They are told that the each child has independently a 50% chance of being born with the disease. If the couple has 4 children, what is the probability that one child will have the disease?
    a. 0.50.
    b. 0.50^4.
    c. $4 (0.50) (1 - 0.50)^3$.
    d. $4 (0.50^3) (1 - 0.50)$.

Data for Question 56

As part of her yearly physical examination, a patient who is entirely well has a 20-screen test performed on a blood sample. In the clinical laboratory to which the sample is submitted, limits for normal are set for each test to include all but the upper and lower $2\frac{1}{2}\%$ of the adult population.

56. What is the probability that this patient will have at least one abnormal test result?

    a. $\dfrac{20\,!}{0\,!(20 - 0)\,!}0.05^0\,0.95^{20\,-\,0} = 0.95^{20} = 0.36$

    b. $\dfrac{20\,!}{1\,!(20 - 1)\,!}0.05^1\,0.95^{20\,-\,1} = 20(0.05)(0.95^{19}) = 0.38$

    c. $1 - \dfrac{20\,!}{0\,!(20 - 0)\,!}0.05^0\,0.95^{20\,-\,0} = 1 - 0.95^{20} = 1 - 0.36 = 0.64$

    d. $1 - \dfrac{20\,!}{1\,!(20 - 1)\,!}0.05^1\,0.95^{20\,-\,1} = 1 - 20(0.05)(0.95^{19}) = 1 - 0.38 = 0.62$

Data for Questions 57 through 59

Amyotrophic lateral sclerosis (ALS) is a disorder caused by degeneration of motor neurons of the central nervous system. Mean survival after diagnosis is 3.5 years, with a standard deviation of 1.2 years. An investigator believes he has identified a dietary oil that blocks this degenerative process and, therefore, increases the survival of ALS patients. In 40 patients to whom this oil is given, mean survival following diagnosis is 3.7 years.

57. Identify the scientific (research) hypothesis.
    a. ALS patients treated with the dietary oil have a mean survival time following diagnosis that is significantly greater than 3.5 years.
    b. ALS patients treated with the dietary oil have a mean survival time following diagnosis that differs significantly from 3.5 years.
    c. A significant difference exists in mean survival time postdiagnosis in two groups of ALS patients, one treated conventionally and one treated with a dietary oil.
    d. In two groups of ALS patients, the mean survival time after diagnosis is significantly greater in patients treated with a dietary oil, compared to conventionally treated patients.

58. Assuming that the relevant distribution of survival times is skewed (nonnormal), which statistical test is appropriate to answer the question of interest?
    a. t test, one mean.
    b. t test, two means, independent groups.
    c. z test, one mean.
    d. z test, two means, independent groups.
59. Identify the appropriate conclusion given the following findings: calculated value of test statistic = 1.05; critical value of test statistic = 1.645; $\alpha = 0.05$.
    a. Dietary oil use in ALS patients contributes to mean survival following diagnosis that is significantly greater than 3.5 years.
    b. Dietary oil use in ALS patients does not contribute to a significant increase in mean survival following diagnosis.
    c. No significant difference exists in mean survival time postdiagnosis between ALS patients treated conventionally and those treated with a dietary oil.
    d. A significant increase in mean postdiagnosis survival accrues to ALS patients treated with dietary oil.

Data for Questions 60 through 62

Monoamine inhibitors are highly effective in treating patients who suffer from panic attacks, providing relief to 80% of individuals who take them. Investigators believe that monoamine inhibitors used in conjunction with behavioral therapy will increase the proportion of patients to whom relief is provided. In a small-scale study, they observe that 9 of 10 patients following this dual regimen experience relief. (M = monoamine inhibitors, MB = monoamine inhibitors and behavioral therapy.)

60. The null hypothesis is
    a. $\pi = 0.80$.
    b. $\pi > 0.80$.
    c. $\pi_{MB} - \pi_{M} = 0$.
    d. $\pi_{MB} - \pi_{M} > 0$.
61. Which statistical test is appropriate to examine the question of interest in this study?
    a. z test (normal approximation to the binomial), two proportions, independent groups.
    b. Chi-square for independence.
    c. Binomial exact test, one proportion.
    d. z test (normal approximation to the binomial), one proportion.
62. In this study, a Type I error would occur if the investigators found
    a. no significant increase, when the true proportion enjoying relief is actually greater than 0.80.
    b. a significant increase, when the true proportion enjoying relief is actually 0.80.
    c. a significant increase, when the true proportion enjoying relief is actually greater than 0.80.

Data for Questions 63 through 66

The results of a study of dementia in 6 elderly nursing home patients are graphed in the figure. Solid lines depict the time each patient was observed and at risk for developing dementia. Dashed lines indicate time observed after diagnosis (Dx) of dementia.

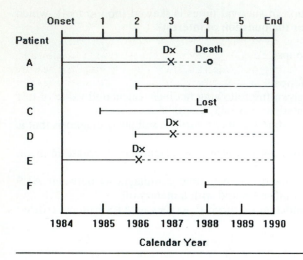

Occurrence of dementia and death in six elderly nursing home patients.

63. The prevalence of dementia in 1987 is
   a. 2/5.
   b. 2/6.
   c. 3/5.
   d. 3/6.

64. Patient E was observed for _____ person-years.
   a. 2
   b. 3
   c. 4
   d. 5
   e. 6

65. The 2-year survival following a diagnosis of dementia is
   a. 2/3.
   b. 2/4.
   c. 2/5.
   d. 2/6.

66. To calculate the incidence density of dementia among these patients, include _____ in the denominator.
   a. total number of patients observed
   b. total number of patients who were followed until the end of the study
   c. total person years for patients B, D, E, and F
   d. total person-years observed for all 6 patients

Data for Questions 67 through 70

The value of diet, exercise, and meditation was studied in 16 hypertensive women. The researchers believe these women will enjoy a decrease in their diastolic blood pressure after 4 months in the experimental program. The pretrial mean diastolic blood pressure of study participants is 120 mm Hg; their posttrial diastolic pressure is 115. Assume normality of the relevant distribution(s).

67. The investigators should use which statistical test to examine their data?
   a. *t* test, two independent means.
   b. *z* test, two independent mean.
   c. *t* test, within-subject design.
   d. *z* test, within-subject design.

68. The researchers conducted the appropriate statistical test with $\alpha = 0.05$ and obtained a p-value < 0.04. The appropriate conclusion is that
   a. severely hypertensive women in the experimental program enjoy a decrease in diastolic blood pressure (pre versus post), but this decrease is not statistically significant.
   b. a significant difference exists between pre- and posttrial diastolic blood pressure among women who participate in the experimental program.
   c. no signficant difference exists between pre- and posttrial diastolic blood pressure among women who participate in the experimental program.
   d. posttrial diastolic blood pressure of severely hypertensive women who participate in the experimental program is significantly less than their pretrial reading.

69. The statistical analysis conducted by these investigators is an example of a _____
   a. two-tailed test.
   b. nondirectional test.
   c. one-tailed, test with pretrial blood pressure greater than posttrial systolic blood pressure.
   d. one-tailed, test with pretrial systolic blood pressure less than posttrial systolic blood pressure.

70. The results of this study are threatened by
   a. a correlation bias.
   b. regression on the mean.
   c. a bogus control bias.
   d. an ecologic fallacy.

Data for Questions 71 through 72

Surgical resection of squamous cell carcinoma of the lung results in a 5-year survival of 35% in women whose tumor is localized at diagnosis. Clinicians tested the hypothesis that surgery, coupled with single-agent chemotherapy following surgery, increases 5-year survival in affected women. Eight of 20 affected women (40%) who undergo surgery and chemotherapy after surgery live 5 years or more.

71. The appropriate alternative hypothesis is
   a. $\pi = 0.35$.
   b. $\pi > 0.35$.
   c. $\pi_{SURG + CHEMO} - \pi_{SURG} = 0$.
   d. $\pi_{SURG + CHEMO} - \pi_{SURG} > 0$.

72. The principal investigator analyzed the data with $\alpha = 0.01$, with the following results: calculated value of the test statistic $= 0.47$, p-value $= 0.32$. Which of the following conclusions is correct?
   a. The null hypothesis is retained because 0.47 is greater than $\alpha = 0.01$.
   b. The null hypothesis is rejected because 40% is greater than 35%.
   c. The null hypothesis is retained because 0.32 is greater than $\alpha = 0.01$.
   d. No conclusion can be made about the null hypothesis without the critical value of the test statistic.

Data for Questions 73 through 76

The health of women after childbirth is studied in women who work full-time outside the home before and during pregnancy. The investigators believe that a significant difference exists between women who took 6 weeks of leave and those who took 3 months of leave after childbirth, with respect to the amount of depression experienced by the new mother. A reliable and valid standardized questionnaire is used to assess depression; the higher the score, the greater the depression. The maximum possible score is 100. Data appear in the table.

Depression scores in two groups of women
after childbirth.

	Length of Leave After Childbirth	
	6 Weeks	**3 Months**
Mean depression score	60	40
Standard deviation	7	6
Sample size	20	20
Relevant distribution(s)	Normal	Normal

73. The null hypothesis is
    a. $\mu_{6\ wks} - \mu_{3\ months} = 0$.
    b. $\mu_{6\ wks} - \mu_{3\ months} > 0$.
    c. $\pi_{6\ wks} - \pi_{3\ months} = 0$.
    d. $\pi_{6\ wks} - \pi_{3\ months} > 0$.

74. The investigators should use a _____ to analyze their data.
    a. t test, matched groups
    b. t test, independent groups, pooled variance estimate, $df = 20 + 20 - 2$
    c. t test, independent groups, separate variances, df_{adj}
    d. z test, independent groups

75. The investigators calculated the appropriate statistic and obtained the following: calculated value = 9.71, critical value = ± 2.02, p-value < 0.001, $\alpha = 0.05$. The appropriate conclusion is that
    a. women who take 3 months of leave after giving birth are significantly less depressed than their counterparts who take 6 weeks of leave.
    b. no significant mean difference in depression exists between these two groups of women.
    c. a significant mean difference exists in the amount of depression experienced by women who take 6 weeks and those who take 3 months of leave after childbirth.
    d. women who take 3 months of leave after giving birth are significantly more depressed than their counterparts who take 6 weeks of leave.

76. Given the information in question 75, the probability in this study of concluding that a significant mean difference exists between these two groups of women when no true difference exists is
    a. less than 0.001.
    b. 0.05.
    c. greater than 0.001, but less than 0.05.
    d. impossible to determine without additional information.

Data for Questions 77 through 79

Clinicians studied survival after the first bout of *Pneumocystis* pneumonia in male volunteers with acquired immunodeficiency syndrome (AIDS). Participants were assigned randomly to receive zidovudine ($n = 100$) or d4T ($n = 100$), a new drug. The researchers wanted to determine if a difference exists in survival between these two groups. After the first bout of *Pneumocystis* pneumonia, 50% of patients receiving zidovudine survived 18 months or more compared to 79% of men taking d4T.

77. This study is an example of a (an)
    a. prospective cohort investigation.
    b. retrospective cohort study.
    c. case-control investigation.
    d. controlled clinical trial.
    e. uncontrolled clinical trial.

78. The scientific (research) hypothesis is
   a. men with AIDS who take zidovudine and men with AIDS who receive d4T differ with respect to the proportion who survive 18 months or more after the first bout of *Pneumocystis* pneumonia.
   b. mean survival time after the first bout of *Pneumocystis* pneumonia differs in men with AIDS who take zidovudine and men with AIDS who receive d4T.
   c. no difference exists between men with AIDS who take zidovudine and men with AIDS who receive d4T with respect to the proportion who survive 18 months or more after the first bout of *Pneumocystis* pneumonia.
   d. no difference exists in mean survival time after the first bout of *Pneumocystis* pneumonia in men with AIDS who take zidovudine and men with AIDS who recieve d4T.

79. Which statistical test is appropriate for analyzing these data?
   a. Chi-square for independence.
   b. Normal approximation to the binomial, two proportions, matched/paired data.
   c. Normal approximation to the binomial, two proportions, independent groups.
   d. *z* test, two means, independent groups.

Data for Questions 80 through 82

The relationship between stress and cholesterol (mg/dL) is investigated in 1000 men. Stress is measured quantitatively, using a reliable and valid instrument. In plotting the data, the investigators observe that stress levels are similar and much higher in men whose cholesterol is either above 240 mg/dL or below 160 mg/dL compared to men whose cholesterol is between these values.

80. If the researchers compute the Pearson correlation to quantify the strength of the association between cholesterol and stress levels, they will
   a. underestimate the strength of the relationship.
   b. overestimate the strength of the relationship.
   c. inaccurately assess the strength of the relationship; but we cannot determine from this information whether they will underestimate or overestimate it.
   d. obtain an appropriate estimate of the strength of the association.

81. Based on their data, the investigators recommend that highly stressed individuals whose cholesterol is above 240 mg/dL reduce their stress level in order to reduce their cholesterol level. This recommendation is
   a. warranted based on the data.
   b. an example of correlation bias.
   c. an example of therapeutic personality bias.
   d. an example of range restriction.

82. Other investigators have consistently found that individuals with low and high cholesterol levels have low serotonin levels. Further, they note that serotonin "fosters tranquillity;" low levels are associated with stress, hostility, impatience, and other similar behaviors. In the analysis of total cholesterol and stress levels
   a. the clinicians should focus on serotonin levels to reduce high levels of cholesterol and stress.
   b. the researchers should focus on the behaviors associated with high stress (eg, impatience) if they want to reduce total cholesterol and stress.
   c. serotonin levels are not important because the researchers are interested in the relationship between cholesterol and stress.
   d. serotonin levels confound the relationship between total cholesterol and stress.

Data for Question 83

Behavioral therapists study the effect of venting anger on the systolic blood pressure of hypertensive women. The initial mean systolic blood pressure of 20 women who participate in the study is 125 mm Hg. The investigators observe that mean systolic blood pressure is 135 mm Hg after study participants vent their anger. Assume the relevant distribution(s) is (are) normal.

83. The investigators constructed a two-sided 95% confidence interval as (pre- − postventing mean) ± standard error x (two-tailed critical value). This interval extends from −15.6 to −4.40. The appropriate conclusion is that
a. no significant difference exists between the pre- and postventing mean systolic blood pressure.
b. a significant differences exists between the pre- and postventing mean systolic blood pressure.
c. the Student's t test for means from matched/paired data should be performed before we can make a conclusion about the null hypothesis.
d. the postventing mean systolic blood pressure is significantly higher than the premean pressure.

Data for Questions 84 through 86

Trigeminal neuralgia is characterized by momentary episodes of sudden lancinating facial pain, lasting typically 10 to 30 seconds per episode. Two drugs, phenytoin and carbamazepine, are compared to determine their effectiveness for controlling these episodes in 100 affected women matched on age at diagnosis. Data appear in the table.

Relief in patients suffering from trigeminal neuralgia.

	Phenytoin		
Carbamazepine	Relief: Yes	Relief: No	Total
Relief: Yes	12	32	44
Relief: No	1	5	6
TOTAL	13	37	50

84. In this study, the dependent variable is the
a. drug therapy.
b. age at diagnosis.
c. disease status.
d. episode control.

85. The appropriate analysis to determine if a difference in effectiveness exists between these two drugs is the
a. binomial exact test for proportions, matched/paired data.
b. normal approximation to the binomial for proportions, matched/paired data.
c. chi-square for independence.
d. t test, two means, matched/paired data.

86. In the analysis of these data, the number of pairs of observations included in the actual calculations is
a. 50.
b. 44.
c. 37.
d. 33.

Data for Questions 87 through 89

Two pediatricians studied the relationship between lead exposure (μg/dL) and performance on a standardized intelligence test in 122 children who lived near a lead-smelting operation from birth to 12 years. Based on previous research, the clinicians postulated an indirect relationship between these two variables. They obtained the following from a linear regression in which test scores are predicted from exposure: $b = -0.40$, $s_b = 0.16$, $t = -2.5$, $t_{crit} = -1.66$, p-value < 0.01, $\alpha = 0.05$.

87. The appropriate conclusion is that
   a. the slope differs significantly from zero, the value in the null hypothesis.
   b. a significant direct relationship exists between lead exposure and performance on a standardized intelligence test.
   c. the slope is significantly greater than zero, the value in the null hypothesis.
   d. the slope is significantly less than zero, the value in the null hypothesis.
88. If lead exposure increases 10 μg/dL, the predicted value of the intelligence score
   a. increases by 4 points.
   b. decreases by 4 points.
   c. increases by an undetermined amount.
   d. decreases by an undetermined amount.
   e. changes by an undetermined amount; but we cannot assess at this point whether the predicted score increases or decreases.
89. If the investigators compute the Pearson correlation to quantify the strength of the association between lead exposure and intelligence test scores, they will find that
   a. the correlation is positive, indicating that increases in lead exposure tend to be associated with increases in intelligence test scores.
   b. the correlation is negative, indicating that increases in lead exposure tend to be associated with decreases in intelligence test scores.
   c. the correlation differs significantly from zero, but its sign cannot be determined before its calculation.
   d. they have to test the null hypothesis of zero correlation to know whether a significant association exists between lead exposure and intelligence test scores in these children.

Data for Questions 90 through 92

In a study to compare streptokinase and tissue plasminogen activator (TPA) to treat heart attack in men, a cardiologist assigns patients randomly to one of the two drug therapy groups. She then follows patients after the administration of drug therapy and charts the development of complications, including severe bleeding, cardiogenic shock, and allergic reactions. Data appear in the table.

Allergic reactions in two groups of male heart-attack patients.

Drug	Allergic Reactions		Total
	Yes	No	
Streptokinase	7	93	100
TPA	3	97	100
TOTAL	10	190	200

90. The null hypothesis is that
   a. the two populations of patients are homogeneous with respect to the proportion experiencing allergic reactions.
   b. the two populations of patients are not homogeneous with respect to the proportion experiencing allergic reactions.
   c. drug type (streptokinase versus TPA) and allergic reaction (yes/no) are independent.
   d. drug type (streptokinase versus TPA) and allergic reaction (yes/no) are associated.
91. To determine if patients taking streptokinase have an increased risk of allergic reactions compared to patients receiving TPA, the investigator should calculate the
   a. odds.
   b. odds-ratio.
   c. risk.
   d. relative risk.

92. The measure that reflects whether patients taking streptokinase have an increased risk of allergic reactions compared to patients receiving TPA is calculated as
   a. **(7/10) / (93/190) = 1.43.**
   b. **(7/100) / (3/100) = 2.33.**
   c. **(7 × 97) / (3 × 93) = 2.43.**
   d. **(10/200) × 100 = 5.00.**

The following questions (93 to 122) are extended matching items. For each description, select the most appropriate response from the lettered choices. Each choice may be used once, more than once, or not at all.

Questions 93 through 102: Characteristics of Clinical Laboratory Tests

   a. Sensitivity
   b. Specificity
   c. False positive
   d. False negative

93. _____ Proportion or percentage of individuals with the disease of interest who have positive test results.
94. _____ Tests with high _____ are helpful during the early stages of a diagnostic workup, when the goal is to rule out disease.
95. _____ Tests with high _____ have few false-positive results.
96. _____ Tests with high _____ are most helpful when their result is positive.
97. _____ Proportion or percentage of individuals without the disease of interest who have a negative test result.
98. _____ Tests with high _____ have few false-negative results.
99. _____ Tests with high _____ are used to identify serious, but treatable diseases (eg, tuberculosis).
100. _____ Tests with high _____ are used to rule in a diagnosis that has been suggested by other data.
101. _____ Proportion or percentage of individuals with the disease of interest who have a negative test result.
102. _____ As the proportion or percentage of false-positive results increase, _____ decreases.

Questions 103 to 112: Types of Studies

   a. Controlled clinical trial
   b. Case series
   c. Case-control
   d. Cross-sectional
   e. Cohort

103. _____ Study in which patients with and without disease are examined to identify factors present in the history of those with disease and absent, or much less common, in disease-free persons.
104. _____ Study from which disease prevalence is estimated.
105. _____ Study in which investigators determine who will and will not be exposed to an exposure or intervention.
106. _____ Study that incorporates the correct time sequence between exposure and disease development.
107. _____ Study in which interesting findings may be due to chance and therefore cannot be generalized.

108. _____ Study that is ill suited to investigating rare diseases or diseases with a long latency period.

109. _____ Study that is heavily dependent on the quality of existing records.

110. _____ Study that helps to describe the frequency of a disease or condition at a particular point in time.

111. _____ Study that is well suited to investigating rare diseases or diseases with a long latency period.

112. _____ Study from which incidence measures are calculated.

Questions 113 to 122: Biases That Affect Medical Studies

a. Admission bias
b. Bogus control bias
c. Contamination bias
d. Correlation bias
e. Detection bias
f. Diagnostic suspicion bias
g. Ecological fallacy

h. Exposure suspicion bias
i. Family information bias
j. Healthy worker effect
k. Nonresponse bias
l. Prevalence-incidence bias
m. Procedure selection bias
n. Withdrawal bias

113. _____ In a study of the effectiveness of mastectomy and lumpectomy to treat breast cancer, the records of women whose breast cancer metastasized or who died during follow-up are removed from the lumpectomy group and excluded from all analyses.

114. _____ Investigators examining the role of dietary fat and breast cancer development find that women whose diets are high in fat have a significantly greater risk of breast cancer than women whose diets are low in fat. They conclude that lowering dietary fat will reduce the risk of breast cancer in women whose diets are high in fat.

115. _____ Psychiatrists studying an experimental drug to treat schizophrenia reassign patients to the standard therapy (control) group when they have psychotic episodes and analyze these patients' data with those of control patients.

116. _____ Epidemiologists studying the effects of workplace exposure to sulfur dioxide observe that exposed men who smoke have higher pulmonary function measurements than comparably aged male smokers in the general population.

117. _____ In an investigation of a new drug, d4T, to treat patients with AIDS, participants for whom zidovudine or ddI has been ineffective are allocated to the experimental group; other participants are assigned to receive zidovudine.

118. _____ Gastroenterologists studying patients with newly diagnosed Crohn's disease note that these patients are much more likely to report a family history of intestinal disorders than family members who are generally healthy.

119. _____ In comparing survival in men with prostate cancer in 1950 and 1994, epidemiologists find that that the proportion of affected men who survive in 1994 is markedly greater than the proportion in 1950.

120. _____ Cardiologists evaluate aspirin versus a placebo to prevent subsequent heart attacks in men who have already had a heart attack. The researchers conclude that no significant difference exists between the two treatments. After the study, they learn that several men in the placebo group were given aspirin by the resident who dispensed the two medications.

121. _____ Based on animal studies, a particular cancer appears to be associated with pesticide exposure. Patients with and without this cancer are compared to determine if pesticide exposure is a risk factor. Disease-free patients are interviewed by the investigator. Patients with disease are interviewed; their job records are searched; and family members are questioned. The study confirms that pesticide exposure is a risk factor.

122. _____ To study specialty choice satisfaction, two researchers sent a questionnaire to 42,000 physicians in different specialties throughout the United States. The researchers find that satisfaction with specialty choice is highest among surgeons and oncologists and lowest among pediatricians ($n_{Total} = 5000$).

Practice Examination Answers and Brief Explanations

For each question on the practice examination, the correct answer is listed, the tested concept is identified, and a brief explanation is provided. In addition, the chapter is noted in which the concept is presented.

Questions 1 through 9

1. *d Study designs* — The starting point in case-control investigations is known disease status. Cases (women with breast cancer) are compared to two groups of controls (women with benign disease and women who are disease-free) to determine if cases are more likely to have a positive p65 test result. [*Chapters 1 and 20*]

2. *d Measures of risk* — The odds-ratio is calculated from case-control studies to quantify the association between disease and exposure. Relative risk is determined from cohort investigations. [*Chapter 4*]

3. *e Cumulative incidence* — Cumulative incidence (CI) is the proportion of new cases of disease, divided by the number of at-risk persons. CI is calculated from cohort investigations. [*Chapter 4*]

4. *c Determining probability from a table* — pr(benign disease) = (number with benign disease/total number of women) = 75/510. [*Chapter 5*]

5. *b Determining conditional probability from a table* — pr(cancer|p65+) = (number with cancer/number of positive results) = 212/246. [*Chapter 5*]

6. *a Identifying joint probability from a table* — pr(disease-free and p65−) is the proportion of women who have these two characteristics, divided by the total number of study participants: 179/510. [*Chapter 5*]

7. *c Reading a table to identify a conditional probability* — 13/246 = pr(benign disease|p65+). Note that we focus on this question: "In women who have a positive p65 test result, what proportion have benign disease?" [*Chapter 5*]

8. *d Odds-ratio* — The association between disease status and test result is examined in disease-free women (control group) and cases. In this study, the odds-ratio is [(212)(179)/(23)(21)] = 78.57. [*Chapter 4*]

9. *d Confounding variable* — Confounding occurs because cigarette smoking is associated with body weight and longevity. In this example, the impact of smoking on longevity cannot be separated from body weight. [*Chapter 1*]

Questions 10 through 13

10. *d Study design* — In a controlled clinical trial, investigators manipulate the experimental maneuver, which in this case is the type of treatment. A control group (patients who receive the conventional treatment) and an experimental group (patients who have a small plastic disc containing radioactive iodine attached to the back of the eyeball) are compared. [*Chapters 1 and 20*]

11. *b Study biases* — Bogus control bias occurs when researchers remove pa-

	tients from the experimental group after patients experience negative outcomes and reassign them to the control group. The intent is to make the experimental treatment appear more favorable than it really is. [*Chapter 20*]
12. *c* *Study biases*	Family history bias occurs because diseased patients are frequently more likely to cite a family history of disease than disease-free patients, even when family members with or without disease are asked about family history. [*Chapter 20*]
13. *a* *Study designs*	Because known disease status is the starting point for case-control investigations, this design is well suited to investigating rare diseases or ones with a long latency period. [*Chapters 1 and 20*]

Questions 14 through 29

14. *c* *Variables*	The independent variable is the factor that is thought to influence the outcome(s) of interest. In this example, the effect of inhaled corticosteroids on bone age, height, weight, height velocity, and pulmonary function is investigated. [*Chapter 1*]
15. *a* *Analysis of means*	A within-subject design is used, in which each patient's status is assessed at the beginning of the trial and again at the end. The independent variables are quantitative. Thus, the investigators are interested in mean differences. [*Chapter 12*]
16. *d* *p-value*	The *p*-value is the probability of obtaining a result as extreme or more extreme than the sample value, assuming the null hypothesis is true. When the *p*-value $\leq \alpha$, we reject the null hypothesis. [*Chapter 10*]
17. *d* *Generalizability (external validity)*	External validity is maximized when important clinical and demographic characteristics of the target and sampled populations are as similar as possible. [*Chapter 1*]
18. *c* *Regression*	The assumption of independence is violated in regression analyses when one of the variables is a repeated measure. [*Chapter 16*]
19. *b* *Study designs*	In experimental studies, researchers manipulate the intervention, such as a treatment or exposure. In observational studies, exposure occurs by choice or happenstance. [*Chapters 1 and 20*]
20. *a* *Random assignment*	Random assignment relies on a chance process and ensures that each study participant has the same chance of being assigned to the treatment or control condition. Matching, in contrast, assures that the treatment and control group are as similar as possible, except for the intervention or treatment. [*Chapter 12*]
21. *b* *Study designs*	Cohort investigations, in contrast to case-control studies, begin with the known exposures of study participants, follow individuals over time, and record the number of *new* cases of disease. [*Chapters 1 and 4*]
22. *b* *Independence and conditional probability*	Two events are independent if the occurrence of one event does not increase or decrease the probability of the occurrence of the other event. If mononucleosis and non-Hodgkin's lymphoma are independent, pr(L+|M+) will equal pr(L+). We find they are not independent, because 15% of individuals who had adolescent mononucleosis develop adult onset non-

Hodgkin's lymphoma. Note that pr(L+) = 0.01. [*Chapter 5*]

23. *a*   *Binomial*   Immunity (adequate versus inadequate) is a binomial outcome. Because we are interested in those who are *inadequately* immunized, we define *p* as the probability of inadequate immunity, which equals 1 − 0.95 = 0.05. [*Chapters 5 and 8*]

24. *b*   *Measures of central tendency*   The distribution of total cholesterol is skewed negatively. Note that 75% of the values fall toward the upper end of the distribution. The median is the preferred measure of central tendency when a distribution is nonnormal. [*Chapter 3*]

25. *a*   *Graphs*   Activity level is qualitative, with categories ranging from heavy to mild or very light exertion. A bar diagram should be used to display the percentage of heart attack victims in each category. [*Chapter 2*]

26. *e*   *Measures of health status*   Computing prevalence or cumulative incidence requires knowledge of the population at risk and served by the hospital. The data provide numerators, but no denominators. From these data, we can determine only that the number of admissions increases between 1975 and 1990 for tumor-related treatment of children with CNS tumors. [*Chapter 4*]

27. *c*   *Graphs*   A frequency polygon, with relative (%) frequency on the y-axis is preferred, because the researchers want to graph three distributions on the same set of axes, sample sizes differ in each group, and HDL levels are measured quantitatively. [*Chapter 2*]

28. *c*   *Graphs and measures of health status*   Neither prevalence nor incidence density can be determined from these data. Prevalence reflects the number of existing cases of a disease or event at a specific point in time, rather than over time. Incidence density reflects new occurrences of a disease or event in a specific interval, divided by total person-time that participants are observed. The percentage of deaths due to accidents is higher in white females than in African-American females. Therefore, only choice C is correct. [*Chapters 2 and 4*]

29. *b*   *Measures of incidence*   Cumulative incidence and incidence density are determined from cohort investigations. Their numerators are identical, that is, the number of new occurrences of an event. Their denominators differ. The number of persons at risk forms the denominator of cumulative incidence density. Units of exposure or length of observation (eg, pack-years of smoking or person-years) are placed in the denominator of incidence density. [*Chapter 4*]

Questions 30 through 34

30. *b*   *Measures of central tendency*   The mean is the sum of all observations, divided by the number of observations. [*Chapter 3*]

31. *b*   *Measures of central tendency*   When the number of observations is odd and observations are arranged in numerical order, the median is the middle-most value. [*Chapter 3*]

32. *a*   *Measures of central tendency*   The mode is the most frequently occurring value. [*Chapter 3*]

| 33. | c | *Measures of variation* | The standard deviation is the square root of the variance; thus, neither a nor b can be considered. The variance of a sample of observations includes $n - 1$ in the denominator; $n = 5$ in this example. [*Chapter 3*] |

| 34. | b | *Measures of central tendency* | The median is the preferred measure of "average" for these data because $8.99 is clearly an outlier. The mean is influenced unduly by its presence. For example, the median cost is $2.14 [($1.99 + $2.29)/2]; the mean cost is $3.25. [*Chapter 3*] |

Questions 36 and 36

| 35. | d | *Measures of variation* | When variables have a different measurement metric, we use the coefficient of variation (CV) to compare relative variation. The CVs are BP, 15.29; weight, 28.57; and cholesterol, 9.63. Thus, the cholesterol measurements exhibit the least amount of dispersion. [*Chapter 3*] |

| 36. | d | *Measures of variation and shapes of distributions* | Measures of variation, by themselves, provide no information about the shape of a distribution—that is, whether it is skewed or normal. Two or more measures of central tendency, such as the median and mean, give information about shape. [*Chapter 3*] |

Questions 37 through 39

| 37. | b | *Normal curve* | The standard normal deviate (z) of 90 is 2.0. Using the area in one tail, we find that approximately 16% of individuals have a diastolic blood pressure of 90 or greater. Thus, the probability is 0.16 that a worker selected at random will have a reading of 90 mm Hg or greater. [*Chapter 6*] |

| 38. | d | *Normal curve* | The value of 70 is one standard deviation below the mean; therefore $z = -1.0$. The area between $z = -1.0$ and the mean is 0.34; the area to the right of the mean is 0.50. The total area is $0.34 + 0.50 = 0.84$. Therefore, 84% of workers have a diastolic blood pressure of 70 or greater. [*Chapter 6*] |

| 39. | d | *Normal curve* | $z_{60} = -2.0$; area between this z value and the mean is approximately 0.48. $z_{90} = +1.0$; area between this z value and the mean is approximately 0.34. $0.48 + 0.34 = 0.82$. 82% of workers have diastolic readings between 60 and 90. [*Chapter 6*] |

Questions 40 and 41

| 40. | b | *Shapes of distributions and measures of central tendency* | A distribution is positively skewed when the mode < median < mean. [*Chapter 3*] |

| 41. | c | *Shapes of distributions and measures of central tendency* | The median is the preferred measure of central tendency for skewed distributions. |

Questions 42 through 45

| 42. | e | *Measures of disease status* | The initial prevalence of disease is the number of existing cases of hypertension at the beginning of the study, divided by the number of adults in the community: 250/1000. [*Chapter 4*] |

| 43. | b | *Measures of disease status* | Cumulative incidence is the number of new cases of hypertension (50), divided by the number of at-risk indi- |

viduals. The number of at-risk individuals are those who are disease free at the beginning of the study ($100 - 250 = 750$). [*Chapter 4*]

44. *a* *Measures of disease status*
Cumulative incidence can be used to indicate risk. [*Chapter 4*]

45. *a* *Measures of disease status, case fatality*
Case fatality of incident cases is the number of deaths (5), divided by the number of new cases of hypertension (50). [*Chapter 4*]

Questions 46 through 61

46. *b* *Laboratory tests, prevalence*
True infection status is defined by the Southern blot, which is considered the "gold standard" in this problem. The true prevalence, then, is the proportion of women with disease (200), divided by the total number of women screened (467). [*Chapter 7*]

47. *c* *Laboratory tests, prevalence*
The prevalence of disease, as estimated by PCR, is the proportion of women with positive tests (213), divided by the total number of women screened (467). [*Chapter 7*]

48. *e* *Laboratory tests, sensitivity*
Sensitivity is the proportion of true positives: $pr(T+|D+)$; in the 200 women who are diseased, 190 test positive. [*Chapter 7*]

49. *b* *Laboratory tests, false positive*
A false positive is $pr(T+|D-)$; it is represented by the proportion of positive results in disease-free women: $23/267 = 0.09$. [*Chapter 7*]

50. *d* *Laboratory tests, specificity*
Specificity is the proportion of true negatives: $pr(T-|D-) = 244/267 = 0.91$. Recall that false positive results are the complement of true negative outcomes. [*Chapter 7*]

51. *d* *Laboratory tests, positive predictive value*
The positive predictive value is $pr(D+|T+)$. It is the proportion of patients who have disease, given the total number with positive test results: 190/213. [*Chapter 7*]

52. *c* *Laboratory tests, positive predictive value*
As noted for Question 51, the positive predictive value is the proportion of patients with disease, given the total number of positive test results. [*Chapter 7*]

53. *b* *Laboratory tests, false negatives*
False negatives are $pr(T-|D+)$; they equal the proportion of patients who test negative, given the total number who are diseased: 10/200. Recall that false negatives are the complement of sensitivity. [*Chapter 7*]

54. *d* *Laboratory tests, prevalence and predictive values*
As prevalence decreases, more and more individuals who are tested are disease-free. Thus, an increasing proportion of disease-free patients will have positive test results. Consquently, the positive predictive value decreases. [*Chapter 7*]

55. *c* *Binomial probability*
Being born with disease (yes/no) is a binomial outcome. The probability of this outcome is 0.50. We use the binomial with $X = 1$, $n = 4$, $p = 0.50$, and $q = 1 - 0.50 = 0.50$ to compute the probability that one child will be affected. [*Chapter 8*]

56. *c* *Binomial probability*
The probability of an abnormal test result is 0.05. The probability that this patient will have *at least* one test result is $pr(X \geq 1|n = 20) = pr(X = 1) + pr(X = 2) + \ldots + pr(X = 20)$. To reduce computation, we recall that $pr(X \geq 1) = 1 - pr(X = 0)$. [*Chapter 8*]

Questions 57 through 59

57. *a* *Scientific hypothesis*
Anticipated or expected findings are stated in prose

form in the scientific hypothesis. In this example, the investigator believes the use of the dietary oil will increase survival beyond the current population value of 3.5 years.

58. *c* *Testing one mean*

The z test for one mean is used because the population standard deviation is known (1.2 years). The shape of the population distribution does not alter our decision when σ is known. [*Chapter 10*]

59. *b* *Retaining and rejecting hypotheses*

The null hypothesis is retained because the calculated value of the test statistic is less than the critical value—that is, the calculated value falls in the region of retention. [*Chapters 9 and 10*]

Questions 60 through 62

60. *a* *Null hypothesis*

In the case of one population, the null hypothesis contains the value of the population parameter. Eighty percent of patients who take monoamine inhibitors experience relief from panic attacks. The outcome (relief) is binomial. Therefore, the null hypothesis is $\pi = 0.80$. [*Chapters 9 and 13*]

61. *c* *Binomial exact test for one proportion*

The binomial exact test is used because one of the rule-of-thumb criteria is less than 5: $n(1 - \pi) = 10(1 - 0.80) = 2$. [*Chapter 13*]

62. *b* *Type I error*

A Type I error is another name for $\alpha = \text{pr}(\text{rejecting } H_0 \mid H_0 \text{ true})$. In this study, a Type I error would occur if we conclude a significant increase when the true proportion experiencing relief is 0.80—the population value in the null hypothesis. [*Chapter 9*]

Questions 63 through 66

63. *c* *Measures of health status, prevalence*

Prevalence is the number of existing cases in the study group at a particular point in time. Two cases of dementia are diagnosed in 1987 and one in 1986. Five patients are observed; note that patient F did not join the study until 1988, and therefore, is not counted between 1984 and 1987. [*Chapter 4*]

64. *e* *Person—years*

Patient E was observed for 6 years. [*Chapter 4*]

65. *a* *Measures of health status, survival*

Two-year survival is the proportion of patients who survive for at least 2 years following a diagnosis of dementia. Patients A, D, and E develop dementia. Patients D and E survive at least 2 years. [*Chapter 4*]

66. *d* *Measures of health status, incidence density*

The denominator of incidence density contains the total amount of time each of the 6 patients was observed. [*Chapter 4*]

Questions 67 through 70

67. *c* *Testing means, within-subject design*

The outcome variable, diastolic blood pressure, is quantitative. Study participants are measured before and after the experimental program. The investigators are interested in whether the posttrial mean is significantly less than the pretrial mean. The Student's t test for the difference between means from a within-subject design is the analysis of choice. [*Chapter 12*]

68. *d* *Retaining or rejecting the null hypothesis, p-values*

Because the obtained p-value is $\leq \alpha$, we reject the null hypothesis. The posttrial mean (115) is significantly less than the pretrial mean (120). [*Chapters 9 and 12*]

69. *c* *Directional significance tests*

Because the investigators believe diastolic blood pressure will decrease after program participation, they conduct a one-tailed test, with the pretrial value being greater than the posttrial measurement. [*Chapters 9 and 12*]

70. *c* *Regression toward the mean*

Regression toward the mean occurs when patients with extremely high or low values on one or more variables of interest are studied. Extremely high measurements tend to be less when measured posttrial. If no control group is included, the researchers cannot separate treatment effects from regression toward the mean. [*Chapter 19*]

Questions 71 and 72

71. *b* *Alternative hypothesis*

The alternative hypothesis is the statistical counterpart of the scientific hypothesis. In this one-group study, the null hypothesis posits a 5-year survival of 35%. The investigators believe that 5-year survival will increase in women treated with surgery and chemotherapy. Therefore, $\pi > 0.35$. [*Chapters 9 and 13*]

72. *c* *Retaining or rejecting the null hypothesis, p-values*

The p-value is 0.32; $\alpha = 0.01$. Because the p-value is $>$ α, we retain the null hypothesis. [*Chapters 9 and 13*]

Questions 73 through 76

73. *a* *Null hypothesis, two means*

An independent groups design is used to study differences in depression as a function of length of leave after childbirth. Depression is measured quantitatively. The null hypothesis states that the mean difference between groups is zero. [*Chapters 9 and 12*]

74. *b* *Testing two means*

Relevant distributions are normal; the homogeneity-of-variance rule-of-thumb is met ($7^2/6^2 = 1.36$). Use the Student's t for the difference between two independent means. The pooled variance estimate appears in the denominator; $df = 20 + 20 - 2$. [*Chapter 12*]

75. *c* *Retaining or rejecting hypotheses, p-values, directional and nondirectional tests*

The investigators believe that a significant difference exists between the two groups; however, it is not known whether one group will be more or less depressed than the other group. Consequently, the test is two-tailed. The researchers conclude from the statistics that a significant difference exists: p-value < 0.001 versus $\alpha = 0.05$. [*Chapters 9 and 12*]

76. *b* *Type I error*

Rejecting the null hypothesis when it is true is a Type I error. The probability of this error equals α, which is 0.05 in this example.

Questions 77 through 79

77. *d* *Study designs*

The study is a controlled clinical trial because (a) the intervention, drug therapy, in manipulated by the clinicians; (b) more than one study group is examined. The study is also randomized because volunteers are assigned randomly to study groups. [*Chapters 1 and 20*]

78. *a* *Scientific hypothesis*

The investigators want to determine if a difference occurs in the proportion surviving 18 months or more in each treatment group after the first bout of *Pneumocystis* pneumonia. [*Chapters 9 and 14*]

79. *c* *Testing two proportions*

The normal approximation to the binomial, two proportions, independent groups is used because two groups are studied, the groups are independent, the outcome is binomial, and rule-of-thumb criteria are met. [*Chapter 14*]

Questions 80 through 83

80. *a* *Pearson correlation and lack of linearity*

The relationship between stress and cholesterol is non-linear; the highest stress levels occur in men with the highest and lowest cholesterol levels. Men whose cholesterol levels are between the highest and lowest values have lower stress levels. The Pearson correlation, which is a measure of linear association, will underestimate the strength of curvilinearly related variables. [*Chapters 18 and 19*]

81. *b* *Study biases*

The investigators err when they equate correlation with causation. An association between stress and cholesterol does not signal that high stress causes high cholesterol. [*Chapter 19*]

82. *d* *Confounding variable*

Confounding occurs because serotonin levels are associated with stress and cholesterol. In this study, the effect of serotonin cannot be separated from cholesterol to examine its independent impact on stress. [*Chapter 1*]

83. *b* *Confidence intervals*

Confidence intervals are well suited to testing hypotheses. If the value in the null hypothesis falls outside the two-sided confidence interval, we reject the null hypothesis and conclude that a significant difference exists. [*Chapters 11 and 12*]

Questions 84 through 86

84. *d* *Dependent variable*

The dependent variable is the outcome of interest. In this study of trigeminal neuralgia, clinicians are interested in episode control (yes/no). [*Chapter 1*]

85. *b* *Testing proportions, matched/paired data*

The outcome is binomial; data are derived from matched pairs. The null hypothesis indicates in the special case of matched pairs a binomial outcome that $\pi = 0.50$. $n\pi = n(1 - \pi) = 33\ (0.50)\ 16.5 > 5$. Therefore, use the normal approximation. [*Chapter 14*] (Why does $n = 33$? See question 86)

86. *d* *Testing two proportions, matched/paired data*

Because pairs in which the same outcome is observed (called *tied pairs*) provide no information about differential effectiveness, we analyze information from the untied pairs (cells 1,2 and 2,1: $32 + 1 = 33$). [*Chapter 14*]

Questions 87 through 89

87. *d* *Regression, testing the slope*

The investigators believe that an indirect relationship exists between lead exposure and performance on a standardized intelligence test. Because the *p*-value (< 0.01) $\leq \alpha = 0.05$, we reject the null hypothesis of zero slope and conclude that a significant indirect association exists, that is $\beta < 0$. [*Chapter 17*]

88. *b* *Slope*

The slope indicates the amount of predicted change in Y, given a one unit change in X. Because the slope is -0.40, we indicate that a 10-unit increase in exposure is associated with a 4-unit decrease in the predicted intelligence test score ($-0.40 \times 10 = 4$ points). [*Chapters 16 and 17*]

89. *b* *Slope and Pearson correlation*

The sign of the slope and the sign of the correlation provide the same information about the direction of the association; for example, a negative slope indicates an indirect relationship—as X increases, Y tends to decrease—and vice-versa. Similarly, a negative correlation describes an indirect association. [*Chapters 16 and 18*]

Questions 90 through 92

90. *a* *Testing frequencies or proportions, independent groups* The null hypothesis indicates that the two treatment populations are homogeneous with respect to the proportion experiencing allergic reactions. Key elements of the study design are: two treatment groups; groups are independent; the outcome is binomial; and the investigators specify no directional hypothesis. [*Chapter 16*]

91. *d* *Study design and measures of risk for a binomial outcome* Although the study is a controlled clinical trial, patients are followed after drug administration (exposure) to chart the occurrence of complications. Relative risk will answer the question about the association between drug and allergic reaction. RR = (7/100)/(3/100) = 2.33. The relative risk of allergic reaction in the streptokinase group is approximately twice that of the TPA group. [*Chapter 4*]

92. *b* *Relative risk* Refer to explanation for question 91

Questions 93 through 102

All questions are referenced to Chapter 7 and focus on interpreting clinical laboratory tests.

93. *a*   98. *a*
94. *a*   99. *a*
95. *b*   100. *b*
96. *b*   101. *d*
97. *b*   102. *b*

Questions 103 through 112

All questions are developed from Chapters 1 and 20 and address types of studies.

103. *c*   108. *e*
104. *d*   109. *c*
105. *a*   110. *d*
106. *e*   111. *c*
107. *b*   112. *e*

Questions 113 through 122

All questions are developed from Chapter 20 and relate to biases that affect studies.

113. *n*   118. *i*
114. *d*   119. *e*
115. *b*   120. *c*
116. *j*   121. *h*
117. *m*   122. *k*

Subject Index

NOTE: Page numbers in bold face type indicate a major discussion. A *t* following a page number indicates tabular material and an *i* following a page number indicates an illustration.